WITHDRAWN

Health Counseling

A Microskills Approach

Richard Blonna, EdD, CHES
Department of Community Health
William Paterson University

Daniel Watter, EdD
Department of Psychology
Seton Hall University

JONES AND BARTLETT PUBLISHERS
Sudbury, Massachusetts
BOSTON   TORONTO   LONDON   SINGAPORE

World Headquarters
Jones and Bartlett Publishers
40 Tall Pine Drive
Sudbury, MA 01776
978-443-5000
info@jbpub.com
www.jbpub.com

Jones and Bartlett Publishers
Canada
2406 Nikanna Road
Mississauga, ON L5C 2W6
CANADA

Jones and Bartlett Publishers
International
Barb House, Barb Mews
London W6 7PA
UK

Production Credits
Acquisitions Editor: Jacqueline Ann Mark
Senior Production Editor: Julie Champagne Bolduc
Associate Editor: Nicole Quinn
Editorial Assistant: Erin Murphy
Senior Marketing Manager: Ed McKenna
Director of Interactive Technology: Adam Alboyadjian
Interactive Technology Manager: Dawn Mahon Priest
Interior Design: Anne Spencer
Photo Research: Kimberly Potvin
Manufacturing Buyer: Therese Bräuer
Cover Design: Timothy Dziewit
Composition: Graphic World
Cover Image: © Photos.com
Printing and Binding: Malloy, Inc.
Cover Printing: John Pow Company

LIBRARY OF CONGRESS CATALOGING-IN-PUBLICATION DATA
Blonna, Richard.
    Health counseling: a microskills approach / Richard Blonna, Daniel Watter.
        p. cm.
    Includes bibliographical references and index.
    ISBN 0-7637-4761-0
    1. Health counseling—Study and teaching. 2. Health counselors—Training of. I. Watter, Daniel. II. Title.
    R727.4.B565 2005
    362.1'04256—dc22

                                        2004022760

Printed in the United States of America
09 08 07 06 05   10 9 8 7 6 5 4 3 2 1

Contents

Foreword ix

Introduction xi

Chapter 1 | **Introduction to Health Counseling** 1

Introduction 1

Health and Wellness Defined 4
The Six Dimensions of Wellness 5

Health Promotion and Health Education 7
Health Promotion 7
Health Education 7

Healthy People 2010 8

What Is Counseling? 9
Characteristics of Effective Counselors 9

What Is Health Counseling? 11
The Practice of Health Counseling 12

The Counselor–Client Relationship 13
The Relationship Itself 13
The Relationship as a Means to an End 14
The Relationship and Outcomes 14

Ethical Issues in Health Counseling 14
Ethical Dilemmas 14

Termination of Counseling 16

Summary 17

Chapter 2 | **The Theoretical Basis of Health Counseling** 19

Health Counseling Theory 19
Health, Illness, and Sick Role Behaviors 20

Behavior Change Theories   21
  Health Belief Model   22
  Social Cognitive Theory   22
  Self-efficacy Theory   25
  Transtheoretical (Stages of Change) Theory   25
  Theory of Reasoned Action   27
  Stimulus Response (Behavior) Theory   28

Counseling Theories   29
  Insight Theories   29
  Behavioral Theories   32
  Microcounseling Theory   32

Compliance and Adherence Theory   34
  Factors Unrelated to Compliance   36
  Factors Related to Compliance   37

Summary   39

| Chapter 3 | **Introductory and Attending Skills** | 43 |

Introductory Skills   44
  Smile   44
  A Firm Handshake   45
  Exchanging Names   46
  Discussing the Nature of Counseling   46
  Description of Roles   47
  Transition to the Client's Story   47

Attending Skills   47
  The Three V's + B: Visuals, Vocals, Verbals, and Body Language   47
  Nonverbal Communication   52

Summary   55

| Chapter 4 | **Observational and Responding Skills** | 57 |

Observational Skills   57
  Nonverbal Messages   57
  Client Orientation   61

Responding Skills   62
  Minimal Encouragers   62
  Questioning   64
  Paraphrasing   70
  Reflection of Feelings   70
  Summarizing   70

Summary   72

| Chapter 5 | Influencing Skills | 74 |

Introduction   74

Confrontation   76

Feedback and Self-disclosure   80
Feedback   80
Self-disclosure   80

Focusing the Narrative   81
Problem and Individual Focus   82
Family Focus   82
Other Individual Focus   82
Mutuality Focus   84
Helper Focus   84
Cultural/Environmental Context Focus   85

Eliciting and Reflecting Meaning   87

Interpretation and Reframing   87
Interpretation of Meaning   88
Reframing   88

Information, Directives, and Instructions   89
Information   89
Directives   90
Instructions   91

Logical Consequences   94

Summary   95

| Chapter 6 | Counseling Persons with Chronic Stress | 97 |

Health Counseling for Primary Prevention   97

What Is Stress?   98
Personality and Stress   101
Psychosomatic Disease and Stress   102
Everly and Benson's Disorders of Arousal   102
The Effects of Stress on Disease   103

The Goals of Stress Management Counseling   104

Counseling Someone with Stress Using Microskills   106
Introductory Skills   107
Attending Skills   108
Responding Skills   110
Influencing Skills   113

Summary   128

Chapter 7	**Birth Control Counseling**	**130**

Introduction   130

Effectiveness: Theoretical and Actual Use   131
Theoretical Effectiveness   131
Actual Use Effectiveness   131
Pregnancy Risk   132

Mechanisms of Action   134

Methods Associated with Each Mechanism of Action   135
Nonpenetrative Behaviors   135
Methods That Prevent Sperm from Reaching Eggs   136
Methods That Provide Barriers Between Sperm and Egg   136
Methods That Prevent Implantation of a Fertilized Egg   141
Methods That Prevent the Release of Ova   141
Methods That Prevent Sperm from Reaching Egg (Surgical)   142
Methods That Terminate an Established Pregnancy   143

Communicating About Sexuality and Birth Control   145
Sexual Vocabulary   145

Counseling Clients About Birth Control Using Microskills   146
Introductory Skills   146
Attending Skills   149
Responding Skills   150
Influencing Skills   153

Summary   161

Chapter 8	**Asthma Counseling**	**163**

Health Counseling for Secondary Prevention   163

Overview of Asthma   164
Epidemiology   164
Diagnosis   164
Treatment   166
Control and Prevention   167

Goals of Asthma Counseling   171

Counseling Clients with Asthma Using Microskills   171
Introductory Skills   172
Attending Skills   173
Responding Skills   176
Influencing Skills   178

Summary   191

Chapter 9   **Hypertension Counseling**   **193**

Overview of Blood Pressure and Hypertension   193
    Diagnosis   194
    Epidemiology   196
    Uncontrollable Hypertension Risk Factors   196
    Controllable Hypertension Risk Factors   198
    Hypertension as a Risk Factor   199
    Prevention and Control   200

Goals of Hypertension Counseling   202

Counseling Clients with Hypertension Using Microskills   203
    Introductory Skills   204
    Attending Skills   205
    Responding Skills   206
    Influencing Skills   209

Summary   224

Chapter 10   **Counseling Persons with Chlamydia and Other Sexually**   **226**
Transmitted Diseases

Introduction   226
    Overall Goals of STD Counseling   227

Overview of *Chlamydia trachomatis*   228
    Epidemiology   228
    Diagnosis   229
    Treatment   230
    Prevention: A Pyramid of Risk for STDs   230

Counseling Clients with Chlamydia Using Microskills   234
    Introductory Skills   235
    Attending Skills   237
    Responding Skills   241
    Influencing Skills   244

Summary   252

Chapter 11   **Injury Counseling: Torn Anterior Cruciate Ligaments**   **254**

Health Counseling for Tertiary Prevention   254

Overview and Epidemiology of ACL Injuries   255

Diagnosis   257

Treatment and Management   258

Serious and Career-Ending Injuries   259
    Applying Kübler-Ross's Model to Career-Ending Injuries   261

Goals for Counseling Someone with a Torn ACL   261

Counseling Clients with ACL Injuries Using Microskills   261
    Introductory Skills   262
    Attending Skills   263
    Responding Skills   265
    Influencing Skills   267

Summary   277

Chapter 12

Sexuality Counseling   279

Introduction   280

Overview of Sexual Concerns   280
    Sexual Disorders   280
    Sexual Problems   282
    Sexual Worries   282

Obstacles to Discussing Sexual Concerns   282

Helping Clients Manage Sexual Concerns   283

The Medicalization of Sexuality Counseling   284

Counseling Clients with Sexual Concerns   285
    The PLISSIT Model   286

Sexuality Counseling Using Microskills   287
    Overall Goals of Sexuality Counseling   287
    Introductory Skills   288
    Attending Skills   291
    Responding Skills   292
    Influencing Skills   294

Summary   298

Glossary   301

Index   309

Foreword

Health counseling has become a central area of practice for a variety of helping professionals, including health educators, nurses, psychologists, psychiatrists, social workers, and mental health counselors. We have finally realized that the medical repair and restorative model, while basic to health, needs to be supplemented with personal approaches that enable and encourage clients to comply with physician recommendations. However, even more important, health counseling can help prevent illness and encourage patients to do a better and more thorough job of taking care of themselves. Effective health counseling enables people to manage their lives more competently and with more satisfaction.

This book by Richard Blonna and Dan Watter is an important and vital contribution to health counseling. They have given us a very clear definition of health counseling and shown us effective techniques and strategies to facilitate client well-being over the lifespan. By reading this book, you'll discover specifics that can make a difference in your work with clients and patients. The examples are clear and to the point and will be used throughout your professional career. I could not endorse this work more highly.

Communication skills of listening to clients form the foundation of competent health counseling. Our first task is to hear the client's story or narrative. As we carefully listen to their thoughts, feelings, and deeper meanings, we can better empathize with them and understand the issues they face. Once we hear their stories, we are then prepared to help them rewrite their stories in new and more positive ways. We can help them to find new answers to old issues, and to live more positively with things that cannot easily be changed.

Blonna and Watter remind us that we live in a multicultural world and that our approach to health counseling must remain aware of individual and cultural differences if our clients are to continue with us. Multicultural competence implies the need to be able to work with patients from many backgrounds and with differences ranging from ethnicity/race to gender and sexual orientation. I believe it is important to be aware that patients who have gone through cancer, endure diabetes, or live with war trauma are also special multicultural populations, each with a common (but also personally unique) history. In that sense, perhaps all health counseling is multicultural.

There is also truth in the saying, "If you haven't been there, you don't fully understand." If you have not been in a family troubled by alcohol or drugs, or by an early parental death, or by constant illness, you as a health counselor will have some difficulty in gaining and maintaining credibility. When you have not had the life experience or do not come from the culture of your clients or patients, you will find that the listening and influencing skills suggested in this book can make an immense difference in your practice.

I'm going to make a special plea that you give extra attention and care to those who are less economically advantaged—the "working poor," the homeless, and the middle-class uninsured. Our medical system in the United States is leveraged to favor those with resources and connections. Our healthcare system is excellent, but we do not offer equal access to all. Evidence is clear that people of color, even when they have financial and insurance resources, receive less competent and careful care than whites. It is also true that those who do not have financial resources often receive inadequate care. I'd ask you to think about these issues constantly while reading this book and when you go into professional work. To ignore the many injustices of our health care system is to support the status quo. At times, this will mean serving as an advocate to ensure that people get the treatment that they need.

This book is practical, it is clear, and it can make a difference to you and those with whom you work. Read it with care, for you can use the book as a basis for practice throughout your life.

Allen E. Ivey, EdD, ABPP
Distinguished University Professor (Emeritus)
University of Massachusetts, Amherst
President, Microtraining Associates, Inc.

Introduction

Health counseling is a psycho-educational process that revolves around two primary functions: (1) helping clients understand and cope with the feelings and emotions associated with their health problems and (2) helping clients develop and adhere to therapeutic regimens designed to treat, cure, or manage these problems. The *psychological* aspect of this process involves the feelings and emotions associated with the health problem. The *educational* part relates to the teaching and learning of information and skills necessary to manage the health problem. The process forges an intensive, interactive relationship between the client and the counselor that centers on the health problem that is the basis of the person's need for counseling.

The major difference between health counseling and generic counseling is the former discipline's focus on the emotional issues surrounding a specific health issue. Often these emotions stand in the way of proper illness and sick role behavior. Sometimes they simply make it more difficult to talk to clients about these problems. The goal of health counseling is to help all types of clients understand and work through their feelings and emotions surrounding their health problems so that they can help develop and adhere to their therapeutic regimens, gain more control over their illnesses, and get better.

Health counseling is a practice that is not distinguished by a recognized professional credential or specialty. Licensed professional counselors, psychologists and psychiatrists, health educators, nurses, doctors, nurse-practitioners, midwives, and physical therapists are among the many helping professionals who engage in health counseling. Health counselors work in a wide array of settings, including private practice, hospitals, outpatient clinics, and community health centers. Health counseling also takes place in the field when public health workers, visiting nurses, and other health professionals visit clients in their homes and other residential locations. This kind of counseling can occur in a single session or multiple sessions, depending on the nature and context of the problem, eligibility for third-party reimbursement, and other issues.

Health counseling, like health promotion and health education, may target any of the three levels of prevention: primary, secondary, or tertiary. *Primary prevention counseling* seeks to teach clients the information, skills, and behaviors they need to reduce their risks of ever developing the health problem. Those engaged in primary prevention activities work with clients who do not have the problem and who may or may not be at risk for developing it. *Secondary prevention counseling* tries to prevent the progression of a health problem through early detection and prompt treatment. Health counselors engaged in secondary prevention activities work with clients who already have the problem and with populations where there is a greater possibility of discovering individuals with the problem. Health counseling associated with screening programs is an integral part of secondary prevention. *Tertiary prevention counseling* focuses on helping clients cope with the disabilities and complications associated with a variety of health problems. This type of counseling is associated with helping clients understand their disabilities, restoring functioning, teaching clients new skills, and assisting them in adapting to challenges associated with their disabilities.

Writing an introductory textbook for such a broad field that cuts across so many professional disciplines poses unique challenges. The book must be able to speak to all of the diverse health professionals involved in health counseling with one voice. It must blend the language of counseling, education, and community health in a meaningful way so that professionals from all of the disciplines represented can relate to the material. It also must present a unifying theoretical framework that cuts across and is accepted by all of the professions involved in training health counselors. Lastly, it must focus on concrete skills that transcend individual health problems and are generalizable to a variety of settings and conditions.

The authors did a preliminary Internet search using the key word "health counseling" and found 347 books identified with this term. Three of the books were entitled *Health Counseling*, and the rest combined the term with an approach (e.g., *Counseling in Health Care Settings*) or a focused topic (e.g., *Counseling People Who Are HIV Positive*). The search revealed two major problems associated with existing health counseling books: (1) they are based on an eclectic theoretical framework and (2) they are too topical for use in training health counselors. Most of the books reviewed blended aspects of many different counseling methodologies but lacked a unifying theoretical framework. This eclectic approach is a problem for entry-level health counselors, who need a strong theoretical framework to guide their skill learning. The topical textbooks offered more specific advice on how to counsel clients but concentrated on only one specific health problem. These books tend to be rather limited for use in training health counselors because of their narrow focus. They also tend to use a more eclectic approach to health counseling.

We felt there was a need for a new book that eliminated these two problems and could be used by all health counselors, regardless of their professional training or the nature of their work setting. *Health Counseling: A Microskills Approach*

eliminates the two major shortcomings associated with other health counseling books. We chose Allen Ivey's microskills model as our theoretical framework when writing the book. The microskills model works well for an entry-level book in health counseling for two reasons: (1) it is a psycho-educational model, and (2) it breaks the counseling process down into discrete skills that can be mastered individually and then combined into a unified counseling approach.

The theoretical framework of Ivey's microskills model is based on a psycho-educational approach to counseling. It suggests that to help people manage their health problems, counselors must aid clients in working through any emotional distress associated with those problems. This endeavor also involves teaching clients new information and skills and helping them develop attitudes and values that support and reinforce healthy behavior.

The perfect way to teach health counseling is to break the process down into discrete skills and ensure that students master each skill before moving to the next one. After the individual skills are mastered, they are assembled together to form a unified approach to working with clients. The microskills model for teaching counseling is based on such an approach.

The examples used to teach this model are drawn from the 10 leading health indicators identified in Healthy People 2010. Throughout this text, we discuss how health counseling is related to these indicators and how counselors can address them as part of their work with clients. Clients will often seek counseling as a direct result of these indicators. For instance, they may seek stress counseling because they are feeling stressed and fear they might be sinking into clinical depression. In some cases, clients seeking counseling for one health problem will afford counselors opportunities to discuss others. For example, in Chapter 9, a client presenting with hypertension also receives counseling about sedentary lifestyle, obesity, and tobacco use. Lastly, clients using public health facilities as their entry point into the healthcare delivery system offer counselors opportunities to empower them to gain broader access to health care by referring them for a range of services such as immunization and nutritional programs for their children.

As educators, we have strived to make this book very student friendly. Its features provide many opportunities for practice, review, and application. We have tried to make key terms and concepts, counseling hints, and diverse, multicultural case studies literally jump off the pages for readers. We hope that students will enjoy reading the book as much as we have enjoyed writing it.

Acknowledgments

We would like to thank the many people whose help, guidance, and inspiration made writing this book possible. First, we would like to thank everyone at Jones and Bartlett for having faith in our project and the opportunity to write this book. We thank Kris Ellis for her initial interest in the project and Jacqueline Mark and Clayton E. Jones for offering us a contract. In addition, we would like to thank all of our reviewers for their careful review of the manuscript and their excellent suggestions for improving our initial work. We appreciate Nicole Quinn's help in editing the manuscript and bringing it to production. Lastly, we would like to thank Julie Bolduc, Senior Production Editor, for the excellent job she did producing the final manuscript. Her careful attention to detail and precise editing helped us craft a book that is both scholarly and useful as a tool for counselors-in-training.

Rich Blonna

First and foremost, I'd like to thank Allen Ivey for his help and inspiration in writing this book. He is truly a living legend in the field of counseling. I've long admired Dr. Ivey for his work in this field, particularly his development and refinement of the microskills model and his efforts to infuse multicultural issues into counseling. These two contributions have been central to my own philosophy of training entry-level health counselors. What is even more remarkable is Dr. Ivey's approachability. I have never had the opportunity to study with Dr. Ivey nor even to meet him in person, yet he generously reached out to me, offered to review the proposal for this book, and encouraged me to submit it to publishers he thought might be interested in publishing it. After I secured a contract, he continued his generous support, offering to review the manuscript and write the Foreword to the book. I cannot express the extent of my gratitude to him for his interest and support. I hope that the book conveys the essence of his work and caring.

I'd also like to thank my co-author Dan Watter for his help in developing this project and contributing to the content. Dan's expertise in writing and reviewing the sections on counseling theory was invaluable. Dan is a master counselor/therapist, and his experience in working with clients put a human face on the many examples, case studies, and counseling hints found throughout the text. It was thoroughly enjoyable to meet with Dan, pick his brain, and bounce ideas off of him. On many occasions, his insights into the nature of human behavior and the counseling process helped me focus my own writing and stay on target. I look forward to the opportunity to collaborate with him on future writing projects.

I'd like to thank all of my colleagues in the Department of Community Health at William Paterson University for their support throughout this project. Their understanding, kind words, and reassurances helped me survive a very trying year that involved juggling a full-time teaching load, normal faculty responsibilities, and writing three textbooks simultaneously. I'd like to give special thanks to Joanna Hayden, my friend and the chairperson of the Department of Community Health at William Paterson University, for all of her help and guidance in developing the proposal and the manuscript. Joanna's critical eye, writing skill, and editorial guidance are evident throughout this book.

I'd like to thank Steven deHaan and Christine Orlowski for their help in researching the chapters on asthma and ACL injuries, respectively. Both provided excellent research on their respective topics as well as identifying and writing clear directives and specific instructions for counseling clients with these conditions. I think both Steve and Christine will make fine health counselors if they choose to pursue that goal. I'm especially indebted to Steve for discussing his own asthma control efforts with me and sharing information about a specific type of medication that he found helpful. After discussing his recommendation with my own physician, I began using this medication and have found it to be a perfect fit for controlling my own asthma. Since using this medication, I have not had a major asthma attack and have felt in control for over one year.

Lastly, I'd like to thank my wife, Heidi, and my sons, Will and Mike, for being so supportive. They gave the encouragement, personal space, emotional support, and love I needed to finish this book.

Dan Watter

What a pleasure it has been writing this book! I would like to thank my co-author (and writing mentor), Rich Blonna, for including me in this project. I have learned a tremendous amount about writing a textbook, and I would never have been able to complete my portion of this undertaking without his support, encouragement, and patience.

There are several people whose work, time, and experience I have valued on my path to becoming a counselor. While I have never met him personally, I want to acknowledge the writings of Irvin Yalom, M.D. There are few writers whose words have influenced my own work so dramatically. Dr. Yalom constantly reminds us of the importance of listening to, and respecting the integrity of, our clients. I urge all present and future counselors to take some time to absorb his thoughts on the therapeutic relationship.

In addition, I would like to express my heartfelt thanks to the many clients who have let me into their lives during the past 20-plus years. I imagine that few endeavors are as rewarding as being a counselor, and I feel both privileged and humbled to have been given the opportunity to have listened to so many "stories." Your trust and confidence in me is genuinely appreciated. I hope you have learned as much from me as much as I have learned from you.

Finally, I would like to thank my wonderful wife, Laurie, and my children, Michael and Emily, for allowing me the time to work on this project. I love you all very much!

Dedication

We dedicate this book to Dr. Allen Ivey. Without Dr. Ivey and his microskills model, there would be no *Health Counseling: A Microskills Approach*. We hope that our book measures up to the long list of books that link to his model.

Chapter 1

Introduction to Health Counseling

Learning Objectives

By the end of the chapter students will:

1. Compare and contrast health and wellness

2. Describe the six dimensions of wellness

3. Explain the similarities and differences between health promotion and health education

4. Define counseling according to Carl Rogers

5. List and describe a variety of characteristics associated with effective counselors

6. Describe the similarities and differences between health counseling and generic counseling

7. Compare and contrast a variety of settings in which health counseling occurs

8. Describe how the nature of health counseling varies according to where it is practiced

9. Describe a few of the ethical principles contained in the American Counseling Association's Code of Conduct

Introduction

Health counseling is a psycho-educational process that revolves around two primary functions: (1) helping clients understand and cope with the feelings and emotions associated with their health problems and (2) helping clients develop and adhere to therapeutic regimens. The *psychological* aspect of this process involves the feelings and emotions associated with the health problem. The *educational* part of the process relates to the teaching and learning of information and skills necessary to manage the health problem. The *process* is an intensive, interactive relationship between the client and the counselor that revolves around the health problem that is the basis of the person's need for counseling.

Gonorrhea can be used as an example of a health problem to illustrate how these three aspects of health counseling work together. Imagine, if you can, what it must feel like to be a man who wakes up one morning and discovers that he has an infection that turns out to be gonorrhea.

When you awake, you discover that your bedding is sticky and wet with patches of a greenish-yellow fluid. You roll out of bed and walk to the bathroom. As you start to urinate, you feel an incredible burning sensation at the end of your penis and notice that more of the greenish-yellow discharge is released in your urine. You continue to urinate, fighting back the pain as your urine washes over your injured urethra.

Panicking because you think that you might have a sexually transmitted disease (STD), you put your clothes, consult the Yellow Pages, and find the nearest STD clinic in your area. You would like to go to your family doctor but are too embarrassed to do so; you worry that he might tell your parents about your visit. You call in and tell your boss you will be late for work this morning. When he asks why, you make up a lame story about needing to take your dog to the veterinarian. You are too embarrassed to tell him the truth. You'll deal with your afternoon college classes later. Right now, your only thought is getting that burning and discharge to stop.

You rush to the clinic, park hastily on the street, and enter the clinic door. The place is jammed. You take a number and have a seat in the waiting room. As you slide into your chair, you're not sure how to act and what to say. Should you make eye contact with the other people in the waiting room and greet them, or should you avoid potentially embarrassing yourself and them by trying to start up a conversation? As you wait for what seems like an eternity, you feel that everyone is looking at you. You hunker down in your seat and wait silently.

The receptionist calls your number and takes you into a cubicle, partitioned off from the four others by walls that are half-glass and extend up about to your shoulders. You can't help but notice how other patients peer over the divider as

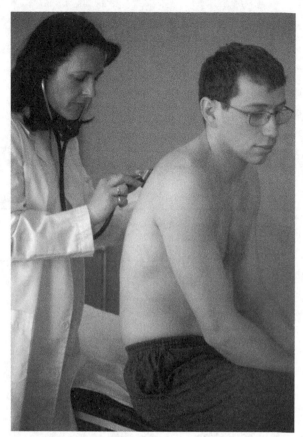

Figure 1.1 Nurse-Practitioner Being examined for an STD by a healthcare provider of the opposite gender can sometimes be embarrassing. (© Pixtal/age fotostock)

they move back and forth from the receptionist's station. The receptionist begins by telling you how everything she will ask you will be kept confidential. She asks for the usual demographic information: name, age, address, and so on. When she asks why you are here today you freeze up, unsure how to answer. You ask yourself, "Should I really tell her everything?" "Should I use the word 'penis'?" "How should I describe this yellow-green stuff coming out of my penis?" The receptionist senses your apprehension and says, "Don't worry, I know you must feel a little strange talking about this. I am not going to examine you. I need to know in general why you are here so I can write it on your intake form for the nurse-practitioner or doctor who will examine and treat you." You quietly tell her, "I have a problem with some kind of discharge." She writes this information down and sends you back to see the clinician.

You can't believe that a female nurse-practitioner is going to examine you. She asks you to explain your problem, and you turn red as you explain what is going on. She asks you to drop your trousers and underwear because she needs to examine you and take specimens. You think to yourself, "Oh boy, specimens. I wonder what the heck that means?" The nurse-practitioner puts on a pair of rubber gloves and adjusts the wall light so she can get a better look at your penis and the discharge. She starts to unwrap a long-handled, cotton-tipped applicator. You begin to sweat: "What are you going to do with THAT?" She explains that she plans to swab the tip of your penis to get a specimen of the discharge, stain it on a microscope slide, and examine it for gonorrhea. Although your symptoms are pretty typical of gonorrhea, she wants to be sure so she will perform a rapid test. The nurse-practitioner explains that it is a very accurate way of diagnosing your problem. She even says that you can look at the sample under the microscope if it is positive. "Great," you say to yourself, "just what I want to do—look at my gonorrhea." You can't remember when you were more embarrassed.

The test is positive. The nurse-practitioner says, "Before I treat you, I will need to take additional specimens from your throat or anus if you use those body parts during sex. I will have to insert additional swabs in those places to get the specimens." You think to yourself, "What? There is no way, lady, that you are going to stick anything up my . . . ." In actuality, you tell her, "That won't be necessary. I don't use those body parts for sex." She tells you to relax while she gets your medication. "Yeah, easy for you to say," you think to yourself.

The nurse-practitioner returns with the medication, explains that it is a tetracycline derivative, and goes into a 10-minute dissertation about how to take it. You are so shell-shocked that you

feign attention, but when she finishes and asks if you have any questions you say, "No. Can I leave now?" She explains that she still needs to discuss your sex partners. "Just great," you think. "Now I have to talk to her about who I am having sex with."

The nurse-practitioner spends the next 15 minutes explaining why it is important for you to get in touch with all of your sex partners from the past month. She goes over strategies for calling them and getting them to see a clinician, then ends by giving you a few referrals for your partners and an appointment at the clinic for a follow-up test. You mumble an inaudible "Thanks" and scoot out of the building like a dog with his tail between his legs.

As you drive to work, you wonder what you will say to your boss and professor about missing work and class today. The last thing you want to do until the discharge and burning stop is go to work or school. You also worry about how you will tell your girlfriend and that other woman you are having sex with about your gonorrhea infection. You start to panic but decide to go home, get some sleep, and deal with your problems later when you wake up.

If you can imagine such a scene, it becomes easy to see how health problems such as gonorrhea never exist in a vacuum for a person. There are always emotions associated with the condition. Often these emotions stand in the way of proper illness and sick role behavior. Other times they simply make it more difficult to talk about these problems if you are the health professional dealing with the client.

For the receptionist and the nurse-practitioner in this scenario to fully serve the client, they must be aware of the interplay between the emotions and the patient regarding his or her health condition. The receptionist must understand how the person might feel being in the clinic with an STD and attempt to put the individual at ease before starting to gather information. The nurse-practitioner must recognize that the client's emotions can stand in the way of a proper examination and follow through with the treatment regimen. For any education to occur, the nurse-practitioner must first work through the emotions the client has regarding the infection. This is why health counseling is best understood as a "psycho-educational" process.

Health counseling is an intensive, exhaustive process because it involves identifying, understanding, and managing clients' complex emotions so as to be able to teach them detailed instructions for managing health problems. Before clients (such as the gonorrhea patient in the illustration) can absorb complex healthcare instructions, they must work through their emotional issues that are related to the problem. Only then will they be able to fully listen to, and become involved in, learning how to manage the health problem.

This chapter explores the origins of health counseling. It also examines the nature of health and wellness, education, health education, and counseling. Finally, it ends with a synthesis of all these disciplines into a working understanding of health counseling.

Health and Wellness Defined

In 1947, the World Health Organization (WHO) defined **health** as "the state of complete mental, physical, and social well-being, not merely the absence of disease" (WHO, 1947). WHO's definition was the first globally accepted conceptualization of health and stood the test of time for more than a decade.

Although multifaceted, this definition of health was flawed, according to members of a new movement called holistic health. The holistic health movement came into being in the 1960s as an attempt to expand the view of health that WHO had promulgated.

One of the early pioneers in the field, Halbert Dunn (1962), believed that WHO's vision of health characterized it as a static state. Rather than call health a state of well-being, Dunn preferred to view it as a continuum **(Figure 1.2)**. Developing and maintaining a high level of health means moving toward high-level functioning along a continuum that starts with low-level well-being and ends with optimal functioning. Health is a conscious and deliberate approach to life and being, rather than something to be abdicated to doctors and the healthcare system. Optimal health is a result of your decisions and behavior.

In addition, Dunn recast the notion of well-being to revolve around how well a person functions. That is, he viewed functioning as evidence of well-being. Although people will have setbacks in their quest for optimal functioning, the direction in which their lives are moving becomes an important criterion for evaluating their well-being. In this movement, daily habits and behaviors, as well as overall lifestyle, assumed primary importance.

Originally, the scope of well-being was limited to three dimensions: physical, social, and mental. Adherents of holistic health argued that the mental dimension has two components—the intellectual (rational thought processes) and the emotional (feelings and emotions). Each of these domains deals with a different aspect of psychological well-being. An additional dimension, the

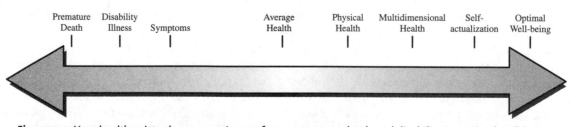

| Premature Death | Disability Illness | Symptoms | Average Health | Physical Health | Multidimensional Health | Self-actualization | Optimal Well-being |

Figure 1.2 Your health exists along a continuum from premature death and disability to optimal well-being.

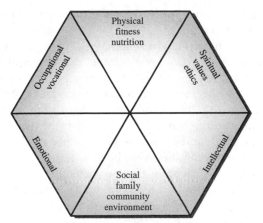

Figure 1.3 Wellness is multidimensional. Achieving optimal well-being is a process of striving toward being the best you can be across all six dimensions. (*Source:* Bill Hettler, MD, Director, University Health Service, University of Wisconsin–Steven's Point.)

spiritual, was added because it was thought that humans could not function optimally in a spiritual vacuum. Therefore, the holistic definition of health has five dimensions: physical, social, emotional, intellectual, and spiritual.

In the 1970s and 1980s, the definition of health was expanded once again by the wellness movement (Ardell, 1985). Wellness is an approach to health that focuses on balancing the many aspects or dimensions (physical, social, spiritual, emotional, intellectual, and environmental/occupational) of a person's life by increasing the adoption of health-enhancing conditions and behaviors rather than by attempting to minimize conditions of illness (AAHE, 2001).

A key element of the wellness model is striving for balance. When all of the six dimensions are at high levels and in balance, we have optimal health and well-being. When the dimensions are out of balance or one is severely lacking, we have lower levels of health and well-being. **Figure 1.3** illustrates this concept.

Another important part of wellness is the process of becoming healthier. The journey (becoming the best one can be) is more important

than the ending. The process of wellness involves becoming increasingly more aware of health and making healthy choices.

The Six Dimensions of Wellness

Physical

The first dimension, physical well-being, is reflected in how well the body performs its intended functions. Absence of disease—although an important influence—is not the sole criterion for health. The physical domain is influenced by your genetic inheritance, nutritional status, fitness level, body composition, and immune status, to name just a few factors.

Intellectual

Intellectual well-being is the ability to process information effectively. It involves the capability to use information in a rational way to solve problems and grow. This dimension includes issues such as creativity, spontaneity, and openness to new ways of viewing situations. To maintain a high level of intellectual well-being, you must seek knowledge and learn from your experiences. Ideally, your college experiences will have added to your intellectual well-being **(Figure 1.4)**.

Emotional

Emotional well-being means being in touch with your feelings, having the ability to express them, and being able to control them when necessary. Optimal functioning involves the understanding that emotions are the mirror of the soul. Emotions help us get in touch with what is important in our lives. Our emotions make us feel alive and provide us with a richness of experience that is uniquely human.

Social

Social well-being involves being connected to others through various types of relationships. Individuals who function optimally in this domain are able to form friendships, have intimate relationships, give and receive love and affection, and accept others unconditionally. They are able to give

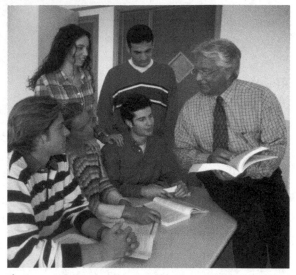

Figure 1.4 Being a college student is a major step in improving your intellectual well-being. (© age fotostock)

of themselves and share in the joys and sorrows of being part of a community. This community includes both formal and informal networks. Formal networks include organizations such as churches, professional organizations, fraternities, sororities, and campus groups requiring official membership, dues, and standards. Informal networks, such as an intramural sports team, do not have rigid rules for membership. In a sense, your social networks are a major part of your environment.

Environmental

Environmental well-being involves high-level functioning on two levels. The most immediate environment, the **micro-environment,** consists of your school, home, neighborhood, and work site. The people with whom you interact in those places link the environment to the social aspects of your health. This environment greatly affects your overall health and personal safety by influencing whether you are at risk for and fear issues such as theft, crime, and violence. The quality of air and water, noise pollution, crowding, and other issues that affect your stress level are also included.

Your social support system is also part of this environment.

The **macro-environment,** the level of well-being at a larger level—state, country, and the world at large—also affects wellness. The wars in Iraq and Afghanistan, the terrorist attacks of September 11, 2001, and other issues such as violence, international disputes, racism, sexism, heterosexism, and ageism—all influence us daily to some extent. When this book's authors were in college, the Vietnam War was going on. College-age men started each day by reading the newspaper to see which draft numbers were being called up (all draft-eligible men were issued draft numbers) and if any of their friends were killed or missing in action. Decisions that our political leaders make, such as engaging in wars or determining where we store radioactive wastes, affect the way we think and live our lives. Our ability to stay focused and whole is constantly challenged by the media, which bring the entire world and its problems into our living rooms each night. We need to learn to think globally, act locally, and be happy despite the myriad of problems in the world.

Spiritual

Spirituality is a belief in or relationship with some higher power, creative force, divine being, or infinite source of energy (Fowler, 1986). This belief is manifested in a sense of interconnectedness, a feeling that somehow, some way, we are all in this together. For people whose spirituality is religion-based, it is ecumenical in scope. It is part of but transcends individual religions. Those whose spirituality is religion-based believe in a supreme being or higher supernatural force and subscribe to a formalized code of conduct. For individuals whose spirituality is secular, it is universal or even extraterrestrial. In a secular sense, spirituality could manifest itself through connection to something greater than oneself. Whether it is being part of a community, working to save the environment, helping to feed the needy, or being committed to world peace, the underlying feeling is a perception of life as having meaning beyond the self (Richards & Bergin, 1997).

Spirituality is a two-dimensional concept. The first dimension relates to one's relationship with the transcendent (a connection with a higher being or power). The second dimension is connected to one's relationship with the self, others, and the environment. A continual interrelationship links the two dimensions. Feeling connected with a higher power or being gives us faith and hope and helps us believe we *can* do things to make life meaningful. Believing in oneself and feeling connected with others and one's community empowers us to act. Those with a high level of spiritual health behave in an interconnected way (Harris et al., 1999). They take part in church and/or community activities. They help others. They get involved in causes and groups that are proactive, whether it involves cleaning up a vacant lot or a beach with an environmental group or visiting the sick and infirm who are hospital bound. It is in the "doing" that some of the greatest benefits of spirituality are derived (Harris et al., 1999; Richards & Bergin, 1997).

Occupational/Vocational

Occupational/vocational well-being involves issues related to job wellness. It encompasses everything from the safety of your particular work site to the nature of your career. Work-site well-being includes both physical (e.g., air, water, physical plant, machinery) and social (e.g., relationships with coworkers, management, health and wellness facilities and activities) factors. Your personal wellness is affected by the health of your work site. Employers and work sites vary tremendously in relation to health. Some strive for optimal levels, encouraging employees to take advantage of a myriad of health-enhancing programs and services. Others merely meet the minimum acceptable standards for health and safety set by the government.

Besides the specific health of the workplace, different jobs pose varying threats to individuals' well-being as a result of the nature of the work. Some

jobs, such as police and military service, are risky because of possible exposure to hostile combatants. Other occupations, such as those of firefighters, emergency medical service workers, coal miners, and oil rig operators, are risky because they place employees in dangerous environments. Still other occupations are characterized by high stress due to deadlines, competition, or other factors.

Health Promotion and Health Education

Health and wellness are best achieved through planned personal and community-level interventions. These are designed to promote health and prevent disease.

Health Promotion

Health promotion is defined as any planned combination of educational, political, environmental, regulatory, or organizational mechanisms that support actions and conditions of living conducive to the health of individuals, groups, and communities (AAHE, 2001). Health promotion activities combine both specific protective measures and health education. Specific protective measures include legislation (e.g., speed limits, smoke-free areas), product design and development (e.g., automatic car seat belts, self-closing pool gates), and other measures. Specific protective measures are often accompanied by health education campaigns designed to educate consumers about the measures (Mausner & Kramer, 1985). Education is traditionally defined as the act or process of providing knowledge or training in a particular area or for a particular purpose. Education focuses primarily on the cognitive domain (knowledge), but can also target attitudes, behavioral intentions, and behavior.

Health Education

Health education is defined as any combination of planned learning experiences based on sound theories that provide individuals, groups, and communities with the opportunity to acquire information and the skills needed to make quality health decisions (AAHE, 2001). Health education usually extends beyond the cognitive domain to include attitudes, emotions, behavioral intentions, and skills/behavior.

For instance, you can teach someone about proper condom use by focusing on information only or by employing a combined approach that touches on attitudes, emotions, behavioral intentions, and skills/behaviors. An information-only approach would cover issues such as condom effectiveness in preventing unintended pregnancy and STDs, types of condoms, lubricants, instructions for use, and storage. A comprehensive condom health education program would start with the assumption that people use or don't use condoms consistently and correctly for a variety of reasons extending beyond what they know about them (information). In addition to what one knows about condoms, how one feels about them and using them with partners influences the decision to use them or not use them. Helping students/clients assess their attitudes and beliefs about condoms is an important first step in getting them to believe the information they need to know to use condoms effectively. In addition to exploring attitudes and emotions, condom health education would cover skill training and behavior modification. These areas would focus on teaching clients exactly how to use condoms and how to work them into one's lifestyle.

Healthy People 2010

Healthy People 2010 is both a vision and a plan of action to improve the health of Americans over the first decade of the twenty-first century. It builds on health promotion and disease prevention initiatives that originated in the 1979 Surgeon General's Report, Healthy People, and Healthy People 2000: National Health Promotion and Disease Prevention Objectives. Healthy People 2010 grew out of the efforts of an alliance of more than 600 federal, state, and territorial governmental agencies; national professional associations; private, public, and nonprofit organizations; colleges and universities; and concerned individuals (USDHHS, 2003).

Healthy People 2010 is based on 467 measurable health objectives derived from the country's 10 Leading Health Indicators (see **Table 1.1**). The 10 Leading Health Indicators are the major health concerns of the United States and are used as benchmarks to measure the health of the country. Throughout this text we will discuss how health counseling is related to these indicators and how counselors can address them as part of their work with clients. Clients will often present for counseling as a direct result of these indicators. For instance, clients may seek stress counseling because they are feeling stressed and fear they might be sinking into clinical depression. Another example is the client infected with *Chlamydia* who attends a public health clinic and receives counseling regarding responsible sexual behavior. In other cases, clients seeking counseling for one health problem will afford counselors the opportunity to discuss other leading indicators. For example, as described in Chapter 9, a client presenting with hypertension might also receive counseling about

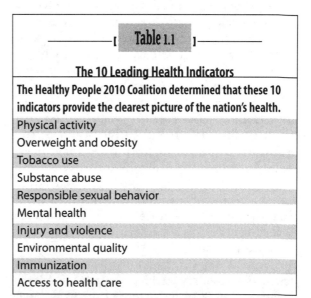

——————[**Table 1.1**]——————
The 10 Leading Health Indicators
The Healthy People 2010 Coalition determined that these 10 indicators provide the clearest picture of the nation's health.
Physical activity
Overweight and obesity
Tobacco use
Substance abuse
Responsible sexual behavior
Mental health
Injury and violence
Environmental quality
Immunization
Access to health care

Source: USDHHS (2003). *The Leading Health Indicators.*
www.healthypeople.gov/Document/html/uih/uih_bw/uih_2.htm#obj.

physical activity, obesity, and tobacco use. Lastly, clients using public health facilities as their entry point into the healthcare delivery system offer opportunities for counselors in these settings to empower them to gain broader access to health care by referring them for a range of services such as immunization and nutritional programs for their children.

What Is Counseling?

There are many ways to define counseling. In Chapter 2, we will explore several counseling theories, including Allen Ivey's microskills theory (Ivey & Authier, 1978). A good working definition of counseling was developed by Carl Rogers (1965). Counseling, according to Rogers, is an intensive interactive process characterized by a unique relationship between the counselor and client leading to change in the client in one or more of the following areas:

- Behavior
- Personal constructs
- Ability to cope
- Decision making (Rogers, 1965)

Counseling by its very nature focuses more on the affective domain (feelings). People come to counseling because they are feeling psychological distress. They are experiencing emotional pain and need help understanding and coping with it.

The opening section of this chapter touched on the intensive nature of counseling. One of the reasons why counseling is such an intense process is because of its interactive nature. Counseling isn't done *to* people, but rather done *with* people. While some educational activities can be performed using one-way communication, counseling demands two-way communication. It entails a dialogue between the counselor and client. The dialogue is based on active listening for the full time during which the client is present. This process can be very exhausting, especially when dealing with highly emotionally charged issues.

A counselor may focus on any or all of the four areas Rogers identified as the primary content of counseling. Clients often come to counseling to understand and work on behaviors that are causing them problems. These behaviors may range from substance abuse to sexual paraphilias. Counselors help people understand their behavior, change destructive behaviors, and reinforce positive behaviors.

Personal constructs are the mental images or story lines clients have regarding a host of issues. They represent how clients view the world and how they think the world should be. Each construct has its own unique script. People have personal constructs about issues such as work, school, taxes, traffic, and money as well as about relationships with family, friends, spouses, lovers, peers, employers, and a host of others. Often these constructs and scripts are not based on logic or realistic expectations and become a source of psychological distress. Counselors help people examine their personal constructs and make them more realistic and logical.

Often, people are in situations that cannot be eliminated or significantly improved at the present time. In such instances, counselors may only be able to help clients cope with the situations rather than help them change or eliminate those circumstances.

Lastly, counselors can often help people make tough decisions. Many people need assistance when evaluating information so as to make informed choices. Counselors help them understand the pros and cons of decisions and make informed choices that best meet the clients' own needs.

Characteristics of Effective Counselors

Counselors are essentially helpers who help facilitate growth in their clients. Egan (2002) differentiates between *smart* and *wise* counselors. Smart counselors are steeped in the theory of helping and applying research findings in their work with clients. Wise counselors integrate the theory of counseling with wisdom, practicality, street smarts, and common sense (Egan, 2002). The following description highlights some of the major characteristics of the wisdom that wise counselors bring to their helping of clients.

1. *Self-knowledge and maturity.* Wise counselors are introspective. They are committed to understanding themselves as well as their clients. They respect the insights gleaned through maturity and value the wisdom that comes with experience and maturity.

2. *A psychological and human understanding of others.* Wise counselors understand the psychological theory of human development and abnormalities. They also understand how the reality of the human condition influences development and how easily problems can occur.

3. *An understanding of cultural conditioning.* Wise counselors understand the effects of culture on psychological development and have a respect for cross-cultural differences. They value and respect cultural diversity, and avoid stereotyping clients based on age, race, gender, ethnicity, sexual orientation, and other variables.

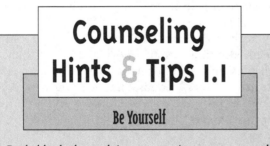

Counseling Hints & Tips 1.1

Be Yourself

Probably the best advice we can give anyone regarding how they should act when counseling someone is this:

Don't act—be yourself!

While the qualities associated with effective counselors are generic and serve as guidelines for practice, clients will respond to you best if you just relax and listen to their stories. If you are worried more about how you are coming across to clients rather than listening to their stories, you will be less effective.

4. *The ability to see through situations.* Wise counselors realize that things are rarely the way they are initially presented. They can tolerate ambiguity as they work through issues to uncover their true meanings. They can synthesize diverse factors and use their intuition to make sense of clients' stories.

5. *A tolerance for "messiness."* Wise counselors realize that people and their problems are rarely tidy and well organized. Rather, people and their problems are usually messy, filled with contradictions and disorganization.

6. *Openness and approachability.* Wise counselors are open to new ideas and new ways to view things. They do not let their experience become a liability by creating blocks or "blind spots." They remain open-minded about nontraditional or seemingly illogical views and behavior presented by clients. They listen, reframe situations, and present options in a nonjudgmental way.

7. *Holistic framework.* Wise counselors understand the many dimensions of life and health that influence their clients. They respect issues such as spirituality that can serve as a source of strength for clients.

8. *An ability to blend seemingly antithetical roles.* Wise counselors realize that to help they sometimes have to get clients to explore painful, troubling issues. Wise counselors accept the responsibility to confront clients and frustrate them so as to assist clients in getting better.

9. *A willingness to take risks.* Good counselors are willing to take risks and leave themselves open to criticism and challenge from clients. They realize that they will make mistakes, have the guts to admit them, and have the sense to learn from their errors.

10. *Genuineness.* Good counselors are real. They are comfortable with themselves and their personal style. They are not pretentious and do not need to be anything but themselves to be effective. They realize that their style may not fit every client and are

willing to help clients find another counselor who better fits their stylistic needs if necessary (Eagan, 2002).

Lastly, good counselors, as Metcalf and Felible (1992) would say, "take their work seriously and themselves lightly." They honor what they do but do not take themselves too seriously. They are not pompous. They know how to lighten up and integrate humor into their work and life. They are not afraid to be self-deprecating and laugh at their own follics.

What Is Health Counseling?

As defined earlier in the chapter, health counseling is a psycho-educational process that revolves around two primary functions: (1) helping clients understand and cope with the feelings and emotions associated with their health problems and (2) helping clients develop and adhere to therapeutic regimens. By nature, health counseling is short term and task oriented. It starts and ends with a specific health problem.

Case Study 1.1
Erica: Health Educator

Erica is 22 and recently graduated with a B.S. in Community Health Education from an approved undergraduate program. She was interviewed by Dr. Blonna regarding the nature of her work since graduating.

Dr. Blonna: Hi, Erica. Can you tell me a little bit about what you have been doing at work since graduating last spring?

Erica: Sure. I have been working as a community health educator for a local health department. I have a wide variety of functions. I plan, implement, and evaluate community health education programs. I develop media pieces to use in promoting our programs and alerting the public to certain health issues, such as getting flu shots. I also do some basic counseling in our health clinics.

Dr. Blonna: Tell me more about the counseling you do.

Erica: First of all, let me just say that I am not a counselor. I realize that I need to get additional training and licensing for that. I do, however, help people who come into the clinics where I work.

Dr. Blonna: Can you give me an example?

Erica: Sure. I work at the STD clinic with a nurse practitioner on Wednesday nights. Clients come in and are seen by the nurse-practitioner, who examines them and treats them based on standing orders from our supervising physician. After she sees the clients, I get to talk to them about prevention, follow-up of sex partners, and anything else they want to talk about. They are often very emotional, and before we can discuss anything I usually need to help them relax and deal with the emotions they have about being infected.

Dr. Blonna: Do you feel comfortable doing this?

Erica: Yes, especially because I know my limits. If I think anyone needs help beyond the basic attending and influencing I am trained in, I refer them to one of our mental health counselors who is a licensed counselor. It doesn't happen that often, but it is important for the clinic to have these referral mechanisms. I feel very comfortable with basic helping skills because we learned these as part of our undergraduate preparation.

The major difference between health counseling and generic counseling is the former's focus on the emotional issues *surrounding a specific health issue*. Each health problem has a unique set of educational and emotional directives. For instance, counseling clients who are HIV positive will be very different from working with clients who are in counseling for help with their obesity. Both sets of clients need to work through the emotional issues they have regarding their conditions. Living with HIV and complying with a weight-loss program, however, are associated with different sets of emotional responses, therapeutic regimens, and adherence issues.

The goal of health counseling is to help all types of clients understand and work through their feelings and emotions surrounding their health problems so they can adhere to their therapeutic regimens, gain more control over their lives, and get better.

The Practice of Health Counseling

Health counseling is a practice that is not distinguished by a recognized professional credential or specialty. Instead, it is practiced in a variety of settings by a variety of helping professionals, ranging from licensed professional counselors, psychologists, and psychiatrists, to health educators, nurses, physicians, nurse-practitioners, and physical therapists.

Licensed professional counselors, psychologists, and psychiatrists work in a variety of settings, ranging from private practice to community health centers. Some of these licensed professionals have a specialized practice that focuses on a particular type of health problem. They help clients with problems ranging from substance abuse to stress management. They typically see clients for multiple sessions and are eligible for third-party reimbursement.

Nurses, nurse-practitioners, midwives, and physicians also work with a variety of clients in many diverse settings. Public health nurses, for example, might counsel new mothers about breastfeeding, child-care issues, and prevention of unintended pregnancy. They typically will see clients for only one or two visits in the field. The same nurses, when working in a public health center clinic, might counsel STD patients, people who are HIV positive, people seeking cholesterol screening, and women learning to perform a breast self-exam, among many other types of clients.

Health educators working in public clinics, private nonprofit agencies, and hospitals will perform counseling duties similar to those carried out by public health nurses. They also might be employed in STD clinics, family planning clinics, HIV testing centers, well-baby and WIC (Women, Infants, and Children) programs, and a variety of other locations where they might be called upon to provide basic counseling services.

Health counseling, like health promotion and health education, can target any of the three levels of prevention: primary, secondary, and tertiary (Mausner & Kramer, 1985). **Primary prevention** activities are designed to reduce the likelihood that the person ever develops the health problem. It consists of teaching people the information, skills, and behaviors they need to reduce their risks of developing the health problem.

Those engaged in primary prevention activities work with clients who do not have the problem and who may or may not be at risk for developing it. A health counselor working in a teen center, for example, might be involved in substance abuse counseling. Such counseling focuses on helping the teens make healthy decisions about substance use. Some of these people may be at high risk for abusing drugs because of their background and lifestyle, while others are not. Some might have experimented with drugs; others have not. All have concerns about their health, substance use and abuse, the law, and a host of other substance abuse–related issues. The counselor works with them, both one on one and in groups, to provide information about substance use and abuse and to teach them how to reduce their risks.

Secondary prevention refers to the early detection and prompt treatment of health problems. The intention of this type of effort is to prevent the progression of the problem. On an individual level, it is designed to halt the progression of the problem within the individual. At a community level, it is designed to prevent the spread of the problem throughout the community.

Health counselors engaged in secondary prevention activities work with clients who already have the problem and with populations in which there is a greater probability of discovering individuals with the problem. Screening programs are an integral part of secondary prevention. Screening tests and examinations are designed to uncover previously undetected health conditions in high-risk individuals. A health counselor in an HIV counseling and testing center, for instance, interacts with those who suspect they may have been exposed to HIV and who need a test to determine their HIV status. The counselor must work through a host of emotions that clients have regarding exposure and possible infection with HIV. Counselors in this setting must educate the clients about HIV, the test, interpretation of results, coping with positive results, and a variety of other issues.

Tertiary prevention consists of limiting disability and premature death of clients who have had the health problem for a while and are suffering from complications associated with it. These clients have lived with their health problem for some time and need help in coping with the complications they are experiencing. A counselor working in a head-trauma rehabilitation center, for instance, will serve clients who have myriad physical, mental, and relationship problems associated with head trauma from intentional and unintentional injuries. They have a host of emotional issues related to their disabilities. To halt the progression of their disability, teach them new skills, and restore functioning, counselors must work through these emotional issues.

The level of prevention that is the focal point of educational and counseling activities will vary depending on the setting and the nature of the problem. For instance, counselors who work in a rehabilitation center will work primarily with tertiary prevention. Counselors who work in an HIV counseling and testing center will focus mainly on primary and secondary prevention, because most of their clients don't have any symptoms of the disease and are coming in to see whether they are infected.

The nature and scope of counseling services are determined not only by the type of practice, but also by legal and professional standards and codes. In some states, strict guidelines regulate who can do what with specific types of clients. In other states, a broader definition of counseling is employed. Throughout this book we will identify and illustrate these and other considerations that guide the practice of health counseling.

The Counselor–Client Relationship

The counselor–client relationship is different from other relationships between two people. Although the theoretical framework of counselors and the individual techniques they use with clients will vary, the *relationship* itself is the most important variable in the therapeutic process. Egan (2002) examines the relationship from three different perspectives: (1) the relationship itself, (2) the relationship as a means to an end, and (3) the relationship and outcomes. This section briefly touches on all three aspects of the counselor–client relationship.

The Relationship Itself

Egan (2002) agrees with Patterson's (1985) earlier assertion that counseling does not merely incorporate the use of interpersonal relationships, but rather that the counseling process *is* a unique interpersonal relationship between two people. In this relationship, two people come together and build a special bond that is central to healing. According to Rogers (1965), the three key elements of this relationship are (1) genuineness, (2) empathy, and (3) unconditional positive regard. Genuineness essentially means being oneself, without facades, pretenses, or defenses. Empathy is feeling things with clients. While counselors do not share clients' experiences and cannot see and feel the world exactly as they do, they can try to put themselves in their clients' places and imagine what it must be like. Unconditional positive regard is similar to what parents feel for their children—the ability to see the good in them despite their flaws. Unlike parent–child relationships, however, counselor–client relationships are not subject to familial and historical biases. Counselors' unconditional positive regard stems from their belief in the inherent goodness of the individual as a *person,* not as a son or daughter.

These three elements create a relationship that is unique among all interpersonal relationships.

The Relationship as a Means to an End

The second way to characterize the counselor–client relationship is to view it as a tool—that is, as a means to an end. It has elements that are crucial to helping clients get to where they want to be. The unconditional positive regard, empathy, and genuineness are important, not in and of themselves, but rather because they facilitate helping the client get better. Without them, clients would not be able to do the other things necessary for growth. For instance, the existence of a warm, trusting relationship built on unconditional positive regard allows counselors to use strategies (e.g., confrontation, role playing) that clients might not agree to in other contexts. It is not the relationship per se that leads to healing and growth, but rather what the relationship allows counselors and clients to *do* that makes this result possible.

The Relationship and Outcomes

The third way to characterize the counselor–client relationship is to view it from a "solution-focused" perspective. This way of viewing the relationship also sees it as a means to an end, but posits that the end is the most important part. Egan (2002) suggests that counselors and schools of counseling that view the relationship in this way focus on helping clients take action as soon as possible without having to spend multiple sessions gaining insight into their problems. That is, the relationship is a vehicle for getting clients to act, but it is the action (and resultant outcomes) that is the major focus and most important part. Wonderful relationships that are full of instructions, strategies, and techniques are interesting, but if they do not result in action they are of little value.

Ethical Issues in Health Counseling

Ethics, according to Greenberg (2003), is a system by which one determines whether an action is moral or immoral. Greenberg (2003) defines **morality** as a judgment about whether an action is good or bad, right or wrong. **Codes of ethics** are formal statements, developed by professional organizations, that prescribe **standards** for practice, state **principles** regarding responsibilities, and define **rules** expressing the duties and behaviors of professionals to whom the codes apply (Greenberg, 2003). Standards set levels or degrees of quality. Counselors can assess how they measure up to the standards set by their codes of ethics. Principles are responsibilities to clients and others that are set by the code of ethics. Principles guide the counselor's behavior toward clients and others. Lastly, rules spell out the actual behaviors deemed appropriate and inappropriate by the code of ethics.

Organizations that govern the practice of health counseling have codes of ethics that are drawn from their missions, philosophy, and accreditation standards. Health education, counseling, and nursing associations—the three professional groups most closely associated with health counseling—all have formal codes of ethics that potential members must pledge to support. Consequently, most health counselors have been required to pledge their support for one or more of the aforementioned disciplines' codes of ethics when joining their respective profession. Failure to pledge support is sufficient grounds for denial of admission into the association. Breaching the code of ethics can lead to dismissal from any professional association with a code of ethics. Loss of licensure and denial of the ability to practice can also result from breaking an organization's code of ethics.

Ethical Dilemmas

Ethical dilemmas arise when two or more ethics and the morality associated with them compete with each other. Many situations create ethical dilemmas. Here we discuss three of the most common types of ethics competitions:

1. Competition between a counselor's differing ethics over the same issue

2. Competition between the counselor's personal ethics (on a single issue, multiple issues, or the entire code) and the organization's code of ethics
3. Competition between the counselor's ethics and the client's ethics

The first type of ethical dilemma might arise, for example, over the counselor's feelings and values regarding personal use of marijuana. Let's assume that the counselor believes that marijuana, as compared to other legal psychoactive substances such as alcohol, is not as significant a personal or public health problem. He believes that people can use marijuana safely and that abuse is more of a legal problem than a health problem. (We won't debate the merits or problems with this viewpoint but just use it for the example.) This counselor has a 16-year-old client who was referred to him as a condition of probation following an arrest and conviction for marijuana use. The client has become a frequent user of the drug and has a long history of school absenteeism and juvenile delinquency.

The counselor finds himself in an ethical dilemma because his personal ethics regarding the use of marijuana conflict with the needs of his client. His client has experienced problems that may be the result of using the drug, is considered by police to be a drug abuser, and is participating in counseling to help him stop using the drug. The counselor wonders whether his personal ethics regarding the drug and its use will interfere with his ability to help his client.

An example of the second ethical dilemma might involve differences between how a counselor's agency views needle sharing as a risk-reduction strategy to prevent the spread of HIV and how she views it. The counselor's professional association has approved an initiative to become actively involved in pressuring local lawmakers to introduce legislation to offer free needle sharing for injection drug users at all public health clinics. The organization believes that this initiative meshes with its code of ethics, which states that the organization will "advocate for the introduction of legislation that promotes the public's health and reduces its risk of disease." The counselor is being pressured to write letters and attend demonstrations promoting the legislation.

The health counselor does not believe that this initiative fits with the association's mission and code of ethics. She believes that needle-sharing programs promote illegal behavior (injecting drugs) and, therefore, go against the standards for professionalism and citizenship set by an association of its kind. She has been soundly criticized for her stance. She does not question the literature supporting the effects of needle sharing in reducing HIV transmission. Nevertheless, she is torn between the effectiveness of this program as a public health strategy and her association's enthusiastic support for it and her own ethics, which do not condone supporting illegal activity.

A final example will demonstrate the competition between a counselor's ethics and morals and those of a client. Suppose that a vulnerable, yet grateful client expresses a sexual or romantic attraction for the counselor. Such powerful reactions are common on both sides of the "therapy couch," yet the acting upon these feelings is considered among the most severe "boundary violations." While the client may develop strong positive feelings for the counselor and desire to extend their relationship beyond the therapeutic, it is incumbent upon the counselor to not let this happen. Most professional disciplines state quite clearly in their ethics code that sexual intimacies between counselor and client are never permissible. The primary reason for this mandate is that it is the counselor's responsibility to ensure that no harm comes to the client as a result of the therapy process. Such a relationship would be considered unethical, exploitive, and harmful to the client. Even if the client clearly expresses a desire and willingness to engage in such a relationship, the counselor must refrain and deal with this issue within the context of the therapeutic environment. All professional counselors should have some training in how to handle these transference/countertransference feelings. If in any doubt, seek supervision at once. These feelings are quite common, but professionalism and ethics must always be the paramount concerns.

Counseling Hints & Tips 1.2

Handling Ethical Dilemmas

All ethical dilemmas have one thing in common: They pit two competing ethics against each other. As mentioned earlier, these can involve the self, professional organizations, or clients. The following hints touch on all three areas.

1. *Know what you value.* Ethics competition evolves out of values conflicts. A key to understanding this point is knowing what you value. Start by asking yourself the following questions:
   - What do I value most about myself as a man/woman?
   - What do I value most about myself as a counselor?
   - What three things would I absolutely never do to a client?
   - What three things do I expect from clients?
   - What do I value most about my professional organization?
   - What are the three values most central to my beliefs about life?

2. *Know your professional code of ethics.* The following three websites link to the codes of ethics for counselors, nurses, and health educators.

American Counseling Association
www.counseling.org/Content/NavigationMenu/
  RESOURCES/ETHICS/ACA_Ethics.pdf

Coalition of National Health Education Organizations
www.nmsu.edu/~hlthdpt/bchethics.html

American Nursing Association
www.nursingworld.org/ethics/code/ethicscode150.
  htm
If your ethics are in competition with any of the organizations' codes of ethics, see whether you can get involved in the committee that reviews and rewrites the code.

3. *Work honestly with clients.* The best way to avoid ethics conflicts with clients is to state your ethics up front.
   - Give your clients your organizations' codes of ethics during their first visit.
   - Explain to your clients that you will let them know if things they discuss or expect during your time together pose an ethics conflict that makes it difficult to work with them.

Explain that you would not rule out referring clients to another counselor if the two of you have serious-enough ethics conflicts.

It is not within the scope of this book to explore the endless types of ethical dilemmas faced by counselors and ways to handle them all. Numerous books, professional workshops, and other resources from professional associations are available for handling them. Counseling Hint 1.2 gives some basic starting points for handling ethical dilemmas.

Termination of Counseling

One of the questions that new counselors most frequently have regarding the counseling process has to do with a simple concern: When does counseling end? While there are few objective ways to answer this question, it is one that must be considered in every counseling relationship.

Health counseling typically ends when the health issue and the emotions associated with it have been resolved. In practice, this is often more complicated than it may sound. The termination of counseling typically involves a gradual process, as opposed to an abrupt termination. In many counseling situations, it is more effective (and more comfortable for the client) to begin by spacing counseling sessions

Susan: Ethical Conflicts

Susan is 23, is married, and identifies as African American. She is a health counselor working in a local family planning clinic. A recent college graduate, Susan has the lowest seniority among the five counselors employed by the facility. As a Certified Health Education Specialist (CHES), she provides individual counseling for women regarding choosing a birth control method. A caveat of Susan's work is the concept of "informed choice"—that is, providing information and helping women work through the emotional issues surrounding which type of birth control is best for them.

Susan is very good at her job. Even though there have been times when she felt a client was making the wrong choice of a method, Susan has remained true to her goal of respecting the client's right to decide what works best for her.

Recently, Susan overheard a discussion between two coworkers regarding counseling their clients about birth control pills. They were referring to young girls (mostly African American teenagers) and knowing what is best for "those kinds of kids." Susan picked up a condescending tone in the way her coworkers were describing these young women. It seems that the two were receiving rewards (cash and other gifts) from their local pharmaceutical sales representative for pressuring their clients to choose the company's brand of birth control pills over other competitors' pills. In addition, they were steering women away from other contraceptive methods that were clearly better choices for them. From the way her coworkers were talking, neither respected the ability of these African American girls to make an informed choice regarding birth control.

Susan has an ethical conflict. She believes that the other counselors' behavior is clearly a breach of their code of ethics as health educators and counselors at the clinic. These counselors' actions clearly violate the principle of informed consent and constitute a blatant misuse of their power over clients. Susan also believes that part of her ethics involves reporting such behavior to her supervisors. Ignoring it would violate her personal and professional ethics.

Susan knows that as the counselor with the lowest seniority it will be her word against that of the other counselors and she might lose her job over this issue. Both of the other counselors are well liked by the other staff members while Susan is still struggling to fit in.

What would you do if you were in Susan's shoes?

---

farther and farther apart, thereby allowing for a more gradual easing out of the counseling mode. Even after the regular sessions have ceased, many counselors recommend the scheduling of periodic "booster sessions" to maximize the likelihood that the gains realized in counseling will be maintained.

The relationship developed in counseling can be quite powerful for many clients. In some ways, it may never completely terminate because clients may decide to return for counseling as other issues may appear in their lives. It is helpful to reassure clients that even though the sessions may be ending for now, the door is always open to return if needed.

Summary

This chapter provided an overview of the field of health counseling. First, health counseling was defined. Its origins can be traced by considering a chronology of the evolution of the concepts of health and wellness.

The next part of the chapter discussed the nature of health education. It emphasized the role of lifestyle change in health education. Health education revolves around people taking more personal responsibility for their health and wellness.

The nature of counseling was the next topic discussed. Counseling, although similar to education, is differentiated from it by its focus on the affective domain rather than the cognitive and behavioral domains (the primary focus of health education). The nature of counseling was described using Carl Rogers' definition, which characterizes it as an intensive, interactive, unique relationship. The qualities of a wise counselor were discussed, noting that counseling, by its very nature, is a helping relationship, so counselors are first and foremost helpers.

The chapter ended with a discussion of the practice of health counseling. Because it is not a professionally regulated discipline, health counseling is practiced by a variety of individuals in a host of different settings.

Study Questions

1. Compare the World Health Organization's 1947 definition of health to the current definition.
2. Describe how health, wellness, and health promotion are similar and different.
3. Describe the six dimensions of wellness. Give an example of each.
4. Why does Rogers characterize counseling as an intensive, exhaustive process?
5. What are the four focal points in Rogers' definition of counseling?
6. List and describe five characteristics of effective counselors.
7. How is health counseling similar to and different from generic counseling?
8. Describe how health counseling varies according to where it is practiced.
9. Pick a health counseling topic and describe one potential ethical conflict that you would associate with it.
10. What is an individual counselor's responsibility regarding the ethical conduct of other counselors?

References

American Association of Health Education (AAHE) (2001). Joint Committee on Health Education and Promotion Terminology.

Ardell D (1985). *The History and Future of Wellness*. Dubuque, IA: Kendall/Hunt.

Dunn H (1962). High-level wellness in the world of today. *Journal of the American Osteopathic Association* 61:9.

Egan G (2002). *The Skilled Helper: A Problem Management and Opportunity Development Approach to Helping*, 7th ed. Pacific Grove, CA: Brooks/Cole.

Fowler JF (1986). *Stages of Faith: The Psychology of Human Development and the Quest for Meaning*. New York: Harper & Row.

Greenberg J (2003). Ethical issues in health counseling. In Donnelly J (Ed.) (2003). *Health Counseling: Application and Theory*. Belmont, CA: Wadsworth/Thomson Learning.

Harris AHS, Thoreson CE, McCollough ME, Larson DB (1999). Spiritually and religiously oriented health interventions. *Journal of Health Psychology* 4:413–433.

Hettler B (2003). *Six Dimensional Model of Wellness*. http://hettler.com/.

Ivey AE, Authier J (1978). *Microcounseling: Innovations in Interviewing, Counseling, Psychotherapy, and Psychoeducation*. Springfield, IL: Charles C. Thomas.

Mausner JS, Kramer S (1985). *Epidemiology: An Introductory Text*. Philadelphia: Saunders.

Metcalf CW, Felible R (1992). *Lighten Up*. Reading, MA: Addison Wesley.

Patterson CH (1985). *The Therapeutic Relationship: Foundations for an Ethical Psychotherapy*. Pacific Grove, CA: Brooks/Cole.

Richards PS, Bergin AE (1997). *A Spiritual Strategy for Counseling and Psychotherapy*. Washington, DC: American Psychological Association.

Rogers C (1965). *Client-Centered Therapy*. Boston: Houghton Mifflin.

United States Department of Health and Human Services (USDHHS), Office of Disease Prevention and Health Promotion (ODPHP) (2003). *Healthy People 2010: A Systematic Approach to Health Improvement. www.healthypeople.gov/Document/html/uih/uih_bw/uih_2.htm#obj*.

World Health Organization (WHO) (1947). Constitution of the World Health Organization. *Chronicles of the World Health Organization* 1:29–43.

Learning Objectives

By the end of the chapter students will:

1. Compare and contrast health, illness, and sick role behavior

2. Describe how counseling varies according to sick role status

3. Describe the key components of a variety of behavior change theories

4. Describe how elements of behavior change theory are integrated into health counseling

5. Draw from the available behavioral change theories to develop a personal theoretical framework regarding client behavior change

6. Compare and contrast the major insight theories in counseling

7. Compare and contrast the major behavioral theories in counseling

8. Draw from the insight and behavioral theories to develop a personal theoretical framework regarding counseling theory

9. Describe how Ivey's microskills theory transcends insight and behavioral theories of counseling

10. List and describe the key factors related to client adherence with therapeutic regimens

Health Counseling Theory

The basis of health counseling is helping clients maintain behaviors that promote health and prevent illness or change behaviors that inhibit the healing process and contribute to illness. To do so, the counselor needs not only to be proficient in using the skills of counseling, but also to have knowledge of the theories used to explain, and change, behavior. Kasl (1966a, 1966b) identified three distinct categories of behaviors that are of concern to health counselors: health behavior, illness behavior, and sick role behavior. For any health problem these three types of behaviors are interwoven with the three levels of prevention discussed in Chapter 1 (primary, secondary, and tertiary) and influence the nature and scope of counseling. For example, a counselor working in a setting that focuses mostly on tertiary prevention, such as a rehabilitation center, will deal mostly with issues related to illness behavior, because the clients served are already ill and have disabling complications.

Health, Illness, and Sick Role Behavior

Health behavior can be defined as the things people do or do not do to promote their health and prevent disease. It includes adopting health-enhancing behaviors (e.g., daily physical activity, use of seat belts, eating more nutritiously) and stopping health-risk behaviors (e.g., smoking,

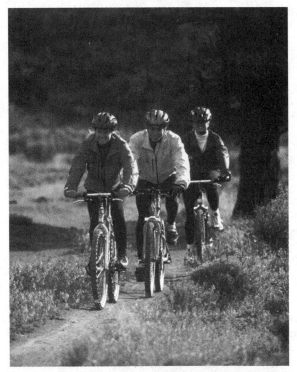

Figure 2.1 Engaging in 30 minutes of moderate or vigorous physical activity daily is a good example of health behavior. (© Photos.com)

nonuse of condoms). The focus of health behavior is on primary prevention. As mentioned in Chapter 1, primary prevention is concerned with preventing the person from developing a disease or illness in the first place. Health counselors working in a variety of settings help clients adopt new health behaviors and maintain existing ones.

Illness behavior comprises the things people do or do not do from the time they suspect that they might be exposed to, infected with, or developing a disease or illness. It includes how people interpret and respond to the presence of symptoms and risk factors. Illness behavior is related to secondary prevention. The intention of secondary prevention is to halt the progression and spread of disease through identification and treatment of early or asymptomatic cases. Some people might have screening tests performed because they have risk factors for a condition and therefore suspect they might be developing disease. Others might experience mild symptoms that they suspect might be related to the disease and therefore seek screening tests as preliminary diagnoses of their conditions. Still others do not link screening tests to risk factors or symptoms, but rather undertake them for a variety of other reasons, ranging from adhering to doctor's orders to habit.

Case Study 5.1
Solomon's Illness Behavior

Solomon, 44, is married and African American. He was infected with gonorrhea and sought treatment as a walk-in patient at a local public STD clinic. He first noticed his symptoms 14 days ago. He had a profuse, yellow-green penile discharge of 14 days' duration. Solomon also had extreme inflammation and swelling of his penis and foreskin, to the point where retracting his foreskin was impossible. Dr. Blonna recounts the interaction between himself and Solomon.

Dr. Blonna: Hello, Solomon. Why don't you tell me what your problem is?

Solomon: I'd rather show you.
Dr. Blonna: I'm not a medical doctor.
Solomon: That's okay. I can't describe it.
Dr. Blonna: Okay, then go ahead.

At this point Solomon removes his trousers and underwear, revealing a homemade "diaper" that he has been using to catch the gonococcal discharge so it doesn't get all over his underwear and groin. Upon removing his clothes, Dr. Blonna is overpowered by the stench of Solomon's infection. As Solomon removes his "diaper," he reveals a severely swollen penis, the head of which is swollen to the size of his fist. His foreskin is extremely stretched and eroded from the discharge. Dr. Blonna is in shock that Solomon can stand the discomfort.

Dr. Blonna: Solomon, how long has this been this way?
Solomon: The swelling started last week.
Dr. Blonna: Why haven't you come into the clinic sooner? It's free.
Solomon: I know, I just haven't had the time.
Dr. Blonna: What do you mean? Hasn't it been painful?
Solomon: Not really until yesterday and today. I just couldn't take the time off work. My boss would have fired me. Today the plant was closed down because they're fixing one of the big machines that broke down. I figured I'd come in, seeing as how I didn't have to go to work.
Dr. Blonna: Well, I'm glad you did. Let's get you some medicine to treat this infection.

The clinic physician prescribed broad-spectrum antibiotics for Solomon's infection, which responded quite well. Upon return for follow-up the next week, his body was almost back to normal.

Solomon's case demonstrates the incredible variability in illness behavior. We should never assume that all clients would respond to their health problems as we do.

Sick role behavior is defined as the things people do or do not do from the time they are diagnosed with a condition to the time they are cured or their condition is in a maintenance stage. It includes such things as taking medication, returning for follow-up tests, adhering to lifestyle modifications (change in eating, exercise, and other habits). Sick role behavior can be a part of either secondary or tertiary prevention. Such behavior connected with secondary prevention revolves around complying with therapeutic regimens designed to halt the development and spread of the newly diagnosed condition. For instance, taking medication and returning for follow-up testing would be routine sick role behaviors for a woman with a newly diagnosed case of *Chlamydia* infection that was uncovered through routine testing during her annual examination conducted by her gynecologist. Sick role behavior related to tertiary prevention refers to behaviors adopted to prevent further disability and help restore functioning to the highest level possible. An example would be adhering to a treatment regimen consisting of medication and physical therapy prescribed as part of the rehabilitation program for a man who recently suffered from a stroke. The medication is designed to help prevent a future stroke by minimizing the risk of blood clotting. The physical therapy is intended to restore all remaining motor function to its highest level.

Behavior Change Theories

A **theory** is "a set of interrelated concepts, definitions, and propositions that presents a systematic view of events or situations by specifying relations among variables in order to explain and predict the events of the situation" (Glanz, Lewis, & Rimer, 1997). Theories help to explain why people do or do not do certain things in a given situation.

When using theory to understand, explain, or change behavior, it is important to remember that each client and each behavior change may be influenced by many different variables and, therefore, may be explained in numerous ways. Hence, there is no one correct theory for each situation.

Instead, any number of theories may prove useful in a given situation. The following are among the most commonly used theories in health education.

Health Belief Model

The health belief model **(Figure 2.2)** explains behavior from the perspective of four perceptions: perceived seriousness, perceived susceptibility, perceived benefits, and perceived barriers (Rosenstock, 1974; Glanz, Lewis, & Rimer, 1997; Dunbar, Marshall, & Hovell, 1999). The perception of seriousness is determined by the individual's beliefs about the significance or gravity of an illness. Not everyone assigns the same weight to a given health condition. Similar to the perception of a stressor, perception of seriousness will vary from person to person.

Perceived seriousness, the extent to which individuals believe an illness to be serious, can significantly alter health behavior. For example, if people believe that the flu is not serious because they have had it before and recovered without incident, then it is unlikely they will get flu vaccinations. However, if the perception is that the flu is serious because it can lead to pneumonia and, in some cases, death, then it is more likely that they will seek such vaccinations. Often, the greater the understanding of a health problem or illness, the more accurate the perception of seriousness is likely to be.

Perceived susceptibility is the extent to which individuals believe they are at risk of contracting a disease or developing a health problem. It is the personal evaluation of risk. For example, if people perceive that they have little to no risk of contracting HIV, then the likelihood of their adopting safer sex behaviors is reduced or nonexistent. In contrast, if they assess their personal risk as being great, then the likelihood of practicing safer sex increases. However, the perception of risk

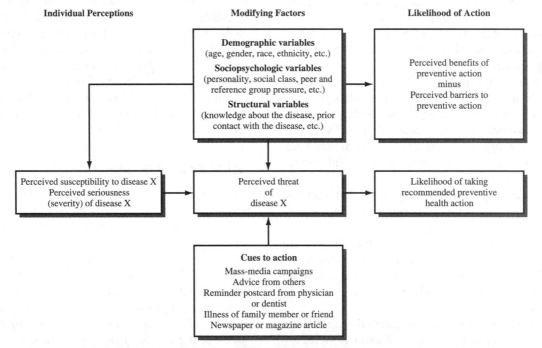

Figure 2.2 The health belief model proposed that the likelihood of health action was influenced by one's perceived susceptibility to and severity of disease. (*Source:* Becker MH (Ed.) (1974). *The Health Belief Model and Personal Behavior.* Thorofare, NJ: Slack, Inc. Reprinted with premission of the publisher.)

may be based on misinformation or lack of information. Sometimes when this information base is corrected, the perceived level of risk changes and the person becomes more open to adopting risk-reducing or health-enhancing behaviors. For example, many Asian American college students perceive HIV/AIDS as being a "white" disease, so they do not practice safer sex behavior.

The last two perceptions relate to benefits and barriers. **Perceived benefits** are unique to individuals. They are the benefits that people feel will come from changing their behavior. For behavior change to occur (whether it is the adoption of a new behavior, such as practicing safer sex, or the suspension of an old behavior, such as quitting smoking), the change must be perceived as being beneficial or advantageous. In the case of tanning, for example, if teenagers perceive skin cancer as being a very serious health problem, and perceive themselves as being at risk of developing this disease, there is a greater likelihood they will avoid tanning booths.

Other benefits from changing behavior may be even greater incentives than decreased risk of disease. For example, a perceived benefit from eliminating one's use of tanning booths may be financial: Tanning booths are expensive. Another might be vanity: Tanning increases the signs of "premature aging"—namely, wrinkles. In other words, the perceived benefit, whatever it is, is determined by clients, not counselors. The counselor's role is to help clients determine for themselves which significant benefits would facilitate behavior change. Even with this identification, behavior is not likely to change unless clients believe that the changes will work (Glanz, Lewis, & Rimer, 1997).

The factors that prevent the adoption of new behaviors constitute **perceived barriers.** The most obvious barrier is the perception that the behavior change will be ineffective. It is highly unlikely that people will adopt behaviors that they feel will not produce the desired results. Other barriers may include the perception that the new behaviors are expensive, painful, complicated, embarrassing, inconvenient, not socially acceptable, and incompatible with religious beliefs. New behaviors will not be adopted unless such barriers are identified, addressed, and removed, if possible. The barriers may be rooted in lack of information or understanding, misconceptions, previous experience, or hearsay evidence on the part of the client. Barriers grounded in culture or religion may not be able to be removed, and other ways of reaching the same outcome may need to be identified.

In addition to these four perceptions, behavior change is affected by **cues to action.** Cues to action are signals or reminders that prompt people to do something. For example, a cue to action to quit smoking may be seeing a picture of lungs streaked with carbon as a result of the person smoking the same number of years as the client. Another example might be a high blood cholesterol reading, or something as simple as a reminder card from the dentist that it is time for a yearly check-up. Health counselors can work with clients to understand their cues to action and incorporate them into their behavior change strategies.

Social Cognitive Theory

According to social cognitive theory (originally called social learning theory), behavior is the result of an interaction among the person (i.e., characteristics, personality), the environment (i.e., physical, social), and the behavior itself (Baranowski, Perry, & Parcel, 1997). A change in one of these factors leads to changes in all of them. This principle is called **reciprocal determinism (Figure 2.3).**

Using this theory to elicit behavior change requires that one or more of the factors (person, environment, or behavior) be modified. Factors that influence behavior include the anticipated outcomes of engaging in the behavior, learning by observing others, self-efficacy, and self-control (Bandura, 1986). Providing opportunities for clients to watch others perform targeted behaviors and mimic or copy them is an example of changing "person factors" and may result in the adoption of the new behavior. Similarly, address-

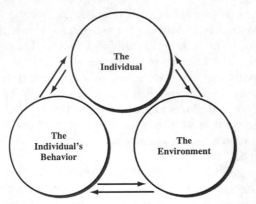

Figure 2.3 Social learning theory is based on the reciprocal determinism of three factors: the individual, the environment, and the behavior of the individual. Any action affecting one influences the others.

ing the concept of self-efficacy—that is, clients' beliefs in their ability to perform new behaviors—may lead to behavior change. If clients do not believe they can do something, they are not very likely to try out new behaviors. By providing opportunities for clients to master new behaviors through skill-building exercises, practice sessions, support group interactions, or learning the new behavior in small parts over time, clients will develop a stronger sense of self-efficacy and perhaps increase their likelihood of changing the behavior.

A person's attitude toward the expected outcomes of the behavior is a personal factor that also plays a role in determining whether a new behavior is adopted. Outcome expectations may be influenced by past experiences in similar situations, through observation of others in similar situations, or through word of mouth or hearing about others in similar situations. These expectations may be either realistic or based on misguided or incomplete information. Consequently, what clients expect to happen as a result of adopting new behaviors may need to be modified for educational interventions to succeed. For example, if overweight persons have tried to lose weight in the past by eliminating complex carbohydrates but always gained the weight back, then the likelihood of them adopting low-carbohydrate diets would be reduced. If the

same people were taught that reducing—not eliminating—carbohydrates was the goal, and they attended group sessions with others who had lost weight and maintained a lower weight by adopting this way of eating, then the change in diet would be more likely to occur.

The value people place on the outcomes of the new behavior also influences adoption. The termed used for this phenomenon is **expectancies.** These expectancies are akin to incentives. Positive expectancies are motivating, as they serve as an incentive to adopt the behavior (Baranowksi, Perry, & Parcel, 1997). To continue with the weight-loss example, if the clients' expectancies were that losing weight was valued (positive expectancy), the likelihood of them adopting the new behavior of reducing carbohydrate portions would be greater. Once the initial weight was lost, the expectancies would shift to the value of maintaining the weight reduction. The same expectancies hold true for keeping the weight off. If the expectancies (i.e., the value of keeping the weight off) are not significant, there is not enough incentive to control portion size, and the weight will be gained back.

Certain characteristics of the behavior itself will affect whether it will be adopted. A significant issue is the extent to which the client has control over the behavior, which is referred to as **self-control.** Self-control allows persons to determine their own goals relative to the adoption of new behaviors. For example, in the case of overweight clients, instead of suggesting that certain foods be eliminated from their diet, such as high-fat and calorie-dense desserts, behavior change may be more successful if they could choose to have a limited amount of the food instead, thereby focusing on the total number of fat grams per day. Thus clients could "spend" their fat grams any way they want. By changing the focus from *telling* clients ("You must do this") to *asking* them ("Here are the parameters—what do you want to do to comply with them?"), you give them control of their own behavior change (Baranowski, Perry, & Parcel, 1997).

In addition to the characteristics of the behavior and the person, the environment in which the behavior takes place is important. The environment obviously includes the physical surroundings, such as the classroom, locker room, soccer field, clinic, physician's office, or work site. It also encompasses the social environment, comprising family, friends, peers, colleagues, and others (Baranowski, Perry, & Parcel, 1997). An excellent example of the role that environment plays in changing behavior can be seen in the workplace when smoking restrictions are implemented (Biener, Abrams, Follick, & Dean, 1989). By changing the environment (i.e., restricting smoking indoors, thereby making smoking during work hours difficult), not only were nonsmokers saved from second-hand smoke exposure, but smokers also cut down on the number of cigarettes they smoked. In the example of the obese clients, changing the environment (i.e., eliminating high-calorie, minimally nutritious foods from vending machines and replacing them with fruits and other healthy snacks) would support a change in eating behavior that supports weight loss or management. To use social cognitive theory as the basis for behavior change in a counseling environment, the counselor needs to learn as much as possible about the clients' beliefs, attitudes, and environment.

Self-efficacy Theory

Self-efficacy is not only a construct in social cognitive theory, but also a theory unto itself. **Self-efficacy** postulates that personal belief in the ability to accomplish something is a determinant of behavior (Bandura, 1989). In short, if you think you can, you will. From a counseling perspective, it entails getting clients to believe they can, so they will attempt to make behavioral changes.

Self-efficacy is based on four factors: performance accomplishments, vicarious experience, verbal persuasion, and physiological state.

Performance accomplishments occur through personal mastery of a particular skill or task. Accomplishments that result from personal mastery are the most powerful sources of efficacy expectations (Bandura, 1977). Simply put, the most im-

portant contribution to behavior change occurs when people learn (master) a new behavior by doing it. Knowing this, counselors need to be aware of and provide opportunities for clients to learn by doing (Hayden, 2002).

Vicarious experience occurs as a result of watching others perform the desired behavior. The "others" demonstrating the behavior are known as "models," because they are modeling, or showing the desired behavior (Strecher, DeVillis, Becker, & Rosenstock, 1986). In a counseling environment, clients might be assisted in identifying a person at their place of employment, a relative, neighbor, former or present teacher, clergy, or other individual who might have accomplished the desired behavior. Having a model not only enables the client to "see" the behavior in action, but also contributes to a sense of self-efficacy: In other words, if this person can master the behavior, so can I.

Verbal persuasion is just that—encouraging the client with words. It is coaching, reassuring clients that they can achieve the desired outcomes. In a sense, it is acting as the client's cheerleader.

Physiological state can also influence how ability is perceived. When people are experiencing fear or anxiety, they will expect failure. Conversely, when people feel relaxed, calm, and safe, they will expect to succeed (Bandura, 1997). For the counselor, this may mean addressing underlying fear or anxiety and establishing a safe, nurturing environment before the real work of changing behavior can begin.

Transtheoretical (Stages of Change) Theory

The transtheoretical model, also known as the stages of change theory, explains that people go through a set of six stages on their way to changing behavior: pre-contemplation, contemplation, preparation, action, maintenance, and termination (Prochaska, Redding, & Evers, 1997).

During the **pre-contemplation stage**, no serious thought is being given to behavior change within the next six months. A projection of six months into the future is used because, in general, it seems to be about as far into the future as people plan for behavior change (Prochaska, Redding, Harlow, et al., 1994). Clients might not give much thought to changing a behavior during this stage because they lack awareness that the behavior is unhealthy. They also may be uninvolved because, although there is awareness that the behavior is unhealthy, it is not seen as very important. Clients might be undecided in that they are still considering the pros and cons—the positive and negative aspects of changing the behavior (Weinstein, Rothman, & Sutton, 1998).

The positive outcomes (pros) are usually perceived as advantages and can act as facilitators of change. Conversely, the negatives (cons) are usually equated to disadvantages and can act as barriers to change (Prochaska, Redding, Harlow, et al., 1994). Logically, it is more likely that clients will move from pre-contemplation to contemplation when the advantages are perceived as being greater than the disadvantages—that is, when the pros outweigh the cons. This sort of decisional balance (Prochaska, Redding, & Evers, 1997) can be useful when working with a client in a counseling setting.

Moving out of pre-contemplation, a person advances to the **contemplation stage.** In this stage, clients are at least aware of the need to change behavior and are thinking about making a change in the next six months. While still weighing the pros and cons of the new behavior, plans are being made for the change. For some clients, however, this stage lasts a very long time. If they do not move forward with a behavior change, but rather continue to weigh the pros and cons of the change, it constitutes behavioral procrastination (Prochaska, Redding, & Evers, 1997).

To enable clients to move from pre-contemplation to contemplation, and to possibly minimize the risk of behavioral procrastination, counseling needs to focus on the positive aspects (i.e., benefits) of the new behavior, rather than the negative aspects. For example, in counseling clients to quit smoking, focus on the positive aspects of quitting, such as breathing easier, walking farther, saving money, and having whiter teeth, rather than on the negative aspects, such as dealing with withdrawal symptoms, weight gain, crankiness, or cravings.

Following contemplation is the **preparation stage.** Once clients have reached this stage (which is also known as the planning stage), planning usually focuses on making the change as quickly as possible. This may occur in the immediate future, or if that is not possible or feasible, within a month (Prochaska, Redding, & Evers, 1997). Planning entails identifying how the change will be implemented. When clients move into the planning stage, they are eager for the change to occur. Consequently, they are receptive to action-oriented suggestions and recommendations because they want to change their behavior, now! Counselors must be ready to take advantage of this willingness to act by being prepared to help clients develop action plans immediately (Prochaska, Redding, Harlow, et al., 1994).

During the **action stage,** people are actively working on changing. Action is necessary for behavior to change, but changing behavior and keeping it changed are two different things. Maintaining a changed behavior is much more difficult than making the change in the first place. Thus the **maintenance stage** is the last phase of change. Beginning after six months of adherence to the new behavior, it represents a period in which constant attention is paid to the new behavior to prevent relapse, although relapse is less likely to occur in this stage than in the previous one. People remain in the maintenance phase for as long as there is temptation to revert to the problem behavior in certain situations (Basler, 1995). These situations, called cues in the environment, can trigger the old behavior (Prochaska, Redding, Harlow, et al., 1994). For example, common cues for smokers are drinking coffee or alcohol, finishing a meal, stress, boredom, driving, and, for some, sex. There is a broad time frame for maintenance, ranging from six months to five years in some cases (Glanz, Lewis, & Remier, 1997).

If using the stages of change theory as the basis for counseling, clients should identify the cues in the environment that might trigger relapse and work to develop strategies for overcoming them. Behavior change is completed and maintenance comes to an end when temptation in problematic situations no longer poses a threat and the ability to resist relapse has developed (Basler, 1995). In some cases, the end of maintenance marks the beginning of the **termination stage.** It is the final stage in the process of change for some behaviors, but not all. Reaching termination means that all temptation to revert to the old behavior has disappeared. It is as if the client never engaged in the behavior in the first place. This stage, if it is reached, more commonly occurs with additive behaviors, rather than with behaviors that are more focused on primary prevention and secondary prevention actions (Glanz, Lewis, & Remier, 1997).

Theory of Reasoned Action

The theory of reasoned action **(Figure 2.4)** proposes that the adoption of new behaviors results from individual intention to engage in the behaviors. **Behavioral intention** is determined by one's attitude toward the behavior and the associated subjective norm (Montano, et al., 1997).

Attitude toward a behavior is affected by beliefs about the outcome or attributes of the behavior. If the belief is that the new behavior will result in a positive outcome, then the attitude toward the behavior will be positive and there is a greater likelihood of its adoption. Conversely, if

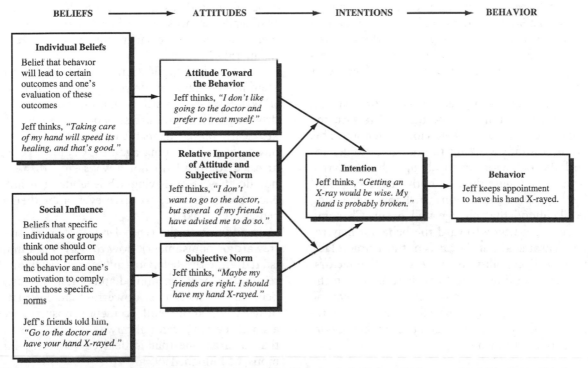

Figure 2.4 The theory of reasoned action asserts that health behavior is the result of a complex interrelationship between individual beliefs and attitudes, social influences and norms, past behavior and behavioral intentions. (*Source:* Adapted from Ajzen I, Fishbein M, (1980). *Understanding Attitudes and Predicting Social Behavior.* Englewood Cliffs, NJ: Prentice Hall, p. 8. Copyright © 1980 by Prentice-Hall, Inc. Reprinted by permission.)

the attitude toward the behavior is negative, the likelihood of adopting the new behavior diminishes (Hayden, 2002).

Subjective norms and important others play a major role in setting clients' behavioral intentions. These "important others" may be family members, significant others, members of a peer group, or colleagues, for example. To effectively use this theory as the basis for behavior change, it is imperative that these individuals be identified. The subjective norm is determined by normative beliefs, or whether important others approve or disapprove of the targeted behavior (Montano, Kasprzyk, & Taplin, 1997).

Simply put, behavior change will result if clients intend to change, if new behaviors are seen as being beneficial, and if the important others in clients' lives value the behavior. If these conditions are met, the likelihood of behavioral adoption increases. Conversely, if clients have no intention of changing their behavior, the behavior is not seen as necessarily being a good thing, or the important other people in their lives do not necessarily value it, then the likelihood of behavior change decreases.

In using this theory as the basis for changing behavior, attention must be directed toward the variables that influence behavioral intention. This may necessitate working to change attitudes toward the behavior or to change the subjective norm. Changing either, or both of these, should affect the client's intentions to change, increasing the likelihood that change will occur. Changing the client's attitude toward the behavior may require learning about the basis of the attitude, lack of knowledge, ability, awareness, or other factors, and then working to address these issues. In the case of changing subjective norms, this may be accomplished through the client, or it may require counseling the client and those other important people as a group.

Stimulus Response (Behavior) Theory

Behavior theory, or modification, was first proposed by B. F. Skinner in 1938. It is based on the premise that behavior occurs because of its consequences (i.e., reinforcements or rewards). Thus, behavior changes when the consequences of the behavior change (Skinner, 1938, 1953, 1974). The consequences of a behavior can be either positive or negative. A positive consequence or **reinforcer** is something that is pleasant or wanted—a reward. Positive reinforcers given after the desired behavior result in the behavior being repeated so that the reward can be received again (Hergehahn, 1994).

Negative consequences are punishments. **Punishment** encompasses giving something that is not wanted or taking away something that is wanted (Hergehahn, 1994). Applying a punishment after a behavior usually discourages the repetition of the behavior, as the consequences are not pleasurable and are not wanted again. Although both rewards and punishment shape behavior, Skinner believed rewards to be preferable. Keep in mind that while rewards strengthen behavior, punishment does not necessarily eliminate it (Hergehahn, 1994).

The practical application of this theory can be seen in the case of driving while intoxicated (DWI). DWI carries stiff penalties, such as loss of driving privilege and arrest. These consequences are clearly punishments meant to prevent this behavior from happening again. Of course, people arrested for DWI do not always stop drinking, nor do they stop driving while under the influence. Some continue to drive even after their licenses are revoked.

In addition to the type of reinforcement given (reward or punishment), how rapidly it is administered after the behavior influences behavior. A reinforcement given immediately after the target behavior occurs is more powerful than one that is delayed. When the reinforcement is positive, even a small reward given right away is more effective than a large one that is delayed (Abrams, Emmons, & Linnan, 1997).

Behavior change, according to this theory, does not result from knowledge, skills, or reasoning, but rather from immediate rewards. To this end, counselors and clients would work toward identifying the positive rewards that are associated with the behavior that needs to be changed, and replace them with positive rewards for the new behavior (Butler, 1997).

For example, if smoking is the unhealthy behavior, which rewards would keep people smoking and prevent quitting? They may be the calming effect felt from smoking, weight management, stress management, or the avoidance of nicotine withdrawal. The healthy behavior is not smoking. The rewards for adopting this behavior might be being able to save the cigarette money for a vacation, better-smelling clothes, being more socially acceptable, reduced risk of lung disease, and reduced risk of heart disease. The positive rewards of the new behavior need to be more important or more pleasurable than the positive rewards of the old behavior if the change is to take place.

Because behavior modification does not provide clients with information, skills, or reasons for them to change behavior themselves, the risk arises that these types of interventions might be seen as manipulative. To avoid this accusation, informed consent should be obtained from clients prior to beginning the intervention (Kothari, 1999). Having signed informed consent documents signals that clients explicitly made a decision to engage in the intervention that is designed to change their behavior. Because the reward is such a powerful determinant of behavior, to further reduce the risk of being accused of behavioral manipulation, clients should choose the reward (or punishment) rather than the counselor (Kothari, 1999).

Counseling Theories

Effective counseling can utilize a variety of **theoretical frameworks** (also known as theoretical perspectives). While several well-recognized and highly regarded approaches to counseling exist, it is worth noting that the actual practice of counseling involves considerable overlap and integration of many elements of the major schools of thought. Counseling theories are important for clinicians because they provide a theoretical framework for client assessment and treatment. They guide our thinking about, and understanding of, client behavior and the factors that interfere with clients' ability to cope. Our theoretical framework also guides our decision making in choosing counseling interventions.

Before discussing specific counseling theories it is worth repeating some general information regarding counseling and the helping process presented in Chapter 1. A counseling theory, like counseling itself, is not about "advice giving." It does not explain the best way to tell people what they "should" do and how they "should" live their lives. Indeed, most counselors would agree that a key element in counseling is to help clients determine what "they" (clients) would like to do so as to live more fulfilling and satisfying lives. Counseling theories merely propose frameworks for helping clients help themselves. All such theories stress that effective counseling involves a helping relationship between a client (someone who is in distress) and a counselor (someone with the training and skills) needed to help the client. While many approaches to counseling exist, most counseling theories can be divided into two major categories: those that focus on insight and those that focus on behavior.

Insight Theories

Insight theories attempt to help clients better understand the "why" of their feelings and behaviors. Insight theorists believe that behavior change comes about only after clients gain some understanding of the origins of their difficulties. Once clients have this insight, they can begin to explore possible solutions to their presenting problems.

Probably the most widely recognized name among the insight theorists is that of Sigmund Freud (Breger, 2000). Freud believed that much psychological distress is caused by unresolved unconscious conflicts from one's childhood. His theory evolved into the practice of **psychoanalysis,** a type of psychotherapy that seeks to probe the unconscious mind and bring these conflicts to light (Freud, 1900). In this type of treatment, the counselor assists the client in better understanding these unconscious conflicts and the **defense mechanisms** the client may be using in an effort to avoid facing these painful memories, which lead to a pattern of maladaptive behavior.

Those who practice psychoanalysis, or psychodynamic forms of treatment, encourage clients to access their unconscious through the techniques of **free association, dream analysis,** and **transference.** The technique of free association encourages clients to express whatever thoughts and feelings come to their minds during the course of a counseling session **(Figure 2.5).** Clients are directed to try not to censor these thoughts because of the belief that the association of these thoughts will provide significant insight into the underlying conflict. Freud and other psychoanalysts also place great emphasis on the importance of dream content. In dream analysis, the analyst helps clients by "interpreting" the symbolic meanings that may be present in the content of their dreams; it is believed that dreams offer a great deal of insight into the dynamics of the unconscious conflict. Finally, transference refers to the unconscious "transference" onto the counselor of traits that may be associated with significant relationships in the life of the client. The practitioner

seeks to help clients understand these conflicts by interpreting what these associations, dreams, and transferences may mean.

While psychodynamic theories and treatments are effective in many situations and with many clients, this approach may not be the most useful choice for those doing counseling in nonpsychiatric health settings. The practice of psychodynamic therapy typically is aimed at helping those who engage in maladaptive patterns of behavior. While this is not to suggest that those problems encountered by health counselors are not related to maladaptive behavioral patterns, most such counselors will assist clients in adjusting to specific health issues and immediate crises. Many health counselors will not have the luxury of the time required to do effective psychodynamic work, as their contacts with clients may be few in number. Nevertheless, it may be useful to be aware of how early life experiences can influence individuals' coping mechanisms in the present.

Of greater utility to most health counselors are the insight theories that have emerged from the **humanistic school** of thought. Humanists such as psychologist Carl Rogers (1961) and psychiatrist Irvin Yalom (1980) emphasize the importance of the counseling relationship as the driving force in healing. Furthermore, they suggest, this relationship, plus a supportive emotional climate, empowers clients to play a major role in determining the pace and direction of their counseling, and thus in developing relevant insights into their feelings and behaviors. In this type of counseling, counselors provide minimal advice and interpretation, but instead assist clients in clarifying for themselves the thoughts and feelings they may be experiencing, and what these thoughts and feelings might mean.

Humanistic counselors do so by helping to create a therapeutic environment that is characterized by **congruence, unconditional positive regard,** and **empathic understanding.** According to Rogers (1961), congruence refers to being aware of whatever attitudes or feelings the counselor is feeling. If the counselor is not able to match clients' feelings with an *awareness* of those feelings, clients will have a difficult time being genuine in their coun-

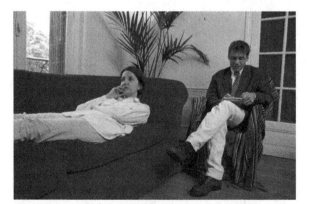

Figure 2.5 A hallmark of psychoanalysis is having clients fully relax and free associate their thoughts and feelings. (© BSIP Agency/Index Stock Imagery)

seling relationships. Unconditional positive regard refers to the counselor's willingness to be warmly accepting of each client, regardless of the counselor's like or dislike for the client's behavior. Finally, empathic understanding refers to the counselor's ability to understand the feelings and personal meanings expressed by the client.

Rogers and many other humanistic counselors suggest that this type of counseling environment is what is most important in facilitating change. Humanistic counseling may be of greater use for many health counselors inasmuch as these techniques can be used effectively in situations in which the counselor has a very limited amount of time to intervene.

In recent decades, another form of insight therapy, **cognitive-behavioral therapy (CBT),** has emerged. While psychodynamic theory focuses on the development of insight through the probing of the unconscious, and humanistic theories urge development of a supportive counseling relationship, CBT targets development of insight through an understanding of how thoughts, or **cognitions,** affect feelings and behaviors. The work of both psychologist Albert Ellis (1973) and psychiatrist Aaron Beck (1976) has been particularly influential in the development of CBT.

Both Beck (1976) and Ellis (1973) believe that much of one's psychological distress results from faulty, or irrational, thinking or beliefs. Cognitive-behavioral theory asserts that humans perceive, or attach meanings, to everything we encounter. According to CBT proponents, all events are essentially neutral; they become meaningful only when we interpret the events, or "talk" to ourselves about them. This process is referred to as **self-talk.** Self-talk can make us feel well or distressed. Many CBT counselors believe that if our self-talk is either exaggerated, overgeneralized, or catastrophic, we will experience significant psychological distress. For example, one of the most common thinking errors we make is using "should" statements. According to Beck (1976) and Ellis (1973), the more we tell ourselves how things "should be" as opposed to how we would "like them to be" or

"prefer them to be," the more angry/anxious/depressed we may feel. Cognitive-behavioral counselors work with clients to identify and challenge such thinking errors, and to allow clients to apply more reasonable or rational standards for their thoughts. Such counselors take a very active role in the counseling process and attempt to "reeducate" clients to better identify these automatic distorted beliefs, then replace them with less maladaptive cognitions. As part of the CBT counseling process, clients are often asked to assume a significant portion of the responsibility for their own treatment, and they may be expected to complete a series of homework assignments that are designed to assist clients in an in vivo type of reality testing. For example, clients who believe that they would just "die" if they were embarrassed in public might be asked to deliberately place themselves in embarrassing situations to test this assumption. By experiencing these situations and not actually "dying," they see that while it may not be "pleasant" to be embarrassed in public, it is not as "catastrophic" as they initially perceived it to be. This type of realization gives clients much more freedom and flexibility to try out new behaviors if they can evaluate the risk of such behaviors in a more reasonable, realistic, and rational manner.

One other insight-based counseling theory worthy of attention is **systems theory.** Systems theory is also referred to as a structural theory, because it tends to look at the structure of human relationships as people relate to others in their environments. This theory suggests that a change in any one member of the social system affects the nature of the social system as a whole (Greene, 1994). Therefore, if one member of a **family system** were to experience a difficulty or illness, it would likely influence or create changes in the entire family, not just for the individual who may be ill. For example, many of us have seen or experienced how the illness of one person in a family requires the other family members to change, to some degree, their day-to-day lives and roles. A recent *New York Times* article (Goode, 2003) emphasized the manner in which the suicide of a family member has substantial implications for the functioning of the surviving family members. Clearly, such an event can be extremely disruptive to the family functioning or equilibrium, and the result may be significant family dysfunction. Counselors who take a systems perspective focus on the entire family system in helping clients understand the effects of their behavior or situation on those around them, and they emphasize that people do not "live in a vacuum." Therefore, interventions tend to be more *structural* in focus and assist clients in adjusting to, or making changes in, their role(s) in the larger system. This focus is particularly important in health counseling.

Behavioral Theories

Behavioral theories differ from insight theories in that behavioral counselors do not strive to help their clients develop insight into the causes of their psychological distress. Rather, behavioral theorists believe that insight is not necessary to produce behavioral/emotional change. Indeed, while insight-based theorists see symptoms as "signs" of an underlying problem, behavioral counselors view the presenting symptoms as "the" problem. Therefore, behavioral counselors will attempt to assist clients by formulating a treatment strategy that is designed to eliminate the symptoms directly.

The most basic premise of behavioral theories is that all behavior is learned (Wolpe, 1990). Whether by **classical conditioning** (Pavlov, 2001) or **operant conditioning** (Skinner, 1974), behavior is learned and continues because it is somehow reinforced **(Figure 2.6)**. According to behavioral theorists, that which can be learned can also be unlearned. Behavioral counseling interventions attempt to assist clients in extinguishing unwanted behaviors and relearning new, more desirable behaviors. In the health counseling arena, most programs that focus on changing behaviors such as smoking and overeating are largely based on the principles of behavioral theory. While debate persists about the effectiveness of behavioral interventions when they are administered alone, even many insight-oriented counselors employ behavioral techniques in their counseling work.

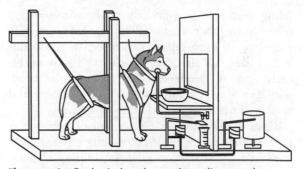

Figure 2.6 Pavlov's dogs learned to salivate at the mere association of a bell or light that signaled that the arrival of food was imminent.

The brief description of the counseling theories presented here is likely to be more confusing than enlightening to new health counselors. In this text, we will focus more on the establishment of the helping relationship as opposed to the use of any particular form of psychotherapy. All of the counseling theories are far more complex than we are able to discuss here. What is most important is that new counselors recognize that human behaviors and emotions result from many complex and interrelated factors, and that human nature can never be reduced to a simplistic mechanical understanding. Nothing we do is as simple as it looks (or as we might like it to be). Effective counselors use many of the theories simultaneously and select counseling interventions to suit a particular client's needs. Remember, the relationship you develop with your clients is the most important determinant of whether you will help them. The warmth, genuineness, and concern that you bring to your counseling will make the difference. Indeed, the most important skill you need to master to be an effective counselor is the ability to listen. People in distress need to be heard and attended to. It is this most important skill that we will turn our attention to as we discuss the process of microcounseling.

Microcounseling Theory

In 1965, while conducting research at Colorado State University, Allen Ivey and his colleagues struggled with the question, "How does one become a helper?" (Ivey & Authier, 1978). They wrestled with the utility of traditional approaches to counselor training that integrated counseling skills into a single theoretical framework. They spent months looking for counseling threads and skills that were common to all theoretical frameworks. They dissected hundreds of counseling sessions into components and then identified specific, discrete skills that were the basis of good counseling practice. Over the years, Ivey and his colleagues refined and renamed these skills. They came up with three sets of "skills"—attending, responding, and influencing—that were universal to good counseling, regardless of the theoretical underpinnings of the counselor (Littrell, 2001; Ivey & Ivey, 2003) **(Figure 2.7)**. Attending skills (including culturally appropriate eye contact; open, approachable body language; verbal following; and vocal tone) were deemed to be critical in establishing a trusting, open relationship that welcomed clients to tell their stories in a safe, caring relationship. Responding skills (including

client observation, questioning, encouraging, paraphrasing, reflecting feelings, and summarizing) were used to keep clients talking and to encourage them to clarify their stories. Influencing skills (including confrontation, eliciting and reflecting meaning, interpretation of meaning and reframing, self-disclosure, feedback, directives and logical consequences, and instruction giving) facilitated helping clients make changes in their lives (Ivey & Ivey, 2003).

Microcounseling is based on a psychoeducator model of helping (Ivey & Authier, 1978) **(Figure 2.8)**. This model moves away from a medical model of helping and focuses on empowering clients to be more competent in their own lives. Rather than view clients' problems as "illnesses" to be diagnosed, prescribed, and cured, the psychoeducator model sees clients' problems as issues with which they are dissatisfied or seek to improve and helps clients master the skills necessary to control them (Ivey & Authier, 1978). The psychoeducator model views the client and the counselor as being on relatively equal footing,

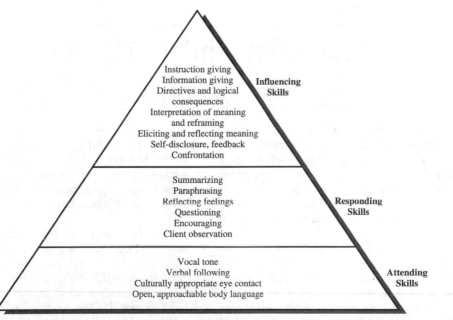

Figure 2.7 A microcounseling approach uses three sets of individual skills that work together and are generic to all counseling and theoretical frameworks. (*Source:* Ivey A, Ivey M (2003). *Intentional Interviewing and Counseling,* Fifth Edition. © 2003 by Thomson/Wadsworth. Reprinted by permission of the publisher.)

Medical Model

Illness ⟶ Diagnosis ⟶ Prescription ⟶ Therapy ⟶ Cure

Psychoeducator Model

Client
dissatisfaction ⟶ Goal ⟶ Skill ⟶ Satisfaction
or ambition   setting teaching or goal
                                    achievement

Figure 2.8 Unlike the medical model, which is based on a healthcare provider curing a sick patient, the psychoeducator model involves a skilled helper teaching clients how to become more satisfied with their lives. (*Source: Adapted from Ivey A, Ivey MB (2003). Intentional Interviewing and Counseling: Facilitating Client Development in a Multicultural Society, 5th ed. Pacific Grove, CA: Thomson/Brooks Cole.*)

with the counselor serving as teacher/trainer more than healer/therapist. Microcounseling is firmly rooted in Rogers' client-centered approach. To get better, clients have to take responsibility for learning new skills and unlearning old ones that contribute to their dissatisfactions.

Microcounseling is an especially useful model for health counseling, because much of it is done by professionals with little or no formal postgraduate counseling training and little background in counseling theory. The individual microskills of microcounseling can be learned and taught by health professionals from a wide variety of backgrounds.

Compliance and Adherence Theory

Compliance and adherence are health behavior terms that are often used synonymously to refer to the theory of following "doctor's orders" and instructions and complying with or adhering to therapeutic regimens. **Compliance** is a term currently out of favor with health professionals. It essentially means getting clients/patients to do what you, the health professional, want them to do. Compliance can be viewed as a continuum (**Figure 2.9**). Patients might comply fully, partially, or not at all. That is, they might comply with some parts of the therapeutic plan but not others.

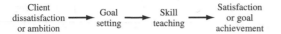

Counseling Hints & Tips 2.1

Developing Cultural Competency

A major focus of the Ivey microskills model is the importance of understanding the role of cultural differences in counseling. These differences affect the perspectives of both counselors and clients, as well as the nature of the counseling. Here are some tips that you can apply right away to help you become more intentional in your use of a more multicultural approach to counseling:

1. *Don't stereotype.* While the very nature of multicultural differences assumes cultural similarities among members, take time to explore how these play out for your clients in their stories.
2. *Look for individual differences.* While members of cultural groups share many similarities, there is still more within-culture variability than between-culture variability.

3. *Don't minimize subcultures.* Although a dominant culture (for example, Italian Americans) exerts a strong influence in shaping attitudes, values, and behaviors, membership in subcultures (for example, lesbian Italian American) can often be stronger or offset many of the influences of the dominant culture.
4. *Don't assume anything.* Try to learn as much about individual cultural groups as you can, but keep an open mind when counseling members of any cultural group. Just because you know about the overall values, attitudes, and behaviors of the group, don't assume that these apply directly to the person in front of you. Let the person tell you his or her story and explain how he or she perceives these cultural influences.

Haynes, Taylor, and Sacket (1979) defined compliance as the "extent" to which a person's behavior coincides with medical or health advice. "Advice" extends beyond taking medications and returning for follow-up tests to include a variety of lifestyle changes, such as eating properly, engaging in regular physical activity, using seatbelts, having regular physical examinations and abstaining from behaviors such as smoking or abusing alcohol. Viewing compliance as a continuum that covers a broad range of behaviors contained in therapeutic regimens and lifestyle modifications helps one understand why it is so hard to achieve **(Figure 2.9)**.

Nonadherence/noncompliance can be direct (the patient refuses to fill a prescription and take medication) or indirect (the patient accepts the prescription but has no intention of filling it). *Partial compliance/adherence* results in incomplete medication taking due to a variety of reasons. Patients may have difficulty getting into the habit of taking their medication. They might take "medication holidays" on weekends or vacations.

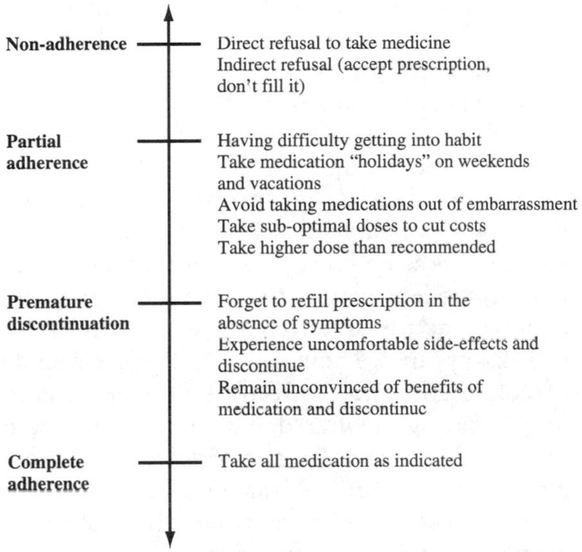

Other partially compliant patients avoid taking medication because of embarrassment of a preconceived stigma associated with it. Still others take a lower dose to save money. *Premature discontinuation,* the next stage on the continuum, results in taking suboptimal doses of the medication because its use is discontinued too early. This can be the result of refusing to refill medications after achieving a certain medication effect. It can also happen because patients forget to refill prescriptions in the absence of symptoms. Sometimes patients experience uncomfortable side effects and discontinue taking their medication. Lastly, some patients may discontinue their treatment because they remain unconvinced that the benefits of taking it outweigh any perceived inconveniences associated with taking it (Patterson, 2001, pp. 7–8).

The term "compliance" fell out of favor in the medical community in the 1980s and 1990s because of its connotation with subservence and was replaced by the term "adherence." Compliance implied blind obedience to therapeutic plans devised by medical professionals for patients. **Adherence** connotes having patients adhere to therapeutic regimens that they are active participants in developing with medical professionals. We'll discuss the theoretical and practical implications of these distinctions later.

Two things must occur for sick people to get better: (1) they must get accurate advice about the diagnosis and therapeutic plan, and (2) they must follow this advice (Brannon & Feist, 2000). Both criteria must be met for a person to get better and to not become reinfected or have a relapse. On the one hand, if a person is misdiagnosed or given an incorrect or ineffective therapeutic regimen, he or she will not get better. On the other hand, the best therapeutic plan available is worthless if the client doesn't follow it.

Most clinicians and counselors greatly overestimate patient compliance (Podell, 1979). Some of the classic studies of compliance uncovered only minimal compliance with therapeutic regimens spanning a variety of diseases and conditions. In a review of the literature, Davis (1966)

Non-adherence	Direct refusal to take medicine
	Indirect refusal (accept prescription, don't fill it)
Partial adherence	Having difficulty getting into habit
	Take medication "holidays" on weekends and vacations
	Avoid taking medications out of embarrassment
	Take sub-optimal doses to cut costs
	Take higher dose than recommended
Premature discontinuation	Forget to refill prescription in the absence of symptoms
	Experience uncomfortable side-effects and discontinue
	Remain unconvinced of benefits of medication and discontinue
Complete adherence	Take all medication as indicated

Figure 2.9 Adherence to a therapeutic regimen exists along a continuum from nonadherence to complete adherence. (*Source:* Adapted from Peterson R (2001). *Changing Patient Behavior: Improving Outcomes in Health and Disease Management.* San Francisco: Jossey-Bass.)

found a 30%–50% rate of noncompliance for the studies he examined. Marston (1970) found noncompliance rates with short-term regimens that were as high as 92%. Sacket and Snow (1979) reviewed more than 500 compliance studies and found that compliance rates varied depending on the nature of the illness. Clients were more likely to comply with therapeutic regimens intended to cure a disease (77% compliance) compared with those prescribed to prevent an illness (63%). Current studies indicate that the overall compliance rate for medical and/or health advice is about 50% (Brannon & Feist; 2000, Haynes et al., 1996; Dimatteo & DiNicol, 1982). Compliance with short-term therapeutic regimens is estimated at about 60%. Estimated compliance with long-term lifestyle changes, such as healthy eating, stopping smoking, and exercising, is about 25% (Brannon & Feist, 2000).

Healthy People 2010 Leading Health Indicators

Access to Health Care
Health Implications of Limited Access to Health Care
Access to quality health care is associated with early intervention in the disease process and with the use of preventive health services such as prenatal health visits and annual physical examinations. Such access is directly related to having health insurance, a higher income level, and continuity in healthcare providers and ongoing health care.

Persons with health insurance are more likely to have a private physician or other primary care provider and to use preventive health care services such as Pap tests, immunization, or early prenatal care. Adults with health insurance are twice as likely to use these services as are those without health insurance.

More than 44 million persons in the United States do not have health insurance. About 11 million of these uninsured people are children. The proportion of persons younger than age 65 years with health insurance has remained steady over the past decade at about 85%. Those most likely to not have health insurance are people living at or below the poverty level and persons of Hispanic origin. Approximately 40% of Mexican Americans are uninsured (USDHHS, 2003).

Objectives for the Nation
- Increase the proportion of persons with health insurance
- Increase the proportion of persons who have a specific source of ongoing care
- Increase the proportion of pregnant women who begin prenatal care in the first trimester of pregnancy (USDHHS, 2003)

Factors Unrelated to Compliance
In general, both demographic variables (e.g., age, sex, race, educational level, income) and individual and personality characteristics (e.g., anxiety, ego strength, intelligence) have been found to be either inconsistent or not significant in their relationship to compliance (Brannon & Feist, 2000; Olsen & Sutton, 1998; Lynch, Birk, Weaver, et al., 1992; Podell, 1979; Dunbar et al., 1999). Decades of research have shown that for every study indicating a positive relationship between either a demographic or a personality variable and compliance, others do not find such associations.

For example, studies examining the relationship between age and compliance have demonstrated mixed results. Lynch et al. (1992), in a study of adherence to an exercise program, originally found a relationship between age and compliance. Initial findings indicated that older subjects complied better than younger subjects. However, as the study continued, this relationship disappeared. Thomas et al. (1995), in a study of colorectal cancer screening in older adults, found that age mattered, but only to a certain point. Adults aged 55 and younger and those more than 80 years old had the worst compliance. The best compliance with routine colorectal cancer screening was found among those who were 70 years old. Brannon and Feist (2000) suggest that younger men probably did not feel that they were at as high a risk for the disease as the 70-year-olds and that the 80-year-olds no longer viewed it as being that important.

Illness factors have also been shown to be unrelated to compliance. The severity of the disease, as perceived by either the clinician or the client, has not been shown to be significantly and consistently related to adherence with therapeutic regimens, although the perception of pain is associated with higher compliance. While pain is not necessarily a true indicator of the severity of an illness, it is often perceived by patients that way. Patients experiencing pain are more likely to comply with therapeutic regimens than those who do not experience it (Brannon & Feist, 2000).

Factors Related to Compliance

While demographic, personality, and illness factors have not been shown to be consistently and significantly related to adherence, certain provider characteristics and educational strategies have been linked with greater compliance. Decades of research have shown the counselor–client relationship to be significantly related to adherence. A warm, caring, friendly clinician/counselor who communicates well is the model for increased adherence (Brannon & Feist, 2000). Specific educational strategies drawn from the fields of health education, health counseling, and behavioral medicine have also been identified as being related to improved patient compliance. Focusing less on the biomedical aspects of health problems and more on the facets of the therapeutic regimen is related to improved adherence (Blonna, Legos, & Burlak, 1989; Davis, 1966).

Several studies have demonstrated that health practitioners who are caring, approachable, friendly, and nonauthoritarian, and who communicate well have the highest levels of client adherence to treatment regimens (DiMatteo, 1994; Russel & Rotter, 1993; Rost, Carter, & Innui, 1989; DiMatteo & DiNicola 1982; Blackwell, 1979). These and countless other studies have shown that little things such as smiling and handshakes demonstrate friendliness and caring to clients. A good "bedside manner" includes such behaviors as open body posture (relaxed, leaning into

client), culturally appropriate eye contact, nonverbal cues (head nods, smiles), joking and laughing, and nonjudgmental language when talking to patients (Ivey & Ivey, 2003). This practitioner style stands in stark contrast to the more "authoritative" demeanor, which includes rigid and noninviting body posture (standing, arms folded); lack of physical contact (handshake); aversion of eye contact; lack of smiling, joking, or other attempts to "loosen up"; and the perception and treatment of clients as inferior (Gastorf & Galanos, 1983; Blackwell, 1978).

Six specific educational strategies have been shown to be related to improved adherence to therapeutic regimens: tailoring, written reinforcement, repetition, expectation citing, patient quizzes, and self-monitoring (Blonna et al., 1989; Davis, 1966).

Tailoring involves scheduling components of the therapeutic plan (e.g., medication taking, engaging in physical activity or exercise) to specific times during the day that best fit the patient's lifestyle rather than to a predetermined schedule (Blackwell, 1978). For instance, some people are "morning people" and are more amenable to exercise when they wake up. Others prefer (and are able) to break up the day and exercise during lunch. Still others prefer to exercise after dinner as a way to finish off their day. Tailoring an exercise program requires knowing such information about clients and scheduling their exercise sessions to coincide with their preferences.

Directives are instructions given to clients about how to comply with parts of the therapeutic plan (Ivey & Ivey, 2003). Clarity and brevity are the two most important characteristics of good instructions. If you want clients to follow instructions, write them down. Written reinforcement involves writing down each instruction that is specifically related to a desired patient behavior. It excludes all other general biomedical information about the health problem (Peck, Neville, & King, 1982).

Repetition involves the planned verbal and written repeating of the specific instructions during the patient's visit (Blackwell, 1979). All instruc-

Joseph: On Defining Culture

Joseph is 52, is married, and identifies as an Italian American.

Culture is an all-encompassing but elusive concept to define. Many people think it is limited to racial/ethnic parameters. To illustrate the scope of culture, we will use the example of Joseph, a colleague of Dr. Blonna's, to illustrate how the many facets of culture evolve and overlap to define who we are.

Joseph's story:

I am a 52-year-old, married, heterosexual, Italian American college professor. I have two sons, aged 17 and 20. I have had asthma all of my life. I was born and raised in Newark, New Jersey, the son of first-generation Italian Americans. All four of my grandparents were born in Italy and their children—my parents—were born in the United States. All of my descendants were blue-collar, working-class people who earned a living in the garment manufacturing industry of the New York metropolitan area. My wife is German American. Both of her parents were first-generation German Americans. Her parents were also working-class people who worked in a brewery and clothing store, respectively. None of our four parents went to college. My wife and I were children of the placid, postwar 1950s, young adults of the tumultuous 1960s, and newlyweds of the Vietnam-era 1970s. We lived through the Cold War (and the end of the Cold War), the Vietnam War, the Gulf War, Woodstock, Watergate, the Chicago Seven, the Hippies, Yippies, Peace Corps, the Me Generation, the stock market crash of 1987, the Clinton/Lewinski affair, and the AIDS epidemic. We grew up in northern New Jersey cities, moved to the suburbs at the edge of the woods, and long for a peaceful life in the country. We've both worked full-time for more than 30 years and have seen our standard of living improve and bank accounts grow as our sanity and physical health have declined somewhat.

To understand how I perceive my culture and the influence it has exerted on shaping who I am and how I view the world, one must look at the interplay of all these variables. Being a son of working-class Italian American immigrants laid the foundation. The combination of lower socioeconomic status and Italian ethnic values and traditions cast the mold for how I would view my world for the first 10–15 years. I was the product of a very warm and loving, if not stiflingly parochial, blue-collar family.

Overlay this foundation with the troubling personal events of my childhood. I was a very sickly child. My asthma kept me from exploring aspects of my world and my self that still linger with me. My most vivid memory of my childhood was standing on a kitchen chair, looking out the window, watching my brother and all of the neighborhood kids have a snowball fight. I could not partake in such fun because of my out-of-control asthma.

My asthma was the driving force for my interest in health and nutrition in high school. I was on a mission to control my asthma despite my parents' lack of understanding and support. I exercised, lost weight, ate sensibly, played high school sports, and started to gain control of my asthma. I developed a lifelong love and respect for health and fitness.

Throughout my high school years, however, my older brother left a legacy that was hard to live down. He was constantly in trouble with the police over alcohol- and drug-related offenses. The effects this had on my parents strongly influenced my desire to live a squeaky-clean life and not add to their grief. It also made me want to escape the yelling, screaming, and depressing gloom of my house. It created a breach in my relationship with my brother and family (whose motto is "Blood is thicker than water") that has never been closed.

I worked my way through college and graduate school without any financial assistance from my parents and distanced myself from my brother and them. I was a serious commuter student and was determined to move out of my house to escape the turmoil. Being in college in Vietnam-era America was a roller-coaster ride, as all of my traditional values and assumptions about life were challenged on a daily basis. I married young and sought the refuge of my relationship with my wife and the quiet of our tiny apartment. Marrying young and growing up together was both liberating and difficult. Being responsible for a marriage at 20 was difficult but we managed to thrive among the demands and challenges of full-time work and school. The 1970s passed into the 1980s, and things began to settle down until parenthood struck in 1983.

Being a father changed my life in so many ways. It renewed my love for my wife, gave me a sense of hope for the future, and connected me with inner feelings and resources I didn't know existed. I thrived as a dad and welcomed the birth of our second son. The early years as a father were difficult financially (my wife stopped working for a few years) but immensely enjoyable. I coached youth sports, got very involved with my kids, and created a new family out of friends. My greatest fears revolved around my sons becoming teenagers and turning out to be like my brother. Fortunately, this never happened.

As a professional, upper-socioeconomic-status, heterosexual, white man, I view the world from a certain privileged position, yet my humble blue-collar roots and history of hard work and personal accomplishments make my perspective on life very different from that of some of my colleagues who come from a more upper-class background. In a sense I resent it when people say I hold a "privileged" position, because I feel that I worked hard and earned everything that I have without ever denying anyone else the same rights.

My cultural inheritance and background are a filter or veil through which I view my clients and their stories. They have shaped the way I perceive everything. I share this with them and ask their help in understanding their cultural backgrounds and how the nuances of their lives have shaped who they are. I find this to be one of the more fascinating aspects of the helping relationship.

Critical Thinking Questions

1. List and describe five aspects of Joseph's culture (or subculture) that have shaped who he is as a man at age 52.
2. Describe five cultural influences on your life up to this point and explain how they will affect the way you view clients.

tions should be repeated at least three times: when they are initially given by the counselor, as the counselor writes them down (incorporated into the written reinforcement strategy), and one more time before the client leaves. Key generic messages (related to any facet of the therapeutic plan) can be written on waiting-room literature, posters, and other office accessories (e.g., paperweights).

Expectation citing seeks to use the power differential in counselor–client or patient–provider relationships in a positive way. Even though the counseling approach advocated in this book (the Ivey Microskills model) utilizes a psychoeducational framework that minimizes power differentials between counselors and clients, differences will still exist. Clients look up to counselors and patients look up to clinicians because, at the very least, they respect their knowledge, training, and ability to help them. They believe that these professionals hold the keys to helping them get better. By stating instructions as "expectations" (what you personally expect the client to do), counselors establish a personal commitment on the part of the client to the therapeutic plan. For instance, it is not uncommon for counselors to ask clients to keep diaries or logs on a variety of issues ranging from eating behavior to stress management. By stating that you "expect" the client to be faithful to this task and bring the diary on the next visit, you increase the likelihood that the client will comply with this instruction (Nathanson & Becker, 1985).

If you want to know if clients understand what you expect of them and what they have to do regarding adhering to their therapeutic plan, ask them. **Patient quizzes** are verbal requests to repeat specific parts of the treatment plan. Patient quizzes are given both for individual segments of the plan and for the entire plan before the patient is allowed to leave. If clients are unclear about the instructions or how to carry out parts of the plan, it will be evident when they cannot repeat them. This gives counselors the opportunity to restate instructions more clearly or to reformulate them (Blackwell, 1979).

Self-monitoring involves the use of devices (e.g., medication packaging, logs) that allow pa-

tients to keep track of components of their therapeutic plan (e.g., pill taking) (Mahoney & Arkhoff, 1979). Oral contraceptive packaging is an example of a simple but effective self-monitoring device that gives quick visual confirmation of pills taken or missed.

Blonna et al. (1989) examined whether the use of an STD educational intervention based on the application of these six strategies influenced patient compliance with a seven-day treatment regimen of tetracycline hydrochloride and patient return for follow-up appointment keeping. Their results revealed that the intervention was significantly related to increasing adherence with return for follow-up testing. It was not related to increased compliance with medication. The latter finding was influenced by the high overall adherence to medication taking by both the control and the experimental groups (the mean pill-taking score for both groups was more than 27 out of a possible 28).

Summary

This chapter reviewed the theoretical basis of health counseling. It began with a discussion of health, illness, and sick role behavior and a consideration of how each of these corresponds with a level of prevention discussed in Chapter 1. For instance, health behavior refers to primary prevention activities—things people do to prevent getting sick in the first place. Each type of behavior (i.e., health, illness, sick role) and level of prevention will affect the nature of the counseling required. Counselors working with healthy clients in primary prevention work settings, for instance, will have different issues and directives to guide their counseling than those employed by rehabilitation facilities engaged mostly in tertiary or rehabilitative services.

The next section of the chapter reviewed the theories used to describe behavior change. These theories ranged from the health belief model, with its emphasis on cognitive factors (beliefs clients have about their health), to behavioral theory, which deemphasizes cognitive factors and focuses on using rewards and punishments to encourage clients to adopt or extinguish behaviors. Ideally, this review will stimulate readers to explore their own philosophical beliefs regarding how and why people change their behavior.

The chapter then described various counseling theories. For the sake of convenience, these theories were organized in two categories: insight theories and behavioral theories. Counselors whose practices are based on insight theories believe that clients can change only after gaining insight into the nature and history of their problems. Behavioral counselors believe just the opposite: that clients don't need to understand the origin of their problems to get better, but rather must know how they feel about their current functioning, how it affects their lives, and where they would like to end up in terms of personal growth and change. Once again, it is hoped that this entry-level discussion of counseling will stimulate readers to pursue additional reading and training while working on establishing their personal theoretical frameworks regarding the nature of counseling and the helping process.

Ivey's microskills model serves as a unifying theory for health counseling. Because it is a skills-based theory, it can transcend all theoretical frameworks regarding health behavior change and counseling, and can be adopted by a variety of practitioners working in diverse healthcare settings.

The chapter ended with a discussion of compliance and adherence theory, merging lessons learned from counseling and health education research.

Study Questions

1. How are health, illness, and sick role behavior similar and different?
2. Match the level of prevention (primary, secondary, tertiary) to the three types of patient behaviors described in Study Question 1.
3. Compare and contrast how counseling clients varies according to their sick role status.
4. How does each of the following theories explain behavior change?
   - Health belief model
   - Social cognitive theory
   - Self-efficacy theory
   - Transtheoretical (stages of change) theory
   - Theory of reasoned action
   - Stimulus response (behavioral) theory
5. Pick two behavior change theories and describe how you could integrate elements of them into counseling someone with a health problem.
6. Which of the behavior change theories best reflects your personal theoretical framework regarding client behavior change? Why?
7. How are the major insight counseling theories similar and different?
8. How are the major behavioral counseling theories similar and different?
9. Which of the counseling theories best reflects your personal theoretical framework regarding counseling clients? Why?
10. Why are all counselors able to use Ivey's microskills, regardless of their theoretical framework (insight versus behavior)?
11. What are the key factors related to client adherence with therapeutic regimens?

References

Abrams DB, Emmons KM, Linnan LA (1997). Health behavior and health education: the past, present and future. In Glanz K, Lewis F, Rimer B (Eds.). *Health Behavior and Health Education: Theory, Research and Practice,* 2nd ed., pp. 453–478. San Francisco: Jossey-Bass.

Bandura A (1977). *A Social Learning Theory.* Englewood Cliffs, NJ: Prentice Hall.

Bandura A (1986). *Social Foundations of Thought and Actions: A Social Cognitive Theory.* Englewood Cliffs, NJ: Prentice Hall.

Bandura A (1989). Human agency in social cognitive theory. *American Psychologist* 44:1175–1184.

Baronowski T, Perry CL, Parcel GS (1997). How individuals, environments and health behavior interact. In Glanz K, Lewis F, Rimer B (Eds.). *Health Behavior and Health Education: Theory, Research and Practice,* 2nd ed., pp. 153–178. San Francisco: Jossey-Bass.

Basler HD (1995). Patient education with reference to the process of behavioral change. *Patient Education and Counseling* 26:91–98.

Beck AT (1976). *Cognitive Therapy and the Emotional Disorders.* New York: Meridian Publishing.

Biener L, Abrams DB, Follick MJ, Dean L (1989). A comparative evaluation of a restrictive smoking policy in a general hospital. *American Journal of Public Health* 79:192–195.

Blackwell B (1978). Counseling and compliance. *Patient Counseling and Health Education* Fall:21–23.

Blackwell B (1979). The literature of delay in seeking medical care for chronic illness. In Haynes R, Taylor DW, Sacket DL (Eds.). *Compliance in Health Care*. Baltimore: Johns Hopkins Press, 1979.

Blonna R, Legos P, Burlak P (1989). The effects of an STD educational intervention on patient compliance. *Sexually Transmitted Diseases.* 16:198–200.

Brannon L, Feist J (2000). *Health Psychology: An Introduction to Behavior and Health,* 4th ed. Belmont, CA: Wadsworth/Thomson Learning.

Breger L (2000). *Freud: Darkness in the Midst of Vision.* New York: John Wiley and Sons.

Butler JT (1997). *Principles of Health Education and Health Promotion.* Englewood, CO: Morton.

Davis DM (1966). Variations in patients' compliance with physicians' orders: analysis of congruence between survey responses and results of original investigations. *Journal of Medical Education* 41:1037–1048.

DiMatteo MR (1994). Enhancing patient adherence to medical recommendations. *Journal of the American Medical Association* 217:79–83.

Dimatteo MR, DiNicola DD (1982). Achieving patient compliance with medical regimens: a social psychological perspective. In Baum A, Taylor SE, Singer J (Eds.). *Handbook of Psychology and Health, Vol. 4. Social Psychological Aspects of Health,* pp. 55–84. Hillsdale, NJ: Erlbaum.

Dunbar J, Marshall G, Hovell M (1999). Behavioral strategies for improving compliance behaviors. In Elder JP, Ayala GX, Harris S (Eds.). Theories and intervention approaches to health behavior change in primary care. *American Journal of Preventive Medicine* 17:275–284.

Ellis A (1973). *Humanistic Psychotherapy.* New York: McGraw-Hill.

Freud S (1900). *The Interpretation of Dreams.* New York: Barnes and Noble.

Gastorf JW, Galanos AN (1983). Patient compliance and physician's attitude. *Family Practice Research Journal* 2:190–198.

Glanz K, Lewis F, Rimer B (Eds.) (1997). *Health Behavior and Health Education: Theory, Research and Practice,* 2nd ed. San Francisco: Jossey-Bass.

Goode E (2003, October 26). And still, echoes of a death long past. *New York Times,* pp. F1, F6.

Greene RR (1994). *Human Behavior Theory: A Diversity Framework.* Hawthorne, NY: Walter De Gruyter.

Hayden J (2002). Motivation and behavior change. In De Young S (Ed.). *Teaching Strategies for Nurse Educators.* Upper Saddle River, NJ: Prentice Hall.

Haynes R, Taylor DW, Sacket DL (Eds.) (1979). *Compliance in Health Care.* Baltimore: Johns Hopkins Press, 335–363.

Hergehahn BR (1994). *An Introduction to Theories of Personality.* Englewood Cliffs, NJ: Prentice Hall.

Ivey A, Authier J (1978). *Microcounseling: Innovations in Interviewing, Counseling, Psychotherapy, and Psychoeducation.* Springfield, IL: Charles C. Thomas.

Ivey A, Ivey M (2003). *Intentional Interviewing and Counseling; Facilitating Client Development in a Multicultural Society.* Pacific Grove, CA: Brooks Cole.

Kasl SV (1966a). Health behavior, illness behavior and sick role behavior 1. Health and illness behaviors. *Archives of Environmental Health* 12:246–266.

Kasl SV (1966b). Health behavior, illness behavior and sick role behavior 2. Sick role behaviors. *Archives of Environmental Health* 12:531–541.

Kothari S (1999). The ethics of behavior modification. *Topics in Stroke Rehabilitation* 5:66–69.

Littrell R (2001). Allen Ivey: transforming counseling theory and practice. *Journal of Counseling and Development.* http://bahai-library.org/newspapers/010101–1html.

Lynch DJ, Birk T, Weaver MT, et al. (1992). Adherence to exercise interventions in the treatment of hypercholesterolemia. *Journal of Behavioral Medicine* 15:365–377.

Mahoney M, Arkoff D (1979). Self-management. In Pomerleau O (Ed.). *Behavioral Medicine Theory and Practice,* pp. 75–99. Baltimore: Williams and Wilkins.

Marston M (1970). Compliance with medical regimens: a review of the literature. *Journal of Nursing Research* 19:312–323.

Montano DE, Kasprzyk D, Taplin SH (1997). The theory of reasoned action and the theory of planned behavior. In Glanz K, Lewis F, Rimer B (Eds.). *Health Behavior and Health Education: Theory, Research and Practice,* 2nd ed., pp. 85–112. San Francisco: Jossey-Bass.

Nathanson C, Becker M (1985). The influence of client–provider relationships on teenage women's subsequent use of contraception. *American Journal of Public Health* 75:33–37.

Olsen R, Sutton J (1998). More hassles, more alone: adolescents with diabetes and the role of formal and informal support. *Child-Care Health & Development* 24:31–39.

Patterson R (Ed.) (2001). *Changing Patient Behavior: Improving Outcomes in Health and Disease Management.* San Francisco: Jossey-Bass.

Pavlov IP (2001). *I.P. Pavlov: Selected Works.* Honolulu: Honolulu University Press of the Pacific.

Peck C, Neville J, King A (1982). Increasing patient compliance with prescriptions. *Journal of the American Medical Association* 248:743–757.

Podell R (1979). *Physician's Guide to Compliance in Hypertension*. New York: Prodist, 20–25.

Prochaska JO, Redding CA, Evers KE (1997). The transtheoretical model and stages of change. In Glanz K, Lewis F, Rimer B (Eds.). *Health Behavior and Health Education: Theory, Research and Practice,* 2nd ed., pp. 60–84. San Francisco: Jossey-Bass.

Prochaska JP, Redding CA, Harlow LL, et al. (1994). The transtheoretical model of change and HIV prevention: a review. *Health Education Quarterly* 21:471–486.

Rogers CR (1961). *On Becoming a Person: A Therapist's View of Psychotherapy*. New York: Houghton Mifflin.

Rosenstock IM (1974). Historical origins of the health belief model. *Health Education Monographs* 2:328–335.

Rost K, Carter W, Innui T (1989). Introduction of information during initial medical visit: consequences for patient follow-through with physician recommendations with medication. *Social Science and Medicine* 28:315–321.

Russel NK, Rotter DL (1993). Health promotion counseling of chronic disease patients during primary care visits. *American Journal of Public Health* 83:979–982.

Sacket DL, Snow JC (1979). The magnitude of compliance and noncompliance. In Haynes RB, Taylor DW, Sackett DL (Eds.). *Compliance in Health Care,* pp. 11–22. Baltimore: Johns Hopkins University Press.

Skinner BF (1938). *The Behavior of Organisms*. East Norwalk, CT: Appleton & Lange.

Skinner BF (1953). *Science and Human Behavior*. New York: Macmillan.

Skinner BF (1974). *About Behaviorism*. New York: Vintage Books.

Strecher VJ, DeVillis BM, Becker MH, Rosenstock IM (1986). The role of self-efficacy in achieving health behavior change. *Health Education Quarterly* 13:730–791.

Thomas W, White CM, Mah J, et al. (1995). Longitudinal compliance with annual screening for fecal occult blood. *American Journal of Epidemiology* 142:176–182.

United States Department of Health and Human Services (USDHHS), Office of Disease Prevention and Health Promotion (ODPHP) (2003). *Healthy People 2010: A Systematic Approach to Health Improvement.* www.healthypeople.gov/Document/html/uih/uih_bw/uih_2.htm#obj.

Weinstein ND, Rothman AJ, Sutton SR (1998). Stages of change theories of health behavior: conceptual and methological issues. *Health Psychology* 17:1–10.

Wolpe J (1990). *The Practice of Behavior Therapy,* 4th ed. New York: Pergamon Press.

Yalom ID (1980). *Existential Psychotherapy*. New York: Basic Books.

Chapter 3

Introductory and Attending Skills

Chapter 2 discussed the variables associated with enhancing adherence to therapeutic regimens. There, the counselor–client relationship was cited as the most important variable related to enhanced adherence. Clients who like and trust their counselors, and who feel comfortable talking with them, are most likely to comply with therapeutic plans. This chapter discusses the initial contact between counselor and client and examines the interpersonal communication skills related to establishing a helping relationship with clients and patients.

Introductory Skills

Although introductory skills are not cited as a separate part of the microskills model, we'd like to pull them out of "attending" skills and present them as a set of skills used to quickly set the tone for the counselor–client relationship in a health counseling setting. Because most health counseling is short-term and revolves around a clearly identified health issue, counselors in these settings often do not have multiple sessions to work with patients. Because of the limited time together, it is imperative that counselors make a good first impression. Six key elements of a good introduction, when used together, create a solid foundation for establishing a helping relationship: a smile, a firm handshake, exchanging names, discussing the nature of counseling, describing roles, and using an open-ended transition to initiate a discussion of the problem.

Case Study 3.1
Entry into the Public Health Care System

Mei Leueng, 28, single, identifies as Vietnamese American. A single mother of two children aged 4 and 3, Mei came into the public health clinic to serve as a translator for her father, Nuygen, who was diagnosed with tuberculosis in the emergency room of a local community hospital. After translating for her father, Mei was asked about her children's immunization status by the clinic counselor. She admitted that because she was still awaiting clarification of her citizenship status, she was afraid to go to the doctor to have her children immunized. She also had little extra money for medical care. The counselor explained to Mei that her children could receive free vaccinations at the clinic despite her current immigration status. Counselors working in public health settings will often use situations such as Mei's to introduce people into the public healthcare system and thereby reduce risks for conditions other than those that were their initial reasons for presenting.

Healthy People 2010 Leading Health Indicators

Immunization
Health Implications of Low Levels of Immunization

The development of effective vaccines has been hailed as one of the greatest public health achievements of the twentieth century. Immunization is a major public health strategy for preventing the development and controlling the spread of infections within communities. Immunization rates for children for communicable diseases such as measles, mumps, and rubella have traditionally exceeded 90% in the United States. The rates for new and illegal immigrants are often well below this level, however, and represent a significant public health risk, particularly where such groups represent a disproportionately high share of the total population. Immunization rates for seasonal diseases, such as influenza, among the elderly and other susceptible segments of our population are also at unacceptably low levels (USDHHS, 2003).

Objectives for the Nation

- Increase the proportion of young children who receive all vaccines that have been recommended for universal administration for at least five years
- Increase the proportion of noninstitutionalized adults who are vaccinated annually against influenza and ever vaccinated against pneumococcal disease (USDHHS, 2003)

Smile

As mentioned in Chapter 2, a show of friendliness is essential to establishing a good client–counselor relationship and enhancing adherence. A smile is a universal sign of friendliness and approachability. Try to remember that clients meeting you for the first time do not know you, are a little apprehensive about being there, and are a little unsure that they can trust you enough to discuss their problem openly with you. A warm (but not excessive) smile is a good icebreaker.

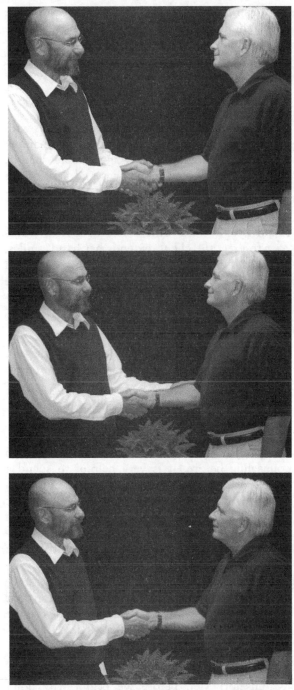

Figure 3.1 These are three common variations on shaking hands. (Photo by Michael Blonna)

A Firm Handshake

A firm handshake, used by both men and women, is an accepted American gesture of warmth and approachability. Although not universally used by all cultures, the handshake is understood as an American sign of respect and greeting. Offering your hand is also a way of establishing "touch" in your counseling. The handshake, combined with a warm smile, is a simple way to establish instant approachability. This consideration is very important in counseling clients with health issues that manifest themselves with physical symptoms that often evoke feelings of shame, guilt, and "feeling dirty." By making skin-to-skin contact with these clients, you can instantly dispel such negative emotions by modeling acceptance (see Case Study 3.2).

Many variations on the handshake exist. Some counselors like to enclose clients' hands with both of their own hands. Others combine a handshake with a touch on the arm or shoulder. Still others combine it with a deferential bow of their head (see **Figure 3.1**).

Case Study 3.2
Dr. X and His Double Gloves

Dr. X, age 60, divorced, identifies as Egyptian American.

In his first career, Dr. Blonna was a counselor in a sexually transmitted diseases clinic in a major metropolitan area in northeastern New Jersey. His job was to counsel people infected with STDs and investigate their sexual partners. Many of the clients were embarrassed about being infected with STDs and uncomfortable discussing their diseases. They often reported feeling "dirty" because their symptoms included genital ulcers, warts, discharges, and rashes on various parts of their bodies. A large part of the counseling involved helping clients cope with these feelings. Dr. Blonna always made it a point to shake their hands and gently touch them when making a point or trying to console them. These gestures helped restore a sense of cleanliness and "normalcy" to their perceived feelings of somehow being unclean.

Dr. Blonna's attending physician in the clinic at this time, Dr. X, had a different approach to dealing with patients. He *never* made skin-to-skin contact with clients. In fact, the only physical contact he ever had with his clients was made when wearing *two* sets of disposable rubber gloves. When a new client would enter his office, Dr. X would sometimes shake the patient's hand if offered it, but *always* with his gloves on. When he finished examining his clients, he would discard the outer set of gloves and put another set on before meeting his next patient.

After a few weeks of working with Dr. X, Dr. Blonna met with him. The following dialogue ensued:

Dr. Blonna: Excuse me Dr. X, but I notice that when you interact with patients you always have gloves on.

Dr. X: Yes, you can never be too careful when dealing with STD patients.

Dr. Blonna: Yes, but I thought that STDs were passed through sexual transmission and that as long as you washed your hands after shaking or touching theirs that the risk of transmitting any disease was infinitesimal.

Dr. X: Well, you never know. Why risk it?

Dr. Blonna: I think it is important to help dispel myths about how these diseases are really spread. I think if we wear gloves it sends inaccurate messages about transmissibility. Besides that, it works against me telling clients that they shouldn't feel guilty or dirty about having STDs. How can I tell them that having an STD is not a stigma, and that they will be treated with respect and dignity here, if you refuse to touch them and treat them as if they had leprosy?

Dr. X: Dr. Blonna, I think you are overstepping your bounds. Let me remind you that I am the physician here, not you.

Shortly thereafter, Dr. X moved on to another job. He was replaced with a more understanding physician who greeted his patients with bare hands and then donned his rubber gloves when he examined them.

Exchanging Names

It is very easy to combine exchanging names with smiling and shaking hands. While remaining standing, smiling, and shaking clients' hands, counselors can give their names and ask for the clients' names.

Example

A client enters the office. The counselor walks over to greet the client, extends her hand, smiles, and says, "I'm Susan, the counselor here, and you are . . . ?" After Susan gets her client's name, she would follow that up with an offer to sit and begin the session.

Example

"So nice to meet you, Mei. Please have a seat. Can I get you a glass of water or a cup of coffee [if available]?"

Discussing the Nature of Counseling

Many clients and patients have never been to counseling before. It is very helpful to spend a couple of minutes discussing the nature of counseling with them so they will understand the process and therefore will be able to participate in it more fully. Many people have the misconception that counseling is something done "to" them rather than "with" them.

Clearing up this misconception sets the stage for clients assuming more responsibility for their treatment regimen. A good way to do so is to use an open-ended statement to assess clients' knowledge of the counseling process.

Example

Counselor: Mei, before we begin, why don't you tell me what you know about counseling.

Client: I really don't know much, other than what I've seen on television. You know, you sit there and the counselor tells you what to do to get better.

Counselor: Actually, Mei, in counseling, we will both work together in developing a plan that works best for you. I will never tell you what to do. I will offer options for you to consider but they are merely suggestions that I think might work for you.

Description of Roles

To further clarify the nature of counseling and explain what will occur during the counseling process, it is important to identify the roles and responsibilities of counselors and clients. It is important to let clients know up front that you intend to discuss very personal issues and that their open and honest discussion of these issues is important if the two of you are to make any progress. It is also important to stress the confidential nature of the relationship. Lastly, it is important to discuss limits. Clients need to know that they have the right to not discuss issues that they are not ready to explore. Over the course of the relationship, they may become willing to revisit issues that they were not initially ready to handle.

Example

Counselor: Mei, my role in this process is to help you find solutions to your problem by listening to you, asking questions, giving information and instructions, proposing options, and helping you organize your thoughts. Your role is to be honest and open, share information, ask questions, challenge me when you feel I am off base, and be an active participant in your therapeutic plan. You must take responsibility for getting better and making choices that are right for you.

Transition to the Client's Story

As Ivey and Ivey (2003) say, every client has a story to tell. The best way to segue into that story, following a solid introduction, is to use an open-

ended statement. We will cover open-ended statements in detail in Chapter 4, but note here that an open-ended statement is one that cannot be answered with a simple yes/no answer. Using an open-ended statement as your transition to their stories forces clients to be descriptive and go into detail regarding the issue(s) that brought them in for counseling. You can focus on either the client or the problem with this statement.

Example: Client Focus

Counselor: So, Mei, why don't you tell me a little bit about yourself.

Client: Well, what do you want to know?

Counselor: You know, things like what you do, where you live and work, your relationships—personal stuff like that so I can get to know you better.

Example: Problem Focus

Counselor: So, Mei, why don't you tell me about the problem that brought you here today.

Client: What do you mean?

Counselor: Tell me a little about what you know about your condition, how you feel about it, some of the concerns you have about it. Things like that.

Good introductions set the stage for good relationships. If clients feel, as a result of your introduction, that you are approachable, that you will listen nonjudgmentally, and that you really care about them, they will tell you their stories and you can begin to help them.

Attending Skills

The Three V's + B: Visuals, Vocals, Verbals, and Body Language

Attending really means "paying attention to." Fully attending to someone means giving that person your undivided attention, being with the individual in the "here and now," listening with an open mind and in a nonjudgmental manner, with no hidden agendas. Attending has visual, vocal, verbal, and body language components (Ivey,

Gluckstern, & Ivey, 1997a, 1997b). When counselors fully attend to clients, they treat them to a rare delight. In the world outside the counseling office, getting someone's full attention is pretty hard to do. In this era of multitasking, stand-up meetings, working lunches, drive-through everything, and incredibly full daily schedules, being able to sit with someone who will give you his or her undivided attention is a luxury. The same trends also make it hard for counselors to divorce themselves from the outside world, close their office doors, step into the worlds of their clients, and give clients their undivided attention. While this isn't always easy to do, it can be achieved through practice and by breaking attending down into discrete skills that can be practiced and perfected.

In 1965, while conducting research at Colorado State University, Ivey and his colleagues did just that. They spent several months dissecting counseling sessions into components and then identifying specific, discrete skills that were the basis of good practice. They came up with sets of "skills" that were universal to good attending (Littrell, 2001). The skills identified by Ivey and Authier (1978) as the basis of good attending were culturally appropriate eye contact, open and approachable body language, verbal following, and vocal quality. Good attending, regardless of the counselor's training or theoretical framework, always included these elements. In fact, these "attending skills" were universal and could be adopted by all counselors regardless of their training (Littrell, 2001).

Visuals: Culturally Appropriate Eye Contact

Making and maintaining eye contact is essential to good communication, whether one is talking to friends and intimate partners or dealing with clients and patients. It is especially important when clients are speaking, because it shows them that you are listening to and understanding their messages. There is much variability in the way different cultures perceive direct eye contact. The dominant U.S. culture places a high value on direct eye contact when speaking. In contrast, Native Americans consider continuous direct eye contact to be insulting and disrespectful. Rules about eye contact also vary by gender in certain cultures. In Islamic cultures, women are taught to avert the eyes, whereas eye contact is acceptable for men. The meaning and acceptability of a myriad of other nonverbal behaviors, such as pointing fingers, shaking hands, and other forms of touch, vary by culture as well (Ivey & Ivey, 2003).

Ivey and Ivey (2003) recommend that counselors employ a "Western European" form of eye contact as an initial standard, because most Americans are familiar with it. Remember, because no universally accepted standard for what is culturally appropriate regarding eye contact exists, intentional counselors will look for nonverbal cues from their clients regarding their eye contact. If clients seem uncomfortable with the

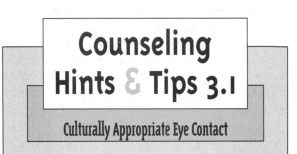

Counseling Hints & Tips 3.1

Culturally Appropriate Eye Contact

You might find the following hints useful for gauging the appropriateness of your eye contact:

1. Remember that a Western European model is just the "starting point" for using eye contact appropriately. You might have to modify this approach as the session unfolds.
2. Client cues such as muscle tension, nonsquared body posture, aversion of eye contact, and facial signs of displeasure or anxiety could indicate problems with the type of eye contact being used.
3. When in doubt, reflect this to the client in a gentle, respectful way. Example: "Excuse me, Mei, but it seems from your body language and eye contact that you are uncomfortable with something I am saying or doing. Could you please let me know what is going on so that I may better help you?"

level or type of eye contact being used, it is the counselor's responsibility to pick this up and correct it.

Vocals

As Ivey and Ivey (2003) remind us, our voices are like instruments that are capable of transmitting a broad range of tones. Clients transmit as much information by *how* they say things as by *what* they actually say. They "underline" key words and phrases in their stories by the pitch, volume, and speed of their speech. Conversely, counselors can intentionally vary the pitch, volume, and speed of their own voices to acknowledge clients and to communicate specific feelings of their own toward the clients. By raising or lowering pitch, we modulate our tone and can show anything from empathy, understanding, and deference to lack of acceptance and authoritarianism. The volume of our vocal tone can combine with the pitch to do the same thing. We can speed clients along by hurrying our pace or slow them down by drawing out

our words and interspersing them with intentional periods of silence (Engen & Albert, 1995).

The key to using vocal qualities effectively is to understand their nuances, be aware of them in our clients and our own speaking, and intentionally alter them to achieve desired effects. Counseling Hints 3.3 discusses the use of videotape to allow students to observe their vocal characteristics in role plays as both clients and counselors. These taped vignettes can serve as vehicles for practicing basic attending skills and for increasing awareness of vocal qualities. Understanding vocal strengths and weaknesses is the first step in being able to use vocal qualities intentionally. It is common to notice things such as speaking too rapidly, speaking too softly, covering the mouth with hands or fingers, or prefacing statements with phrases such as "Well, ah" or "okay." Once such habits are noticed, counselors must practice correcting them. When you feel that you are in control of your vocal qualities, rather than having them control the way you communicate, you can intentionally begin to use them.

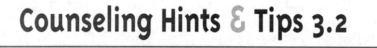

Counseling Hints & Tips 3.2

How to Listen

There are two types of listening—passive and active. Although both are acceptable, counselors need to sharpen their active listening skills.

1. In **passive listening**, the counselor merely absorbs what the initiator of the message is sending. Passive listening is what we do when watching television or a movie, listening to the radio, and so on. It is one-way communication. Although passive listening can be an effective way to receive information, it is not the most effective form of listening to another person when trying to establish or maintain a dialogue.

2. **Active listening** is much better than passive listening for dealing with interpersonal communication because, by definition, it requires feedback. Active listeners show that they are listening by providing both nonverbal and verbal feedback. For this rea-

son, active listening is demanding. It takes a lot of energy and concentration, and the listener can easily get distracted and lose interest.

3. Get ready to listen actively by preparing yourself mentally before your session begins.

- Get away from your desk; walk around for a few minutes and stretch.
- Have a glass of water.
- Splash some cold water on your face.
- Take a few deep diaphragmatic breaths.
- Contract and relax any tight muscles you have in your body, particularly your head, neck, face, arms, and shoulders (the parts most noticed by clients).
- Free your mind from your previous client by consciously telling yourself, "The last session is over—time to renew for my next client."

Counseling Hints & Tips 3.3

Videotaping Skills Sessions

Many counseling students remain oblivious to the pitch, volume, and speed of their speaking until they see themselves on videotape. The best scenario for videotaping is a classroom setting where students are more likely to take the taping seriously and carefully act out the roles of counselor and client.

Instructions

1. Set up class with two chairs in the middle and the rest of the chairs surrounding them in a semicircle. Make sure the outer chairs are at least 8–10 feet away from the chairs in the middle. Set up the video camera at the open end of the circle so that it focuses on both volunteers in a profile view.
2. Have one of the volunteers play the counselor and the other the client. The remaining students will form a semicircle out of camera view and serve as observers.
3. Instruct the students in the audience to remain silent, be respectful, and treat the two volunteers as they would want to be treated when it is their turn.
4. Give the client a topic to discuss for 10 minutes. It can be as generic and nonintimate as "for the next 10 minutes I want you to discuss what you really like and dislike about your college/university" or as specific and personal as "for the next 10 minutes I want you to discuss a problem you are facing in your life at the present time." You may also use prearranged role plays with scripts and characters you develop in advance.
5. Videotape the role play of the counselor practicing basic attending skills and the client discussing a personal issue or role playing for 10 minutes.
6. After 10 minutes, rewind the videotape and tell the class that as a whole you will be reviewing the tape for the purpose of helping the participants improve their use of basic attending skills.
7. Before showing the videotape go around the circle and ask the following questions: What was one thing the counselor did very well? (Get at least 3–5 positive comments). What was one thing the counselor could have done better? (Get at least 3–5 comments).
8. Explain that the next step in this learning process is to review the videotape so that the volunteers can review their skills and see how they are perceived by other people. The latter point is a valuable source of objective feedback that many students never get regarding their skills.
9. Review the tape, stopping frequently to illustrate both the positive and negative aspects of the counselor's session.
10. When reviewing the videotape, be sure to ask the volunteers how they thought they did. Have them critique their strengths and weaknesses so they take an active role in the process.
11. Conclude by thanking the volunteers and the class and by explaining how although this can be a painful and somewhat artificial process, it is an invaluable tool in improving their skills.

There are two basic goals when using vocal qualities intentionally: (1) to stop creating communication problems because of vocal imperfections and (2) to start attending better by using vocal qualities to strengthen relationships with clients.

The best way to accomplish these two goals is to try to match clients' pitch, volume, and speed as much as possible. For instance, clients will often lower their pitch and volume when dealing with sensitive information that evokes strong feelings. They will often slow the pace, use frequent pauses, and intersperse their words with sighs and shallow inspirations. This pattern of speaking and breathing sends a distinct message regarding their vulnerability. Effective counselors will see and hear this message and adjust their own vocal qualities to match the clients' pattern.

By matching their clients' pitch, volume, and pace, counselors demonstrate empathy for their clients. Counselors who do not sense these vocal qualities and respond with a different pitch, volume, or pace show clients that they are not sensitive to these issues and will not create the same bonds with their clients. Clients will often perceive them as aloof, uncaring, insensitive, or poor listeners.

Verbals

The key verbal attending skill is tracking (also known as following). Verbal tracking literally means "following clients' stories." The goal of verbal tracking is to keep the dialogue going where clients lead rather than where counselors want to go. This consideration is especially important at the beginning of counseling, because this period is when clients form their initial impressions of counselors. Counselors need to resist the temptation to cut clients off, ask questions, and redirect stories (Engen & Albert, 1995; Ivey et al., 1997b). There is ample time to do these things once trust is established and clients have had the initial opportunity to tell their stories.

The hardest thing for new counselors to learn is patience. It is very difficult to sit quietly, listen actively, and stay focused when learning attending skills. Often, counselors-in-training will begin to formulate questions in their minds regarding clients' stories and actually miss dialogue that could prove helpful in understanding the entire story. The best listeners make speakers feel like they are the only people in the world at that moment. Counseling Hints 3.4 provides suggestions on how to stay focused and minimize distractions during this critical initial phase of counseling sessions. By following these tips, you can join the ranks of good listeners.

Verbal tracking is critical in helping clients tell their stories. Clients must feel free to fully explain their stories. Counselors can encourage them by listening actively, asking very directed questions, and providing the minimal amount of encouragement necessary to keep clients talking. Chapter 4 discusses these "minimal encouragers." At this point in the counseling process, clients should be doing most of the talking. A balance of about 80%–20%, client to counselor, a 4:1 ratio, is a good standard to strive for. While this is very hard to learn, it will

Counseling Hints & Tips 3.4

Minimizing Distractions

1. Don't judge the messenger. Try not to let your thoughts about clients interfere with their stories. It is easy to tune out clients whom you don't initially like.
2. Watch out for emotion-laden words. Clients often use words and phrases that push our hot buttons. Vulgar, sexist, racist, and insensitive words and remarks can throw us off from hearing the entire story. Be ready for them, acknowledge them, but don't let them distract you.
3. Don't just listen for the facts. Pay attention to the way things are said as much as to what is being said. The true meanings of clients' stories are often conveyed in the way they tell their stories.

4. Maintain eye contact with clients when they speak. This practice will help you assess clients' nonverbal messages.
5. Avoid distracting mannerisms. Habits such as hair twirling, fingernail inspecting, and similar behaviors convey boredom and disinterest.
6. Resist the temptation to let your mind wander. It's easy to do considering that we can think much faster than clients can speak. It is not difficult to think at a rate of 1000 words/minute while most people speak at a rate of 125 words/minute.

ensure that the client is doing most of the talking, with the counselor providing encouragement.

The main skill of verbal tracking is picking up where clients leave off. Once clients pause or complete part of their stories, counselors must resist the temptation to ask too many questions or redirect the stories until clients have had the opportunity to fully complete them. The best way to do so is to stay focused on where they left off and simply urge them to continue by nodding your head, acknowledging them with an "uh, huh," or asking a simple question.

Example

Counselor: So, Mei, tell me what brings you here today.

Client: Well, I'm here to find out more about having my children immunized.

Counselor: Okay, tell me more about this.

Client: I'm not sure how to do this or if it is safe.

Counselor: (Maintains eye contact and leans forward) Uh, huh.

Client: It's just that I haven't gotten my final citizenship papers yet. I am worried that if I go to a clinic they might hold me and my children or send us back home.

Counselor: Tell me more about this.

Client: I came here with my husband who is an American soldier. He was recently sent to Iraq and was killed in action. I am not sure if I can still get my citizenship papers. He was supposed to take care of it.

Counselor: I am so sorry to hear about your husband. What is the status of your citizenship now?

Client: I don't know.

This type of following and focusing on having clients continue to tell their stories is the essence of verbal tracking.

Nonverbal Communication

There are many ways to convey information nonverbally. Nonverbal communication strategies can be used either to supplement verbal techniques or by themselves. This type of communication can transmit messages as effectively, and in some cases more effectively, than verbal techniques.

Body Language

How we say things is just as important as *what* we say. **Body language** describes the nonverbal messages we send through posture, gestures, movement, and physical appearance, including adornment. Our body language intentionally or unintentionally sends messages to receivers (Andersen, 1999). Positive, or open, body language is demonstrated by a relaxed posture, steady eye contact, nods of the head, and an occasional smile or happy expression. These cues signal that you are an approachable sender or a receptive receiver (see **Figure 3.2**) (McGinty et al., 2003).

Negative, or closed, body language has visible signs of tension, such as clenched fists or tight jaw muscles, a closed posture (arms folded, body shifted sideways, and the like), and facial expressions ranging from anger to disbelief. Negative body language can indicate either apathy or disturbance about something (see **Figure 3.3**) (McGinty et al., 2003).

Physical Appearance

Physical appearance can convey a variety of messages. A messy, sloppy, or ungroomed appearance may send encoded messages ranging from positive ("I'm comfortable enough in your presence to relax") to negative ("I don't care enough about you or myself to pay attention to my appearance"). Clothing and adornment might intentionally or unintentionally be erotic and seductive. This can affect both the encoding process and the decoding process, as the sender might be trying to convey one message ("I'm trying to look my best") while the receiver may perceive another ("This person is trying to manipulate or come on to me sexually").

Time Frame and Silence

Our perception of time provides the context in which clients frame their stories. The perception

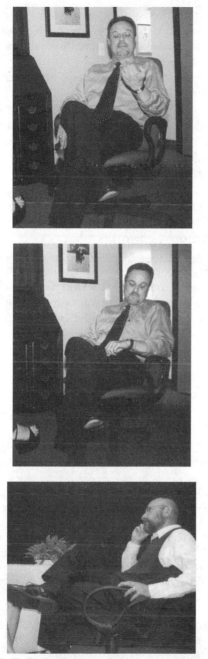

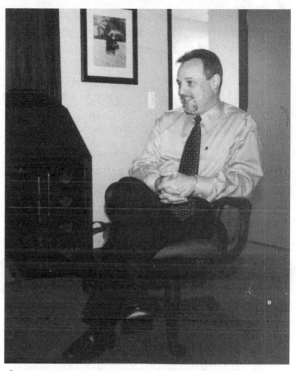

Figure 3.3 Leaning in slightly, looking relaxed, and having an open body position are good ways to show clients you are interested. (Photo by Michael Blonna)

Figure 3.2 Looking at your watch or your hands, and leaning back staring off into space are common tip-offs to clients that the counselor is either bored or disapproving. (Photos by Michael Blonna)

of time and the relationship of the past, the present, and the future vary by culture. The predominant culture in the United States is time urgent and future oriented. Being aware of the present and doing something now to plan for the future (such as exercising now to prevent heart disease in the future) are commonly accepted. In daily life, people are oriented to specific times of the day and strict schedules. Some other cultures are much less interested in time and are not as oriented to specific schedules. Many Native American homes do not even have clocks, as people of some tribes are more concerned about the present and live one day at a time (Ivey, D'Andrea, Ivey, & Simek-Morgan, 2002).

The perception of time also factors into how we deal with silence. Beginning counselors often have a hard time dealing with silence because even short periods of quiet time are perceived as "endless" or "interminable." We often need to learn or relearn ways to deal with periods of silence. Becoming more intentional in our use of silence is a major skill in attending.

Silence is a form of nonverbal communication that can be either a source of stress or a sign of comfort. It can also be used to hurt and control people. Silence is a stressor when wordless pauses are perceived as signs of a breakdown in communication. Conversely, it communicates comfort and acceptance between counselors and clients who understand that a helping bond is present despite a lack of conversation. Silence is a necessary part of effective communication that is often overlooked. We need time to listen, digest, and understand messages. Silence allows us time to reflect as we formulate our thoughts and words.

Touch

A firm handshake, a reassuring touch on the arm, and a gentle squeeze of the shoulder all convey messages without speaking a single word (McBurney, 2002). Appropriately used, touch adds another dimension of communication that sometimes reaches deeper than mere words.

When used inappropriately, however, the effects of touch can be devastating. A pat on the head can be a sign of endearment to a child but can embarrass or infuriate another adult. A squeeze on your friend's shoulder can show him you understand his problems and care about him; the same squeeze on your secretary's shoulder can convey an entirely different meaning. A pat on a teammate's buttocks can show appreciation of a great play or an extreme effort; the same pat on a coworker's buttocks can be perceived as sexual harassment. While using hand gestures, squeezing an arm, and giving other nonintimate touches are examples of behaviors common to everyday interactions among Americans, they would be consider major gaffes when used by Americans with clients from such places as China and Japan (Dou & Clark, 1999).

diverse perspectives 3.1

Multicultural Issues in Verbal and Nonverbal Communication

The following general suggestions can be helpful in verbal and nonverbal communication with people from cultures different from one's own:

1. *Slow down.* People for whom English is a second language sometimes have a hard time keeping up with and understanding English when it is spoken too rapidly.
2. *Minimize nonverbal distractions.* Be conservative rather than flamboyant in your use of gestures, personal space, and other nonverbal communication.
3. *Look for feedback.* People who don't understand, can't keep up, or are uncomfortable with something you do or say often give nonverbal or verbal cues.

These cues can be as overt as asking for clarification or as subtle as a turned head or lack of eye contact. Seek clarification of these cues.
4. *Avoid talking louder.* Sometimes, when we are not sure we are being understood, we raise our voice, assuming that the person can't hear us. Talking too loudly can be perceived as threatening or condescending and is rarely helpful.
5. *Show respect.* Being humble and respectful of cultural differences conveys the message that you care and want to understand and improve communication.
6. *Use an interpreter.* If necessary, get someone to translate your message into the person's primary language.
7. *Seek information.* Take advantage of opportunities to learn more about cultural differences in communication (e.g., read, travel, go to workshops).

Space

The space between sender and receiver also affects communication. Four space zones are common to communication in North America:

1. Intimate space (less than 18 inches)—space reserved for communication between intimate partners
2. Personal space (18 inches to 4 feet)—space appropriate for close relationships that may involve touching
3. Social-consultive space (4 feet to 12 feet)—space for nontouching, less intimate relationships that may involve louder verbal communication
4. Public space (more than 12 feet)—space used for formal gatherings such as addressing a large group (Andersen, 1999)

Although these categories provide a good baseline for understanding space parameters for Americans, their dimensions will vary from culture to culture. That is, cultures differ in their norms for territoriality and personal space. In general, people of Arabic, southern European, and African origins sit or stand relatively close to one another when talking. People of Asian, northern European, and North American countries are more comfortable being farther apart when they are talking (Ivey et al., 2002).

Stress and tension can arise when we violate culturally accepted space parameters. For example, we may find ourselves backing up to reclaim our violated space when a nonintimate person gets within the boundaries of our intimate space. Sometimes we place objects as barriers between us and other people to define our space and set allowable communication zones. Culture plays an important part in determining what is acceptable and unacceptable concerning space.

Summary

This chapter introduced the first stage of the Ivey microskills model, attending skills. Attending skills are the central behaviors used in paying full attention to clients. A strong introduction is the foundation of attending and gets the client–counselor relationship off to a good start. Introductory skills—having counselors and clients introduce themselves, discussing roles and responsibilities, smiling, and shaking hands—establish good initial impressions and build trust.

The chapter described the three V's (visuals, vocals, and verbal tracking) and B (body language) of attending. Visuals encompass the fundamental principles of culturally appropriate eye contact. Using eye contact effectively, especially when clients are speaking, is central to establishing trust. Vocals include variations in pitch, volume, and speed. Modifying these three variables intentionally allows counselors to parallel clients' vocals as well as to express and emphasize elements of the story they want to highlight. Verbal tracking refers to following clients' stories. Learning verbal tracking requires discipline, as it is very easy to allow one's mind to wander as clients weave elaborate webs in their stories. Body language comprises the nonverbal messages counselors and clients send as they tell and listen to stories. Often, the nonverbal messages sent through body language say as much as the actual words used when telling these stories.

Study Questions

1. What is the purpose of a good introduction?
2. What are the key elements of a good introduction?
3. How does the introduction set the stage for developing trust?
4. What are the three V's + B?
5. Describe a Western European approach to culturally appropriate eye contact.
6. What are the three components of "vocals"?
7. Why would a counselor want to modulate pitch, volume, and speed intentionally during a counseling session?
8. List and describe the key elements of verbal tracking.

9. What are some of the common barriers to verbal tracking?
10. Describe three key elements of approachable body language.

References

Andersen PA (1999). *Nonverbal Communication: Form and Function*. Palo Alto, CA: Mayfield.

Dou WL, Clark W (1999). Appreciating the diversity in multicultural communication styles. *Business Forum* 24:54–62.

Engen H, Albert M (1995). *Microcounseling* (four-part videotape series). Iowa City, IA: University of Iowa.

Ivey AE, D'Andrea MD, Ivey MB, Simek-Morgan L (2002). *Theories of Counseling and Psychotherapy: A Multicultural Perspective*, 5th ed. Boston: Allyn & Bacon.

Ivey AE, Authier J (1978). *Microcounseling: Innovations in Interviewing, Counseling, Psychotherapy, and Psychoeducation*. Springfield, IL: Charles C. Thomas.

Ivey AE, Gluckstern NB, Ivey MB (1997a). *Basic Influencing Skills*, 3rd ed. North Amherst, MA: Microtraining Associates.

Ivey AE, Gluckstern NB, Ivey MB (1997b). *Basic Influencing Skills*, 3rd ed. (videotape). North Amherst, MA: Microtraining Associates.

Ivey AE, Ivey MB (2003). *Intentional Interviewing and Counseling: Facilitating Client Development in a Multicultural Society*. Pacific Grove, CA: Brooks Cole.

Littrell J (2001). Allen Ivey: transforming counseling theory and practice. *Journal of Counseling & Development*. http://Bahai-library.org/newspapers/010101–1.html.

McBurney L (2002). Touch me—not there! How to be sensual without necessarily being sexual. *Marriage Partnership* 19:26–29.

McGinty K, Knox D, Zusman ME (2003). Nonverbal and verbal communication in "involved" and "casual" relationships among college students. *College Student Journal* 37:68–72.

United States Department of Health and Human Services (USDHHS), Office of Disease Prevention and Health Promotion (ODPHP) (2003). *Healthy People 2010: A Systematic Approach to Health Improvement*. www.healthypeople.gov/Document/html/uih/uih_bw/uih_2.htm#obj.

Chapter 4

Observational and Responding Skills

Learning Objectives

By the end of the chapter students will:

1. Describe three nonverbal indicators of client behavior

2. Compare and contrast the three different client observational styles

3. List and describe the nonverbal minimal encouragers

4. List and describe the verbal minimal encouragers

5. Give examples of appropriate use of verbal and nonverbal minimal encouragers

6. Describe the positive uses of questioning

7. Describe some of the problems associated with questioning

8. Describe and give examples of open-ended statements and questions

9. Describe and give examples of yes/no questions

10. Describe and give examples of forced-choice questions

11. Explain the appropriate use of the various types of questions

12. Describe and give examples of the three key elements of effective paraphrases

13. Compare reflection of feelings to paraphrasing

14. Describe and give examples of effective summaries

Observational Skills

Nonverbal Messages

Chapter 3 discussed the essentials of non-verbal communication. We considered how closed body language can transmit a lack of approachability and why it is important for counselors to be aware of subtle nuances in their own eye contact, body position, tension, spacing, and use of silence. This chapter focuses on observing and responding to these qualities in clients and using them to understand their stories and to frame responses that will help clarify issues and discrepancies in their stories.

In Chapter 3, we suggested that counselors use a European-American model for culturally appropriate eye contact. If clients respond to this type of eye contact in a dissimilar way (e.g., avoid eye contact, stare at the floor, or stare into space), it might indicate misunderstanding, confusion, disagreement, discomfort, or some other problem (Ivey, Gluckstern, & Ivey, 1997b; Engen & Albert, 1995). Counselors are responsible for observing these responses and dealing with them at the appropriate time.

Counselors are also responsible for noting and responding to clients' closed body positioning, muscle tension, use of silence, and space requirements. Clients who show excessive muscle tension (e.g., clenched fists, furrowed brows) and a closed body posture (see the numerous examples in Chapter 3) might also be demonstrating signs of their misunderstanding, confusion, disagreement, discomfort, or some other problem. Sometimes, as in Case Study 4.1, this discomfort can be resolved very simply. At other times, it is symbolic of deeper issues that must be addressed to help clients.

Case Study 4.1
Alberto

Alberto, 22, is single, gay, and Mexican American. Infected with syphilis, he was attending a public STD clinic. Dr. Blonna, a counselor in the clinic, had just met Alberto and was starting to counsel him regarding his syphilis infection. After reviewing Alberto's medical chart, Dr. Blonna began by saying, "Hello, Alberto [extending hand and smiling]. My name is Rich Blonna. I am one of the STD counselors here at the clinic. It is my job to talk to you about your infection and how to cure it. We are going to have to discuss a lot of intimate, personal issues regarding your sexuality,

and I want you to know that everything we discuss is confidential. I also want you to know that I am not here to judge you, just to help you get better. Your job is to be as open and honest with me as you can be. We are quite different. I am an older, married, Anglo guy and you are a young, single, Mexican American man. If this makes it hard for us to work together, please let me know."

As he was saying this, Dr. Blonna noticed that Alberto was not facing him squarely, seemed tense, and averted his eye contact. Dr. Blonna continued, "We can talk about anything you wish to, but before you leave I must talk to you about five things: (1) how to follow your treatment plan, (2) how to take care of your sex partners, (3) when and why to return for follow-up tests, (4) what to do in the future if you think you are exposed to another STD, and (5) how to reduce your risk of future infections."

Once again, Dr. Blonna noticed that Alberto was tense (his legs were tightly squeezed together, his arms folded tightly across his chest). He was sitting sideways, and still avoiding eye contact. Rather than proceed, Dr. Blonna decided to confront him.

"Alberto, you seem very tense and distracted. What have I said that makes you so uncomfortable?"

Alberto replied, "I just really have to go to the bathroom. I am about to burst."

Several minutes later, a relieved Alberto returned to the interviewing room and turned out to be a very cooperative, interesting client.

Experiences such as these show us that clients' body language can transmit all kinds of messages, some easier to discern than others. When in doubt, it is our responsibility—not the clients'—to find out what they mean.

Clients vary in their needs for silence to process information, formulate their thoughts, and express themselves verbally. It is important for counselors to allow clients ample time to do this and not rush them along. Counselors need to practice dealing with periods of silence and to become sensitive to judging lapses in time so as not to rush clients in formulating and telling their stories. Attending properly provides opportunities to observe clients' verbal abilities and their use of silence.

Changing spacing when communicating is sometimes like a chess game, as clients and counselors readjust their body positions, chairs, desks, and tables to modify space parameters. In particular, counselors and clients will lean into and move their chairs closer to the other person when they feel safe and are open to communicating. Conversely, they will lean back or move their chairs away when they are feeling uncomfortable and do not want to communicate (see **Figure 4.1**). Often, people will combine body tension with increasing distance as they tense up and lean away in a show of discomfort and increased unapproachability (Andersen, 1999; Engen & Albert, 1995).

Counselors need to pay attention to what clients are saying verbally as they communicate these nonverbal messages. The linking of uncomfortable, closed nonverbal messages with specific parts of the stories provides information about the stories and areas that need to be clarified and confronted at the appropriate time. It is important that counselors pay attention to these linkages between *what* is being said and *how* it is be-

Counseling Hints & Tips 4.1

Learning How to Deal with Silence

The ability to tolerate (and encourage) intentional periods of silence is a skill that can be learned. Many counselors are caught up in the hectic pace of living and have an inability to deal with the silence of their clients. Counselors must be role models for serenity and the ability to enjoy silence. Here are some simple hints for becoming more comfortable with silence.

Instructions for Classroom Activity 1

1. Designate one student to be the timekeeper. Make sure this person has a watch that measures seconds.
2. Form a circle and sit quietly while looking at one another. No one is allowed to talk or look at his or her watch.
3. The timekeeper will announce the start of the silent period. He or she should not announce how long the silence will continue.
4. The timekeeper will continue this period for 15 seconds.
5. After 15 seconds, have students guess how long the silence lasted.

6. The timekeeper should repeat this activity for 30 seconds and then for a full 60 seconds.
7. Have students describe how they felt sitting silently for that long while attending to their classmates.

Instructions for Classroom Activity 2

1. Set up triads with a counselor, client, and observer in each group.
2. Have students playing counselor and client roles advise independently and instruct them to intentionally build silence into their role plays.
3. Tell observers to record how counselors and clients respond to each other.
4. Have observers provide feedback to counselors and clients regarding their behavior during the intentional periods of silence. Pay particular attention to counselors who cut into silent periods because of their own discomfort.

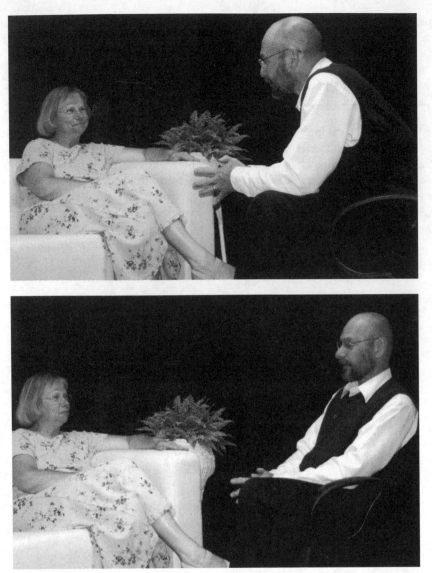

Figure 4.1 People generally lean in when they are interested and approving, and lean away when they are disinterested and disapproving. (Photos by Michael Blonna)

ing said, because they may not be congruent. Such discrepancies constitute one of the major reasons to use the skill of confrontation, which will be discussed in detail Chapter 5.

We will use Susan as a Case Study example throughout this chapter to illustrate the various responding skills.

Case Study 4.2
Susan

Susan is 29, single, heterosexual, and identifies as African American. A professional woman, she is attending graduate school to obtain a master's degree in social work. She works full-time as a social worker for a local hospital and has been seeing a counselor for about a month because of an eating disorder. In addition to her eating disorder, Susan needs help in working through her relationship problems with Hassan, her boyfriend of six months. Susan is not a real person, but rather a composite of three or four clients with whom the authors worked and one client who was portrayed in an Engen and Albert (1995) video.

Example of Verbal/Nonverbal Mismatch

Counselor: So, Susan, how did you enjoy the wedding you went to with Hassan last weekend?

Susan: (Looking away from the counselor, averting her eyes, and responding in a faint voice) It was fine.

The counselor immediately saw the mismatch between what was actually said ("It was fine") and how it was said (body turned away, aversion of eye contact, and faint volume in her speech). These verbal and nonverbal reactions to the counselor's question were obvious signs that something is wrong and will need to be addressed at some point (if not immediately) in the session.

Client Orientation

Clients have three primary orientations to how they experience their world: **visual, auditory,** and **kinesthetic** (Engen & Albert, 1995). People who are primarily visual in their orientation to life describe their world in terms of sight. They are more attuned to the myriad pictures that make up their day-to-day interactions with others and the world around them. People who are primarily auditory in their orientation to life describe their world in terms of sound. They are more sensitive to sounds, music, and the words contained in their daily interactions with others and the world

around them. Lastly, people who are primarily kinesthetic in their orientation to life are acutely aware of feelings and movement. Their orientation to the world around them and other people is primarily physical.

While everyone uses all three orientations in their daily interactions with others, most people tend to favor one of these orientations over the other. Attending to this and being able to identify the primary orientations of clients is quite helpful in establishing bonds with them and responding to them more intentionally and accurately. Clients will tip you off about their primary orientations to the world with the words and phrases they use when telling their stories.

Example: Visual Client

Counselor: Susan, why don't you tell me a little bit about what went on last week when you went with Hassan to his friend's wedding.

Susan: I can remember it in vivid detail. When he arrived to pick me up, he had on a dark gray suit with just the slightest hint of pink striping running vertically through it. He had a dark pink shirt with a very starched white collar and cuffs and had very elegant gold initial cuff links and shirt studs. He had a silk foulard tie in swirling patterns of gray, white, and black. He had on black patent leather shoes and carried a black cashmere topcoat over his left arm. He was very elegant looking.

Example: Auditory Client

Counselor: Susan, why don't you tell me a little bit about what went on last week when you went with Hassan to his friend's wedding.

Susan: It was very strange. From the moment he rang my doorbell, he had this tone in his voice. He was all dressed up, and I commented on how gorgeous he looked. He said, "Yeah, right." The way he said it just cut right through me. When I finished getting dressed, he said, "Don't you look nice," but said it with the slightest little emphasis on "you" that made me feel he was mocking me.

The whole ride consisted of him throwing little barbs at me.

Example: Kinesthetic Client

Counselor: Susan, why don't you tell me a little bit about what went on last week when you went with Hassan to his friend's wedding.

Susan: It's hard to explain, but the whole night I just felt this bad vibe from him. Like everything he said just cut me to the bone and made my stomach churn. I can't even remember what he said, but I felt on edge the whole night and my stomach never quite settled down.

Responding Skills

Responding skills are used to keep clients talking and to clarify issues in their stories. There are several categories of responding skills, ranging from simple ways of offering clients encouragement to detailed summaries of their words and feelings.

Minimal Encouragers

Minimal encouragers work by using the "minimum" amount of feedback necessary to encourage clients to keep talking. They are designed to be used in consort with verbal tracking to keep clients focused when describing their stories. Minimal encouragers can be either nonverbal or verbal. Both types of encouragers are often used together. For instance, counselors might combine head nods or hand gestures with key words from clients' stories (Ivey, Gluckstern, & Ivey, 1997a, 1997b).

diverse perspectives 4.1

Multicultural Issues in Language Level

The level of language we use plays an important part in effective verbal communication. The four levels of language are childhood, street, everyday discourse, and scientific/professional language (Mandel, 1981).

1. *Childhood language* is simple, cute, and fun and often is used to disguise embarrassment. People also use childhood language when they make mistakes and seek forgiveness. "Ooops, sowwy about that," we might say in mock childhood tones.

2. *Street language* is tough, expressive, and emotional. It can be disarming and often is used to level the playing field when communicators do not share equal power or prestige. Tough talk can convey power and superiority. Street language also serves to create bonds between members of subcultures who share a language that members of mainstream society do not understand **(Figure 4.2)**. Rap music incorporates the power and raw sensuality of street language into a unique art form.

3. *Common discourse* is the language level of mainstream society. It is the generally accepted form of language with which most of us communicate. Most people use its words, expressions, and speech patterns in communicating information that is neither intimate nor scientific. Common discourse is the language taught in schools and used in most communications.

4. *Scientific/professional language* is the discourse of the work world and professional community. It is the language that professional peers use as they communicate about the subtleties of their chosen professions. Like street language, it usually is understood only by those who share its culture. Counselors, along with computer programmers, doctors, and members of other professions, have unique vocabularies, complete with acronyms only they understand.

When we communicate with our clients, it is important to understand that they will communicate using the level of language with which they are most comfortable. Counselors may have to adjust their language levels to improve understanding if they sense problems occurring. Miscommunication can arise when the language levels of counselors and clients are not the same.

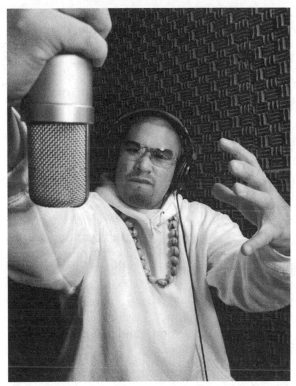

Figure 4.2 Many people find rap music threatening because of the combination of street language and "in your face" theatrics. (© Digital Vision/age fotostock)

Nonverbal Minimal Encouragers

Nonverbal minimal encouragers include the following: (1) overall relaxed open body posture, (2) facial expressions (e.g., nods, eyes, smile, eyebrows), and (3) hand gestures (roll hands to indicate "continue"). As mentioned previously, a relaxed open body posture with culturally appropriate eye contact encourages clients to continue talking by setting an accepting, inviting tone (Engen & Albert, 1995; Ivey et al., 1997a, 1997b).

Encouraging facial gestures include smiling, arching of the eyebrows, and nodding or tilting the head. These nonverbal gestures indicate that you are listening, hear what clients are saying, and want them to continue. Turning the hands over (rolling) indicates that you want clients to continue. This simple, nonverbal gesture alone can keep clients talking or encourage them to go into greater detail on a subject. Effective counselors combine nonverbal encouragers—for example, pairing head nods with arching eyebrows or rolling hands.

Verbal Minimal Encouragers

Verbal minimal encouragers include minimal verbal utterances such as "ummm" or "uh huh," key words, and mirroring. Simple "ummms" and "uh huhs" show clients you are paying attention and understand their stories. Repeating key words and mirroring are techniques intended to get clients to expand on words and themes contained in their stories without asking them direct questions (Engen & Albert, 1995; Ivey et al., 1997a, 1997b).

A **key word** is the most important word in the sentence. It captures the essence of the sentence. Key words can be either cognitive (thoughts) or affective (feelings) words and capture the key thoughts and feelings inherent in the sentence. Counselors use key words by merely repeating them back verbatim.

A powerful technique for providing feedback and keeping clients talking is **mirroring,** restating the person's exact words while mimicking the body posturing. This is done intentionally for impact. Mirroring is useful when clients say something that has strong emotional connotations. It highlights content that is so powerful that counselors don't want to risk weakening or misinterpreting it. As with using key words, mirroring involves direct repeating of the exact phrase or group of words.

Example: *Verbal Minimal Encouragers*

Counselor: Susan, why don't you tell me a little bit about what went on last week when you went with Hassan to his friend's wedding.

Susan: I can remember it in vivid detail. When he arrived to pick me up, he had on a dark gray suit with just the slightest hint of pink striping running vertically through it. He had a dark pink shirt with a very starched white collar and cuffs and had very elegant gold initial cuff links and shirt studs. He had a silk foulard tie in swirling patterns of gray, white, and black. He had on black patent leather shoes and carried a black cashmere topcoat over his left arm. He was very elegant looking.

Counselor: Tell me what else you saw. (Counselor responds to Susan in a "visual" way because this is her primary orientation)

Susan: Well, I don't know if it is my imagination or not, but I could swear that his friends were all staring at me the whole night.

Counselor: (Nods head, rolls hands) Uh huh. (Nonverbals and simple utterance)

Susan: Well, I'm not sure but I couldn't see very well. When we walked into the reception hall, a beautiful place with elaborate cornice molding and tapestries etched in gold, Hassan dumped me at a table in the farthest corner of the room, kind of behind a support column. I was so angry.

Counselor: Angry? (Key word)

Susan: Yeah, I was fuming. I couldn't see a thing, and on top of that he left me at a table of strangers by myself for about 20 minutes.

Counselor: (Leans in and shakes his head) Ummm. (Nonverbal change of position plus simple utterance)

Susan: I couldn't believe it. I just wanted to get up and run away.

Counselor: Get up and run away? (Mirroring)

Susan: Yes, I was so embarrassed. I didn't know any of these people. They all were couples. I couldn't see Hassan at all. I really didn't know what to do. I was so embarrassed. It felt like everybody was staring at me.

Counselor: (Nods head in agreement)

This simple example demonstrates how the use of minimal encouragers is often enough to get and keep clients talking. They also can be used, in lieu of questions, to get clients to expand or clarify their stories. New helpers often rely too heavily on questions to accomplish this goal and run the risk of turning clients off before they get to know them well and establish trust. Minimal encouragers can be used at any time during the counseling intervention but are particularly important in the beginning stages, when counselors want to get to know clients and establish the trust that is essential to the influencing that occurs in the later stages.

Questioning

Positive Uses of Questioning

Being able to use questions intentionally and appropriately is an invaluable, but often overused, counseling skill. Questions serve a variety of functions. Counselors must be aware of the intended uses of questions, their appropriateness at different times during counseling sessions, the potential risks of using specific types of questions at specific times, and ways to be more intentional in their use of questions. The section describes the major uses of questions and issues that might arise when using them.

1. Questions can start counseling sessions. Questions can be used to start the interview after introductions are made. Open-ended questions such as "Can you tell me a little about what brought you here?" or "What would you like to talk about?" are examples of questions used to start an interview. These types of questions are intended to give clients considerable room in deciding how and where to start their stories, especially when the reasons for their visits aren't clearly established (Ivey & Ivey, 2003).

In health counseling situations, where counselors know what brought clients in to see them, a questioning approach can be used to narrow and direct clients' starting points. In this approach, counselors combine open questions with **primacy** to allow clients to start with issues that are most important to them. For example, counselors working with STD patients in clinic settings have limited time and five key issues they must address. Consequently, they might start their counseling sessions with the following kind of open-ended question: "Today we have to discuss five issues related to your STD: (1) how to take your medication, (2) when and why to return for follow-up, (3) how to take care of your sex partners, (4) what to do in the future if you think you've been exposed to this disease again, and (5) how to reduce your risk for future infection. Which one of these five issues would you like to start with?" Using a more directive approach limits the starting points available to the client but also focuses on the key issues that must be addressed in the limited time STD counselors have with their clients.

2. Questions can help enrich and elaborate on clients' stories and bring out specific details. Clients do not always have an easy time describing their stories and going into enough detail to allow counselors to get a sense of what they are thinking and feeling. Questions can be used to help clients to elaborate on their stories (Ivey & Ivey, 2003). Using simple open statements such as "Tell me more about what happened" or "Please go into a little more detail regarding that" are examples of open-ended questions designed to get clients to expand and elaborate on their stories. Questions can also be used to bring out *specific* examples that are helpful in clarifying stories. "Can you give me a specific example of how that played out?" is a way of asking for specific details in clients' stories. Ivey and Ivey (2003) also describe this strategy as becoming more concrete. It is especially helpful for clients who are very abstract in their thinking. The farther clients move up the abstraction ladder (**Figure 4.3**), the more difficult it is for them to describe specific, concrete examples.

The bottom rungs of the abstraction ladder represent clients who are the most concrete/situational in their orientations. These clients are very skilled in providing elaborate detail (to the point of minutiae) in describing situations. Their strength lies in giving counselors lots of information about their stories from their point of view. They have difficulty with self-analysis, however, and tend to not dig too deeply beneath the surface of their own stories. Concrete/situational clients have difficulty understanding the divergent viewpoints of others. They tend to view things simplistically as being black and white, either/or.

The top rungs of the ladder represent clients who are the most abstract/formal operational in their orientations. Their strength lies in their self-

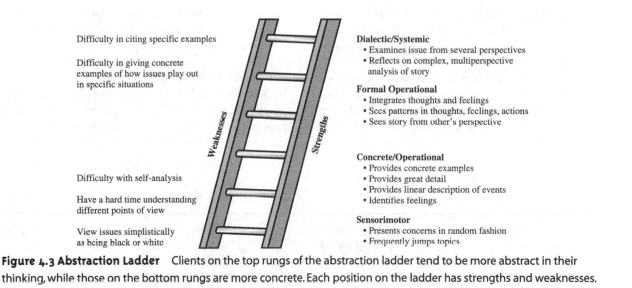

Figure 4.3 Abstraction Ladder Clients on the top rungs of the abstraction ladder tend to be more abstract in their thinking, while those on the bottom rungs are more concrete. Each position on the ladder has strengths and weaknesses.

analysis and ability to reflect on the meaning of their stories. They are very good at seeing the patterns in their behaviors and reflecting on how these patterns play out in their world. They like to use metaphors for describing their lives and the ways their stories relate to the world. While these clients are excellent at seeing broad patterns in their behavior, they have difficulty citing specific examples. Getting them to describe concrete examples of how issues played out in specific situations is difficult. Helping them work on specific problems becomes difficult when they cannot isolate these problems and give concrete examples of how they manifest themselves in specific situations.

The rest of the ladder is populated by clients who blend concrete/situational and abstract/formal operational styles. Clients who fall in the middle are able to move from one style to the next freely, citing specific, concrete examples when necessary, and being able to tie together the broad themes of their lives to understand the meaning of patterns in their behavior (Ivey & Ivey, 2003).

3. Questions are essential in assessment.
   Assessment is a key component of counseling, especially health counseling. Questions are critical in assessing clients' problems, symptoms, and history. Ivey and Ivey (2003) suggest a *who, what, when, where, why* approach for using questions to assess problems. *Who* is the client? *What* is the problem? *When* did it begin? *Where* (physical or under what circumstances) is it or does it occur? *Why* does it occur? The answers to these questions will usually cover most of the information necessary for assessing problems.

4. Questions can help clients identify their strengths and positive assets.
   Although clients come to counseling to get help with problems and overcome weaknesses, they bring with them strengths that can be perceived as assets (Ivey & Ivey, 2003). To get better, they need to get stronger. Helping them identify strengths that they already possess can help them change the way they perceive themselves and their problems and lay the foundation for developing even greater strengths and getting better. Questions can help them search for strengths.

Example: Searching for Strengths

Counselor: Susan, I know you are struggling with your eating disorder but you are an intelligent, hard-working woman who has overcome a lot of obstacles to get where you are today. Can you give me an example of some obstacle you've overcome in your life, and the strength you developed as a result of this?

Susan: Well, I had a problem with alcohol and marijuana while I was in college. It was a struggle to get through college. I worked my way through undergraduate and graduate school while maintaining an A− average. I used alcohol and marijuana to deal with the stress. After a while, I knew I was starting to rely on the drugs too much, so I cut back on their use. Eventually, I just stopped using them.

Counselor: Susan, with that kind of determination and work ethic, I'm sure you will have success overcoming your eating disorder. Are you sure you don't still need help with your alcohol and drug use?

Potential Problems with Questioning

In addition to having many beneficial applications and positive outcomes, questions can create problems if not used correctly. The following are examples of problems associated with questions.

1. Questions can foster mistrust in cross-cultural situations.
   Because questions place the direction (and therefore the power) of the interview in the hands of the counselor, they need to be used judiciously. Using too many questions together and too early in the counseling session can place clients on the defensive (En-

Alcohol and Other Substance Use

Health Implications of Alcohol and Other Substance Abuse

The abuse of alcohol and use of other illegal psychoactive substances are associated with many serious problems, including violence, injury, and HIV infection. The annual direct and indirect economic costs to the United States related to use and abuse of these substances are estimated to be $167 billion for alcohol and $110 billion for illegal psychoactive drug use (USDHHS, 2003).

Alcohol abuse is a risk factor for motor vehicle crashes and fatalities, homicides, suicides, date rape, child and spousal abuse, and drowning. Long-term abuse can lead to heart disease, cancer, alcohol-related liver disease, and pancreatitis. Alcohol use during pregnancy is known to cause fetal alcohol syndrome, a leading cause of preventable mental retardation. Alcohol abuse and the use of other illegal psychoactive drugs are associated with sexually transmitted diseases, including HIV infection; teen pregnancy; school failure; motor vehicle crashes; escalation of healthcare costs; low worker productivity; and homelessness. Both alcohol abuse and illicit drug use can result in major disruptions in family, work, and personal life (USDHHS, 2003).

Objectives for the Nation

- Increase the proportion of adolescents not using alcohol or any illicit drugs during the past 30 days
- Reduce the proportion of adults using any illicit drug during the past 30 days
- Reduce the proportion of adults engaging in binge drinking of alcoholic beverages during the past month (USDHHS, 2003)

gen & Albert, 1995). This is particularly true of clients from different cultural groups than those of counselors. Cultural (and subcultural) differences can be associated with race, ethnicity, gender, age, sexual orientation, disability status, and socioeconomic status, to name a few of the more common sources of breakdowns. Mismatches between counselors and clients across any of these cultural divisions can create suspicion, mistrust, and discomfort. Counselors who are not aware of this potential and fire away with question after question will often meet resistance from clients who feel threatened by this type of onslaught. The best way for counselors to deal with this problem is to admit it upfront and assess clients' reactions.

Example: Stating Cultural Differences

Counselor: Susan, with me being a 52-year-old married white male and you being a young single African American female, we are quite different. I will be asking you questions throughout our sessions together. How do you feel about answering these questions and working with me? (Alternative: What problems do you foresee with me being able to help you?)

2. "Why" questions put some people on the defensive.
   "Why" questions are fraught with problems. They are designed to help clients search for the reasons behind their actions and outcomes of these actions. They are also used to search for historical antecedents in clients' stories that may have led to the problems they are experiencing today. Not all counseling theoretical frameworks rely on understanding the "whys" of client behavior to help clients get better. Behaviorists, for example, have little use for the "whys" of problems, whereas psychoanalysts spend months and years trying to help clients gain insight into the "whys" of their behavior.

"Why" questions are often perceived by clients as threatening and put them on the defensive. Many clients view questions such as "Why did you do that?" or "Why do you feel that way?" as forms of attack. They may feel that counselors are asking them to justify their behaviors and feelings and go on the defensive.

Lastly, "why" questions are usually unanswerable. Counseling Hints 4.2 describes why these questions cannot often be answered.

3. Questioning shifts the counselor–client balance of power.

The microskills approach to counseling is a psycho-educational model that assumes a fairly equal balance of power and responsibility for getting well between counselors and clients. Questioning takes power away from clients and places it in the hands of counselors, who then use it to direct sessions rather than follow the directions set by clients. Counselors need to be intentional in their use of questions so as to keep the balance of power as equal as possible (Ivey & Authier, 1978).

Open-Ended Statements and Questions

Open-ended statements are queries that cannot be answered with a simple yes or no. To respond to them, clients need to go into detail. They are excellent ways to initiate a dialogue because they cannot be answered with a simple yes/no response. Some people refer to open-ended statements as *open-indirect questions* (Engen & Albert, 1995). We prefer to use the word "statements," rather than "questions," because these queries do not end with a question mark.

Examples: Open-Ended Statements
"Tell me more about that."
"Describe that in more detail for me, please."
"Explain how you feel about that."
"Clarify that for me a little more."
"Expand on that a little more."

Open-ended questions are similar to open-ended statements except that they end with a

---

Counseling Hints & Tips 4.2

Three Reasons to Avoid "Why" Questions

Here are three good reasons to avoid, or at least minimize your use of, "why" questions:

1. Why clients feel or think anything at any given point in space and time is a result of myriad factors: their genetic inheritance, their cultural upbringing, their educational level, their socioeconomic status, the number of hours they slept the night before, their nutritional status, their level of fitness, the nature of their interpersonal relationships, the last time they had an orgasm, their use of psychoactive substances in the past 24 hours, their memory, the interaction of all of these factors, and a host of other factors too numerous to list. In short, clients can't explain *why* they feel, think, or behave the way they do. They can describe *how* they would prefer to feel, think, and behave. It is much more productive, and less threatening, to focus on these issues.

2. You can get the same information and help create the same insights by asking other, less threatening questions. "What factors do you think contribute to your thinking/feeling this way?" will bring out the same information without making clients as defensive.

3. Regardless of how skillful counselors are in asking "why" questions, they usually are interpreted by clients as asking for justification for how they think or feel, which immediately puts clients on the defensive.

---

question mark. They are often referred to as *open-direct questions* for this reason. They generally fall into the *who, what, when, where, why* categories of questions previously mentioned.

Examples: Open-Ended Questions
"What did you do then?"
"How did you feel after that?"
"When did all of this happen?"
"Where were you going when this happened?"
"Why do you think you were singled out for this?"

A separate category of open-direct questions are called **permission-asking questions** because they end in a question mark and are asked in such a way that clients perceive that they are being asked permission to explore these sensitive, potentially distressing areas of their lives (Engen & Albert, 1995; Ivey et al., 1997a, 1997b). If asked in a respectful, gentle way, clients usually respond with detailed answers even though they technically could answer this type of question with a yes/no answer. This is an example of where counselors' vocals (tone, volume, and speed) are critical in modulating voice quality to convey the appropriate effect. These questions use the words "could," "can," and "would."

Examples: Permission-Asking Questions
"Could you please explain that more fully?"
"Can you please give me another example of that?"
"Could you go over that one more time for me, please?"

Closed (Yes/No) Questions
Closed questions are queries that can be answered with a simple yes or no and typically don't motivate clients to answer with much more detail. The weakest way to initiate and continue a dialogue (and the way most people start conversations) is to ask direct yes/no questions. Such questions don't require explanation or enrichment of the

story in the same way that open-ended statements and questions do. Although they are useful for verifying facts (example: "Do you still work there?" or "Does it still bother you to speak in front of groups?"), when they are overused, they can shut down a dialogue (Ivey, D'Andrea, Ivey, & Simek-Morgan, 2002; Engen & Albert, 1995).

Forced-Choice Questions
Forced-choice questions limit clients' range of options for responding but are valuable for helping them make decisions **(Figure 4.4)**. These questions should be used intentionally in situations where counselors want clients to pick from a variety of options. They are very helpful when working with clients who tend to be scattered and abstract in their decision making. Forced-choice questions can be used at any point in the counseling process but tend to be most helpful during the influencing stage, when counselors are trying to get clients to make decisions and adopt treatment plans.

Examples: Forced-Choice Questions
"You seem to vacillate between wanting to continue this relationship with Hassan and

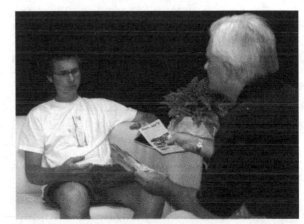

Figure 4.4 Giving teens too many options can be confusing. Forced-choice questions help young people focus and make better choices. (Photo by Michael Blonna)

wanting to end it. Which one would you prefer?"

"Based on what you have told me, it seems that there are four issues in the relationship you want to work on: improving the level of communication between the two of you, doing more things together, spending more time with mutual friends, and spending less time with his friends. Which one do you want to work on first?"

Paraphrasing

Paraphrasing is a responding skill used to keep clients talking and to clarify information in their stories. It gives clients feedback regarding how counselors interpret their stories. Paraphrasing differs from mirroring in that it does not directly quote clients, but rather phrases things in the counselor's words. Effective paraphrases include three elements:

- A shortened restatement of the client's statement in the counselor's words
- The use of a key word from the client's story
- The use of a "check it out" strategy by counselors (Engen & Albert, 1995)

Paraphrasing is used to cover a single thread in the discussion. Frequent paraphrasing shows clients that counselors hear what they are saying and understand their stories. It also provides opportunities for clients to let counselors know that they do not understand their stories without those misunderstandings becoming too great. This opportunity for feedback ensures that counselors and clients are both in sync regarding the facts and feelings of the stories.

Example: Paraphrasing
Susan: Yeah, so I am really disgusted with the way things are working out between us. I am an avid skier and the thought of this happening in our relationship in late October, just as the weather is getting cold and ski season is approaching, just depresses me. I'm not sure if

I'll be able to get any skiing in with Hassan this winter. I've already been planning a big ski trip out west during the New Year's holiday.

Counselor: It seems that this setback in your relationship has really put a damper on your enthusiasm about the approaching winter. I sense that you are very depressed about possibly losing your New Year's holiday ski trip. Is that accurate?

In this paraphrase the counselor complied with the three guidelines for an effective paraphrase:

- Restated the essence of what was being said in his own words
- Used the key words "depressed" and "ski trip"
- Checked it out by asking "Is that accurate?"

Be careful about paraphrasing all short statements from clients. Let clients finish their trains of thought regarding threads in their stories before jumping in and paraphrasing. Too many paraphrases diminish their effectiveness.

Reflection of Feelings

Reflection of feelings is similar to paraphrasing except the focus is on feelings (the affective domain) instead of thoughts and facts (cognitive domain). When counselors reflect clients' feelings, they are essentially identifying or interpreting what the clients are feeling and paraphrasing the emotions instead of the facts. New counselors often confuse this skill with asking clients what they are feeling. They are two separate skills. Questioning skills can be applied to either thoughts or feelings. The same rules for asking questions about facts and thoughts apply to asking about feelings. Reflecting feelings differs because the onus for identification of the feelings is on the counselors, not the clients.

The more counselors are able to label clients' emotions accurately, the easier it will be to understand their stories and be able to help them. Being an intentional counselor doesn't necessarily mean reflecting all the feelings clients seem to be experiencing. Often, it is best to make a mental note of

Counseling Hints & Tips 4.3

How to Reflect Feelings Effectively

The following five guidelines will help you organize your thoughts regarding reflecting feelings effectively.

1. *Use a sentence stem.* Introduce your reflection with a sentence stem. The following stems are simple and easy to use:

   "I hear you feeling . . ."

   "It seems that you are feeling . . ."

   "I get the impression that you are feeling . . ."

2. *Label the feeling.* Use the most accurate word possible from your feeling vocabulary.

   "It seems you are feeling *relieved.*"

   "You seem to have *mixed* feelings."

   "I get the impression that you are feeling *angry.*"

3. *Put the feeling into context.* Finish the sentence stem by placing the feeling into context.

   "It seems you are feeling *relieved* over not having to make this choice anymore."

   "You seem to have *mixed* feelings about your parents getting divorced. On the one hand, you are glad they are no longer fighting every day; on the other hand, you're going to miss not living with both of them."

   "I get the impression from what you are saying and how you are saying it that you are feeling *angry.*"

4. *Use the correct tense.* If the feelings are related to past events, label them that way. If they are related to current feelings, be sure to indicate this.

   "Right now you seem to feel *relieved* over not having to make this choice anymore."

   "Back when this happened, you seemed to have felt *relieved* over not having to make that choice."

5. *Check it out.* As with good paraphrasing, effective reflection of feelings requires a checkout.

   "Is that right?"

   "Is that how you feel?"

   "Am I accurate in assuming that's how you felt?"

   (Ivey & Ivey, 2003)

the feeling and get back to reflecting it at an appropriate time. This is very similar to paraphrasing too frequently. Counselors don't want to cut clients off or distract them from finishing their stories by reflecting feelings at inappropriate times.

Summarizing

Summarizing is similar to paraphrasing in that it is a restatement of the story with some interpretation. It differs from paraphrasing in that it covers more information and a longer span of time. Summarization is different from both paraphrasing and reflection of feelings because it combines the two into a statement of both fact and feeling. Good summaries tie clients' thoughts and feelings about issues together into more meaningful wholes than can either paraphrases or reflections of feelings used independently.

Use summarization to weave together multiple threads of dialogue (or multiple paraphrases) and emotions. Summarization typically occurs in the beginning, middle, and end of the session. In the beginning, counselors want to summarize to make sure they are on the right verbal track. In the middle segment of sessions, counselors want to summarize to confirm that they understand the broad themes in the story and how clients feel about them. At the end, counselors want to summarize to wrap things up, tie the disparate threads (cognitive and affective) of the story together into a more meaningful whole, and give clients the opportunity to correct misinterpretations that may have been made (Engen & Albert, 1995).

Lastly, summarization can serve as a fallback position when counselors get stuck and don't know how or where to proceed. A good motto for counselors regarding summarization is "When in doubt, summarize."

Effective summarization includes several key elements:

- A shortened restatement of the client's story up to this point in the counselor's words (this will tie together multiple threads)

- A linking of the major issues in the story to the client's emotions related to these issues
- Use of a "check it out" strategy

Example

Counselor: So, Susan, let me see if I understand what is going on between you and your boyfriend. You are very upset because the whole experience from last week seems to be symbolic of your current relationship with Hassan. On the one hand, he is a charismatic and handsome guy to whom you are attracted. On the other hand, he doesn't seem to treat you with the kind of caring and attention you desire. You seem torn between wanting to end this relationship because it is not providing you with what you are looking for and wanting to continue it because it is safe, and a crummy relationship seems better to you than no relationship at all. Is this accurate?

Susan: Yeah, pretty much. I just wish it were better and I didn't feel so bummed out by it.

The summary ties together Susan's thoughts and feelings about all of the threads.

Summary

This chapter began with a discussion of client nonverbal messages and observation. In general, clients' body language tells counselors a lot about how they feel and the meaning of what they say. A variety of key nonverbal indicators can be observed. In addition to sending nonverbal messages, clients tell us how they view the world verbally. There are three primary client orientations: visual, auditory, and kinesthetic. Relating to clients through their primary orientations helps connect counselors to clients in more meaningful ways than treating all clients the same.

Minimal encouragers are techniques involving the minimal amount of counselor activity necessary to keep clients talking. Both verbal and nonverbal minimal encouragers were discussed in this chapter.

Questioning has both pros and cons. A warning was issued about counselors' tendencies to overuse questions. Various types of questions were described and examples of their appropriate uses were given. The remainder of the chapter was devoted to paraphrasing, reflecting client feelings, and summarizing—all responding skills used to weave together the threads in clients' stories.

Study Questions

1. What are three nonverbal indicators of client behavior?
2. What are the key features of the three client observational styles?
3. How can counselors use clients' observational styles to facilitate more effective counseling sessions?
4. What are minimal encouragers, and why are they used in counseling?
5. What are verbal minimal encouragers, and why are they used in counseling?
6. What are appropriate uses of verbal and nonverbal minimal encouragers?
7. List and describe the positive uses of questioning.
8. How can questioning create problems when counseling clients?
9. How do open-ended statements differ from open-ended questions?
10. When is the use of yes/no questions most appropriate in counseling?
11. What is the best use of forced-choice questions in counseling?
12. What are the three key elements of effective paraphrases?
13. How is reflection of feelings similar to and different from paraphrasing?
14. What are the key elements of effective summaries?

References

Andersen PA (1999). *Nonverbal Communication: Form and Function.* Palo Alto, CA: Mayfield.

Engen H, Albert M (1995). *Microcounseling* (four-part videotape series). Iowa City, IA: University of Iowa.

Ivey AE, D'Andrea MD, Ivey MB, Simek-Morgan L (2002). *Theories of Counseling and Psychotherapy: A Multicultural Perspective,* 5th ed. Boston: Allyn & Bacon.

Ivey AE, Authier J (1978). *Microcounseling: Innovations in Interviewing, Counseling, Psychotherapy, and Psychoeducation.* Springfield, IL: Charles C. Thomas.

Ivey AE, Gluckstern NB, Ivey MB (1997a). *Basic Influencing Skills,* 3rd ed. North Amherst, MA: Microtraining Associates.

Ivey AF, Gluckstern NB, Ivey MB (1997b). *Basic Influencing Skills,* 3rd ed. (videotape). North Amherst, MA: Microtraining Associates.

Ivey AE, Ivey MB (2003). *Intentional Interviewing and Counseling: Facilitating Client Development in a Multicultural Society.* Pacific Grove, CA: Brooks/Cole.

Mandel B (1981). Communication: a four part process. *Hotliner* 1:6.

United States Department of Health and Human Services (USDHHS), Office of Disease Prevention and Health Promotion (ODPHP) (2003). *Healthy People 2010: A Systematic Approach to Health Improvement.* www.healthypeople.gov/Document/html/uih/uih_bw/uih_2.htm#obj.

Chapter 5

Influencing Skills

Learning Objectives

By the end of the chapter students will:

1. Explain how influencing skills are used to help clients change their personal constructs, behavior, coping skills, and decision making

2. Describe the six major focal points for exploring clients' stories

3. Explain how changing focal points influences clients

4. Understand how confrontation can be used as a supportive challenge

5. Compare and contrast various types of client discrepancies

6. Describe appropriate and inappropriate uses of self-disclosure

7. Explain how counselor self-disclosure influences clients

8. Compare and contrast reflection of meaning and interpretation of meaning

9. Describe how the meaning of a health problem influences subsequent therapeutic regimens

10. Describe how reframing influences clients and helps them formulate alternative endings to their stories

Introduction

The final set of microskills comprises the influencing skills. Influencing skills are, by definition, those skills used by counselors, in consort with clients, to change one or more of the four goals of counseling proposed by Carl Rogers (1965) and discussed in Chapter 1:

- Personal constructs
- Behavior
- Ability to cope
- Decision making

Because health counseling revolves around a disease, infection, or condition, the changes that clients make in their personal constructs, behavior, ability to cope, or decision making will primarily focus on the health issues that brought them into counseling. We say "primarily" because although clients' initial entry into counseling may have been related to their health problems, other issues will often surface when working through the emotions associated with their health problems.

For instance, STD patients, as part of their therapeutic regimens, have to devise plans for getting their sex partners evaluated and treated. As a result of this endeavor, they will often gain insight into the nature of their intimate relationships and their sexual lifestyles. Such insights may help them make changes in STD-specific personal constructs and behavior. In addition, counseling often uncovers other relationship and sexual lifestyle issues that transcend their STD risks. Examination of issues related to lack of assertiveness, gender role stereotyping, low self-esteem, and a host of other factors often emerge as a by-product of taking care of the initial concern—that is, treating the STD (Blonna et al., 1989).

The same is true for patients who are fighting life-threatening illness such as cancer. They may enter counseling seeking help in making decisions related to cancer treatment and learning how to cope with changes in their bodies and body image. Often, as a result of surviving a life-threatening disease, they leave counseling with new personal constructs about life and health and a blueprint for behavior change shaped by their counseling experience. Many report having an entirely new perspective on life. They no longer take life for granted. It is as if their near-death experience has opened them up to the beauty and potential of their lives (Case Study 5.1).

Case Study 5.1
Heidi: Leukemia Survivor

Heidi is a 52-year-old married heterosexual female, who identifies as Caucasian. She was rushed to the emergency room one winter evening after suffering from what she initially thought were symptoms associated with asthma—shortness of breath, difficulty breathing, low endurance, and fatigue. After spending the entire evening in the emergency room hooked up to tubes, probes, and monitors, Heidi was diagnosed with acute adult leukemia. She was told that her chest cavity was filled with fluid that blocked her lungs, making breathing difficult. Her blood pressure and heart rate were life-threateningly high, and her immunity was so compromised that she would have to be hospitalized and begin treatment immediately.

On Christmas Eve, after being in the cancer intensive care unit for nearly a month, Heidi was released. For the next two and one-half years, she participated in an aggressive experimental treatment program that consisted of a daily regimen of three oral chemotherapeutic agents, an oral steroid, an antinausea agent, and an injection (administered by her husband) of a drug designed to boost her immunity. This combination of drugs left Heidi exhausted, nauseated, and with damage to her balance and equilibrium. In addition to this daily, home-based regimen, Heidi received weekly intravenous chemotherapy treatments and blood tests on an outpatient basis. To ensure that the cancer did not spread to her brain, Heidi had cranial radiation treatment.

Heidi went back to work part-time after about six months and gradually increased her hours to full-time after about nine months. After two and one-half years, her cancer was thought to be in remission. Five years later, she is still in remission. We talked to Heidi about her ordeal.

Authors: Heidi, what went through your mind the evening you were brought into the hospital?

Heidi: I was so afraid. I had never even stayed overnight in a hospital. Both of my sons were born in a birthing center. I felt so helpless.

Authors: How did you feel when you were diagnosed with leukemia?

Heidi: I was afraid, but I never thought I was going to die. I couldn't believe that God would let me die knowing I had two beautiful sons to care for. I had faith that I could make it.

Authors: What gave you so much faith?

Heidi: I really believed in my doctors and the nurses. They explained everything to me, answered all of my questions, and made me feel I was getting the best care possible. They made me believe that they were doing everything possible to give me the best care they could. All I needed to do was give the same effort and not fight them. I knew that God was looking out for me. I just felt that if Rich [her husband] was with me and I could get out of the hospital by Christmas, I would make it. He stayed with me almost every night, sleeping on a cot. On Christmas Eve, I was strong enough to go home. I knew I was going to make it after that.

Authors: Did you ever lose that faith?

Heidi: Yes, a couple of days before Christmas, my blood counts were so low I got depressed. Rich came to me and told me to hold his hands and feel his strength. We held hands for a long time, and I really did feel his energy coming into me. I can't explain it but that day and the next, my blood count rose and I was released.

Authors: When you were going through your ordeal did you seek counseling?

Heidi: I talked to the oncology social worker and the minister. They both recommended that I join a cancer support group, but that wasn't for me. I am not a group person. My sister, who had breast cancer, helped me a lot. My main therapy came from talking things out with Rich every day. He, and my sons, helped me cope.

Authors: Can you tell us how this experience has affected you?

Heidi: I guess I don't think about the future as much. I try to live in the present as much as possible and do little things to enjoy each day. I have a garden and a pool and try to spend as much time in each as possible. I always have appreciated the little things, but I think I appreciate them even more. Rich and I try to take advantage of every opportunity to do the things we enjoy and to not put too much off until tomorrow. We like to hike in the woods and go canoeing as well as just hang out by the pool. Lately we have been going to a lot of midday movies. We both really enjoy that. I guess my experience made both of us realize how fragile life really is and how quickly you can lose it all. It just doesn't make sense any more to defer life's pleasures.

As the case study demonstrates, the insights gained from working through the emotions associated with a life-threatening illness can have a profound influence on clients' lives after their ordeals are over. We will turn our attention to the major influencing skills, starting with confrontation.

Confrontation

Most counselors-in-training are uncomfortable with the thought of **confrontation**. When asked to free-associate about this term, they typically mention things such as "fight," "anger," "strong disagreement," "agitation," "stress," "catch someone at something," and "call someone on something." Most of the associations are negative. When asked whether they like confrontation, the overwhelming majority of students say "no." Confronting people is not very high on most people's lists of things they enjoy doing. Given this mindset, a considerable amount of unlearning and relearning must go on for counselors to become comfortable with the notion of confrontation as a positive skill that can help clients be more genuine and assertive (Engen & Albert, 1995). To actually get counselors to enjoy helping clients through confrontation requires even more time and practice.

Throughout the rest of the chapter, we will use Doris (Case Study 5.2) to illustrate influencing skills.

Case Study 5.2
Doris: Young and Suffering from Hypertension

Doris is 22 years old, is a single heterosexual female, identifies as African American. A college junior, she lives at home with her mother, two younger brothers, and an older sister. Her father died last year of alcohol-related cirrhosis of the liver. The family resides in a modest home, and everyone in the family works and contributes toward living expenses. Doris's mother is in her late fifties and works full-time during the day as an x-ray technician in a local hospital and part-time on weekends for a company that cleans offices.

Doris, an attractive young woman, is about 80 pounds overweight and suffers from recently diagnosed (about three weeks ago) high blood pressure. She takes antihypertensive medication and has been in counseling for a few sessions to help manage her hypertension and the lifestyle changes recommended by her physician. Doris is very worried about having high blood pressure because her father, besides being an alcoholic, had hypertension. She is also very self-conscious of her weight and has had problems maintaining healthy body composition her whole life. Her mother and older sister Sonya are also overweight and have hypertension. Doris does not exercise and does not eat a well-balanced diet. She likes fast foods (particularly fried foods) and is always on the go between school, work, church, and home. When she is not busy with school, work, or other responsibilities, Doris likes to read, watch TV, and go to the movies. She is a self-described "couch potato."

Ivey and Ivey (2003) stress that the first step in getting counselors to embrace confrontation is changing the way they think about it. To do so, they suggest redefining confrontation as "supportive challenge." Rather than view confrontation as a harsh tactic of "going against" clients, it

Healthy People 2010 Leading Health Indicators

Physical Activity
Health Implications of Physical Activity
Daily physical activity is important for maintaining a healthy body, enhancing psychological well-being, and preventing premature death. In 1999, 65% of adolescents engaged in the recommended amount of physical activity. In 1997, only 15% of adults performed the recommended amount of physical activity, and 40% of adults engaged in no leisure-time physical activity (USDHHS, 2003).

Moderate levels of daily physical activity are associated with lower death rates for adults of any age. They also decrease the risk of death from heart disease, lower the risk of developing diabetes, and are associated with a decreased risk of colon cancer. Likewise, they help prevent high blood pressure and help reduce blood pressure in persons with elevated levels.

In addition, moderate levels of daily physical activity are associated with the following health benefits:

- Increased muscle and bone strength
- Increased lean muscle and decreased body fat
- Better weight control and improvement of any weight-loss effort
- Enhanced psychological well-being and perhaps a reduction of the risk of developing depression
- Reduced symptoms of depression and anxiety and improved mood

Objectives for the Nation
- Increase the proportion of adolescents who engage in vigorous physical activity that promotes cardio-respiratory fitness three or more days per week for 20 or more minutes per occasion
- Increase the proportion of adults who engage regularly—preferably daily—in moderate physical activity for at least 30 minutes per day (USDHHS, 2003)

can be viewed as a gentle means of "going with" clients by seeking their help in clarifying any **discrepancies, incongruities,** or **mixed messages** in their stories. Gently and respectfully pointing out discrepancies in their stories and asking for clarification forces clients to rethink their behavior (Ivey & Ivey, 2003). Confrontation helps clients become more congruent. In time, over the course of counseling clients learn that such incongruities, discrepancies, or mixed messages will not go unnoticed by counselors. They also relearn how to be more genuine by becoming less and less discrepant in their thoughts, feelings, and actions (Ivey, Gluckstern, & Ivey, 1997a, 1997b; Engen & Albert, 1995). This growth, which begins in relation to how they deal with their health problems, carries over into the way they deal with all issues in their lives. Confrontational counselors serve as positive role models for the client by offering direct, honest, open confrontation.

Discrepancies can be either internal or external. Those that are internal to clients comprise incongruities in what is being said (different versions of the same story), how it is being said (words versus nonverbal messages such as body language, tone, pace, or volume), or what is being said and what actually is being done (words versus actual behavior). Discrepancies that are external involve incongruities between clients and other people or clients and situations in their environments (Ivey & Ivey, 2003). Such discrepancies, whether internal or external, send mixed messages to counselors that must be confronted and clarified if clients are to grow and become more genuine in their lives.

Four main categories of discrepancies exist:

1. *Thoughts/beliefs and actions.* Clients believe one thing but behave in ways that are inconsistent with their beliefs.
2. *Feelings and actions.* Clients behave in ways that are incongruent with how they feel about something.
3. *Thoughts/beliefs and feelings.* Clients say one thing but feel another.

4. *Versions of the story or parts of the story.* Clients describe their stories one way but describe it differently at a later point (Ivey & Ivey, 2003).

The first type of client discrepancy revolves around behaving in ways that are inconsistent with previously stated beliefs. The second type of

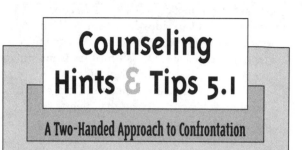

Counseling Hints & Tips 5.1

A Two-Handed Approach to Confrontation

Ivey et al. (1997b) recommend a "two-handed" approach to confrontation **(Figure 5.1)**. This approach combines body language with words to identify discrepancies, incongruities, and mixed messages in clients' stories. Here are simple instructions on use of this highly effective technique.

1. Call the client by name and put the confrontation in gentle, supportive context.
   "Doris, I know this is difficult for you to talk about and I want to help you, but something about your story troubles me."
2. Use the "first hand." Introduce the discrepancy by extending one hand as you speak.
   "On the one hand, you stated last week that you were excited about the new diet and exercise plan we devised and that you were going to stick to it."
3. Use the "second hand." Leave the first hand extended and extend your other hand as you continue the description.
   "On the other hand, you just told me that you neither exercised nor watched your diet this past week."
4. Finish with a gentle, probing, open-ended clarifying statement.
   "Can you please explain this to me?"

The two-handed approach is easy to remember, uses body language to reinforce the confrontation, and provides a simple cue for clients to remember your point outside of counseling.

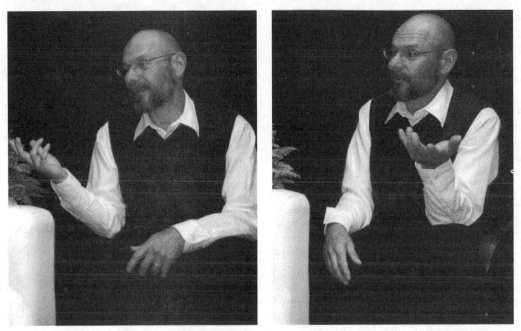

Figure 5.1 Use the one hand, other hand technique for pointing out discrepancies in the client's story.

(Photos by Michael Blonna)

incongruity is very similar but deals with mismatches in previously stated feelings and behavior. Clients often describe feelings that don't match the appropriate behavior associated with such emotions. For example, Doris behaves in ways that are very different from her previously stated verbal commitments and excitement about wanting to change her dietary and exercise behavior. If she was being consistent in her behavior, she would have maintained her diet and exercise regimen. Counseling Hints 5.1 demonstrates that by gently confronting her on this discrepancy, the counselor can empathize with Doris on the difficulty of maintaining such a regimen but show her that such discrepancies will not go unnoticed.

In the third type of discrepancy, clients say things that don't match the nonverbal behavior associated with their words. That is, the actual words they use don't match the appropriate body language or vocal tone, pitch, and volume for the statements. If Doris says she is excited, for instance, the counselor would expect to see her show signs of excitement such as expressive body language or a rise in volume or pitch of her voice. If these signs were missing, or if Doris seemed closed or tense instead and her voice was quiet and timid, this would be a mismatch between her words and feelings.

Example

Counselor: How are things going since we mapped out your new diet and exercise program?

Doris: (Averting eye contact, slightly turning away, and speaking in a hushed voice) Everything is fine.

Counselor: (Noticing these clues) Doris, it doesn't seem like everything is fine. You say this, but the way you say it leads me to believe that you are upset.

The fourth type of discrepancy is the easiest to pick up if counselors are actively listening. In this discrepancy, clients give two different versions of the same story. This might occur within the same counseling session or on two different occasions.

Example

Counselor: Hold on a minute, Doris. I'm confused. Five minutes ago, you said you were excited about your new diet and exercise plan. Now you are saying that you are afraid it is too difficult. Can you explain this for me, please?

By gently and respectfully pointing out Doris's incongruities and mixed messages, the counselor helps her sort through her thoughts, feelings, and behavior. This exercise can help her become more congruent. It can also help her reconstitute her therapeutic plan. Perhaps the plan the counselor and the client worked out is too aggressive. Perhaps these mixed messages and incongruities signal that it is time to rethink and fine-tune the treatment plan. Pointing out the discrepancies creates a window of opportunity to redefine the plan (Engen & Albert, 1995).

Feedback and Self-disclosure

Feedback and self-disclosure are subtle influencing skills that are used to help clients gain new insights into their own behavior and their counselors' experiences. Often, clients do not get objective feedback about their behavior and how they come off to others. Such information, when presented in a supportive way in the comfort of the counseling session, can prove very helpful in helping clients see how their behavior is perceived by others and can either contribute to their problems or serve as a source of strength in overcoming these problems (Ivey & Ivey, 2003). When counselors self-disclose information about their own struggles and successes with similar problems, they help clients see that these issues can be overcome and don't have to permanently stand in the way of achieving their goals. In a sense, this practice levels the playing field between clients and counselors. It humanizes counselors and helps facilitate empathy (Engen & Albert, 1995).

Feedback

Feedback entails giving objective information about how the client is behaving. It differs from paraphrasing and summarizing in that the information counselors "feed back" to clients isn't about their stories, but rather about how they act and appear to others when telling their stories. Feedback can be positive or negative in nature. "Feeding back" can be a very powerful technique when clients hear things about themselves and the way they come off to others that they might never have considered or are new to them. Counselors need to remember that even the most careful attempts to provide objective feedback are tainted by their own perception of clients' behavior.

Example

Counselor: Doris, you have been sitting here for the entire session complaining about everything. It is very hard for me to follow you when you complain about everything instead of focusing on the topic we started to discuss. What is going on?

Counselor: Doris, did you ever notice how you end most of your sentences with a change of inflection and a question mark? It's almost as if you have to ask permission to say what is on your mind.

Counselor: Doris, you have a really nice way of using words to paint a beautiful picture of what is going on in your life. That is a rare ability.

Self-disclosure

Self-disclosure is counselors' *intentional* disclosing of information about themselves as part of their effort to connect with clients in a deeper, more personal way. It should not be confused with the unintentional self-disclosure that goes on simply as a result of being who we are as people. We all have a personal style that comes across in the way we speak, dress, and present ourselves to clients. Part of this is a result of our background, experience, lifestyle, and culture. We must always remember that despite our best efforts to remain neutral in the way we appear to clients, we must be honest with ourselves and true to this personal style if we are to be genuine and effective as helpers. In essence, the issue isn't whether we self-disclose, but rather how we intentionally use this skill to influence clients (Engen & Albert, 1995). When self-disclosure is used inappropriately, counselors' stories begin to take precedence over those of their clients. This happens most often when counselors have irrational needs to be liked, seek to control and direct clients, or are uncertain about how to proceed. When this happens, counselors go into too much detail or begin talking about issues that are not directly related to their clients' situations (lack of parallelism). Counseling Hints 5.2 describes appropriate uses of self-disclosure.

Example: Appropriate Self-disclosure

Counselor: Doris, I know how difficult it is to lose weight and keep up a program of regular exercise if your family doesn't really support it. I was overweight and very unfit as a young

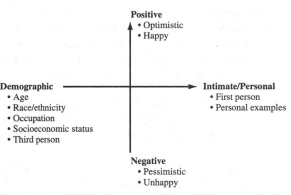

Figure 5.2 Self-disclosure works best if the counselor's self-disclosure is parallel to the client's.

person. I come from an Italian American family where everything revolved around food. Neither of my parents exercised, and both were overweight and suffered from high blood pressure. I never received any encouragement from them to lose weight and get in shape.

Doris: You seem to be in very good shape now.

Counselor: It took a couple of years to take control of my eating and exercise behavior. I started making the big changes like you, when I was in college.

Focusing the Narrative

Focusing the narrative influences clients by helping them see their problems from a variety of focal points or perspectives. Often, when we are struggling with a problem, we see it only one way. Sometimes it is almost as if we have blinders on and cannot see the issue from any other perspective except from our current one. Changing the focal point forces us to take the blinders off and consider the problem from a different perspective. Changing the perspective "influences" clients because it exposes them to the reality that there are several ways (other than their own) to view the problem. Even if they do not accept any of these different viewpoints, acknowledging the fact that they exist is itself a change (Ivey & Ivey, 2003).

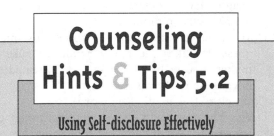

Counseling Hints & Tips 5.2

Using Self-disclosure Effectively

The following guidelines make recommendations for the appropriate use of self-disclosure:

1. *Be intentional.* Use self-disclosure to create a more trusting relationship, to model appropriate behavior, to increase mutuality between counselors and clients, and to influence clients' perceived ability to change.
2. *Keep it simple.* Be concise; share only what is necessary to achieve your goal.
3. *Stay parallel.* Limit sharing to the same demographic–intimate and positive–negative dimensions (see **Figure 5.2**) used by clients.
4. *Do not lie.* Clients will sense when your self-disclosure is not genuine, and the lie will undermine any trust already built up in the relationship.

Focusing the narrative is a subtle influencing skill that helps clients open their minds to different ways of viewing their world. Seven major focal points can be used to help clients see their problems from a variety of perspectives:

- *Individual focus:* the client's perspective on the story. It focuses on clients' thoughts and feelings about how the problem affects their lives.
- *Main theme or problem focus:* the client's perception of the problem. It focuses on the major theme or nature of the problem as seen through the eyes of clients.
- *Family focus:* the family's perspective on the problem. It focuses on the effects of the problem on the family.
- *Other individual focus:* the perspective of other key individuals in the story. It focuses on how other key individual(s) are affected by the problem.
- *Mutuality focus:* the perspective on the problem as it exists between the counselor and the client as a partnership devoted to helping resolve the issue.
- *Interviewer/counselor focus:* the counselor's perspective on the story. It focuses on counselors' self-disclosure about their experiences with the problem.
- *Culture/environmental context focus:* the cultural/environmental basis of the problem. It focuses on the dynamics of the problem within clients' cultural and environmental frameworks (Ivey & Ivey, 2003).

Problem and Individual Focus

In the previous chapters, we spent a considerable amount of time describing skills and strategies for helping counselors explore clients' problems and the effects of these problems on their (the clients') lives. The first two focal points (the problem and the individual) are the usual starting points for most clients' stories. By the time the interview reaches the influencing stage, most counselors will have a relatively good sense of these first two focal points because they have been the major focus of the interview and have been explored in sufficient depth. They will be explored again as part of reframing the story once clients have had the chance to explore the remaining focal points. Doris's problem and individual focus are described in her case study summary.

Family Focus

Getting clients to change the focal point to that of other family members in the story helps both clients and counselors hear about the story from a new frame of reference. Exploring how family members view the problem and play a role in it can help influence clients to change for the better.

Example

Counselor: Doris, you mentioned that your older sister and mother also suffer from high blood pressure and have problems with their weight. How does this relate to your problem? (Focus on mom and sister)

Doris: I never really thought about this but I guess it makes me really afraid because it makes it seem like I am kind of destined to have these problems myself.

Counselor: Destined? (Key word)

Doris: You know, like it is predetermined or something. For the longest time I felt that all of the women in our family were fat and had heart problems, and it was my fate to follow them.

Counselor: I sense that maybe you don't feel that way anymore.

Doris: I am confused about it. I've seen my mom and sister being so weak and just kind of giving up to the weight problem, like there is nothing they can do. I mean they don't even *try* to watch their diet or exercise. I haven't given up yet.

Counselor: No, you haven't, and that is why you are here. You are stronger than them and can gain control over this. (Strength statement) Doris, I'd like you to imagine using your sister or mother as a visual image to keep yourself motivated as you continue with your hypertension control.

Doris: What do you mean?

Counselor: I mean to literally keep a picture of either one or both of them in your mind, or even a real one in your wallet, and use it to motivate yourself to stay on your medication, diet, and exercise program. You could combine looking at it or thinking of them and saying something like, "I'm not going to be like mom and Sonya. I am strong and in control." What do you think of that?

Doris: I think that might help. It's worth a try.

Other Individual Focus

Getting clients to change the focal point to that of other key individuals in the story helps both clients and counselors hear about the story from a new frame of reference. Exploring how friends, coworkers, siblings, and other individuals view the problem and play a role in it can help influence clients to change for the better.

Example

Counselor: You spoke of being involved in clubs at school and in your church. Tell me a little more about your friends at school and church.

Doris: Although I know a lot of girls and am pretty active in my church group and sorority on campus, I'd say that my two best friends are Sharese and Lynette.

Counselor: Tell me about them.

Doris: Sharese is my best friend from the neighborhood and high school. She goes to my church, and her family and mine are really tight. Her daddy and mine were best friends. She is a single mom and has a little girl. I'm trying to get her to go back to school and come to my college. She is really smart. Lynette is my best friend from college. We met in our freshman year and just clicked. We joined the sorority together and hang out at school. I am always on my cell phone with that girl.

Counselor: How do you think Sharese and Lynette view your health problems?

Doris: They are like night and day. Lynette is always trying to get me to go to the gym with her and get on the latest diet. She is in terrific shape. She ran track in high school and never fell out of shape. In my freshman year, when I lived on campus, I actually used to run with her. Do you believe that?

Counselor: Absolutely, I think you could do anything you put your mind to. Tell me more about Sharese.

Doris: Now that girl is the anti-Lynette. She is more like me. She has never met a pizza she didn't like. That girl loves her fried chicken. The two of us spend a lot of time watching old movies and our soaps on TV. She could stand to lose about 50 pounds herself.

Counselor: It seems that Lynette and Sharese are like the two sides of your own personality—the disciplined, hard-working side, and the not-so-disciplined, couch-potato side. Does that seem pretty accurate?

Doris: Well yes. I kind of gravitate to them at different times for different things.

Counselor: How do you think that influences your health problems?

Doris: I guess I use Sharese as my example of how hard it is to get and stay in shape and my excuse for not doing it. I look at Lynette as some lovable freak of nature. She has so much discipline.

Counselor: What do you think about using her as an example of someone, who, like yourself, is a hard worker and has a lot of discipline? She is just different in that she has applied some of this work ethic and discipline to staying fit and healthy.

Doris: I guess if I did that, rather than thinking of her as some freak of nature, maybe I could see myself getting slimmer and eating better.

Counselor: Exactly.

Mutuality Focus

This perspective concentrates on the problem as it exists between the counselor and the client as a partnership devoted to helping resolve the issue. It is a very powerful tool, as it focuses directly on the counselor–client relationship and can expose problems in that relationship. By highlighting the mutuality of the responsibility for getting better, it levels the power balance between counselor and client. This leaves counselors open to criticism and blame if the relationship is not a good fit (Ivey & Ivey, 2003).

Example

Counselor: Doris, we've been working together on this problem and I think we are making progress. I'd like you to take a minute and think about your feelings toward me, and toward our relationship. How are these working to help or hinder you in making changes?

Doris: I feel funny talking about this.

Counselor: Funny?

Doris: Yes. On the one hand, I really think you are trying to help and care about me. On the other hand, I wonder if you really have a clue about me.

Counselor: Could you explain that more, please?

Doris: We are so different. I am a 22-year-old single African American woman who lives at home and is really not in control of her life. You are a well-to-do older married white man who can do whatever you want, when you want. You have money, power, and experience—all of the things I don't. Sometimes I wonder if I should even be listening to you.

Counselor: Doris, I understand what you are saying and how you feel. If you think these differences are barriers to you getting better or if you would be more comfortable with a different counselor, I will help you find someone you might work better with.

Doris: I'll have to think about it. Part of me really likes talking to you because you are coming from such a different place from me and

maybe you can be more objective than somebody more similar to me.

Counselor: How can I change to work better with you?

Doris: Maybe just keep asking how our differences affect me and how I feel about what you have to say. Maybe I just need to keep hearing that you are open to discussing our differences.

Counselor: Okay, I'll try to bring this up more often.

Doris: Thanks.

In a sense, even if these kinds of discussions don't help Doris or the counselor achieve their health-related goals, they are valuable in achieving other, more generic outcomes. Exchanges that focus on mutuality help both Doris and the counselor realize that differences in perceptions of power and privilege can affect how clients and counselors perceive helping advice. In other situations in both of their lives, these differences in race, ethnicity, gender, and social class will affect how they receive and transmit information with people outside of the counseling session. Ideally, working through how to deal with them in the safety of the counseling session will generalize to real-world situations that have nothing to do with the health problem.

Helper Focus

In the helper focus, counselors use self-disclosure to empower clients by showing them that they are not alone with their problems. By shifting the focus to themselves, in essence counselors are saying, "I have been there, know what you are going through, and am proof that you can work through this."

Example

Counselor: Doris, I know what you are going through and how hard it is to change your lifestyle given your family background and friends. Both of my parents were overweight, didn't exercise, and had cardiovascular disease. My mom also had diabetes. They were not supportive of my efforts to improve my health at all.

Doris: Really, you look like you have always been in good shape.

Counselor: Not really. I was a chubby kid with pretty bad asthma. I had to work at getting healthy. It took me years to change the way I thought about diet and exercise and to go from being a chubby, out-of-shape adolescent to a reasonably fit young adult. I used my parents as motivation by considering them to be an example of what I did *not* want to become. I felt a little guilty about using them that way, but I had to.

Doris: Wow, it took years.

Counselor: Yes, but like you, I had dreams and didn't want my health to hold me back. You have many of the same characteristics I had as a young adult: You are smart, a hard worker, and very self-sufficient. I'm sure you can do this if you really want to. It won't be easy and will take years to fully change your lifestyle, but I know you can do it.

Cultural/Environmental Context Focus

The cultural/environmental context focus highlights the dynamics of the problem using the clients' cultural and environmental frameworks. Changing the focus to have the client examine this framework will often provide insights into the barriers to change. It will also identify cultural and environmental factors that can foster change, thereby enabling clients to improve their health.

Major cultural factors that influence health behavior include race, ethnicity, religiosity, education, occupation, and income (the latter three are components of socioeconomic status). In addition to these broad cultural parameters, membership in subcultures such as a sorority/fraternity, sports team, or youth group/gang will exert influence (some good, some bad) on health behavior.

The environments in which clients live, work, and play all exert effects on health behavior. Demographic variables ranging from population density, to crime rate, to weather, to location (urban, rural, suburban) influence everything from the availability and accessibility of resources to

diverse perspectives 5.1

Exercise in African American Women

Increasing physical activity among all people is a national focus. Regular physical activity is part of a healthy lifestyle that contributes to weight management, hypertension control, cardiovascular risk reduction, and reduction in risk for type 2 diabetes and certain cancers.

For African American women, 50% of whom are considered obese (Allison, Edlen-Nezin, & Clay-William, 1997) and whose rates of hypertension are the highest among all groups, physical activity is of special concern (USDHHS, 2003). For these women, however, culture greatly affects on their likelihood of adopting a regular exercise regime.

Among the more salient cultural concerns related to regular exercise is the tendency of African American women to have been raised to put their needs last, and the needs of their families and communities first (Banks-Wallace, 2000). Family responsibilities pose a real barrier to the adoption of a regular exercise routine (Walcott-McQuigg & Prohaska, 2001). The intense commitment to helping those around them often leaves these women physically exhausted and with very little spare time. Because setting time aside for themselves is not an accepted behavior (Banks-Wallace, 2000), mainstream exercise recommendations, such as joining a gym or following a set routine, are incompatible with their cultural commitments. Methods for increasing physical activity may need to be individualized, taking into account each woman's family and community responsibilities and enhancing the activity she is engaging in already.

personal safety. These factors can serve as enabling factors for change or barriers to change (Blonna & Levitan, 2005).

Example

Counselor: Doris, tell me a little bit about your culture and how it relates to your health problems.

Doris: What do you mean?

Counselor: Things like your race/ethnicity and religion—you know, things like that.

Doris: Okay. Both my parents are—were—from big African American families. My mom's side, the Johnsons, are from North Carolina. We have a big family reunion down near Raleigh–Durham every July. My mom was one of eight children. Most of her brothers and sisters left the South, but three of them still live in that area. My dad's family, the Bassettes are from Jamaica. I'm not sure how many of them are down there, but I know he had four brothers and one sister at least. We don't stay in contact with them much. My dad was the only one to stay in the United States. His brother stayed with us for a while but moved back—he couldn't take the cold weather in the winter.

Counselor: Sounds like you have a big, wonderful family, Doris.

Doris: Oh yeah, they're fun, especially around the holidays and reunion time. I can't say much about what all this has to do with my health, except to say that the Johnson side of the family really likes to eat. There is so much food at these reunions and holiday get-togethers that it could feed a small city. My uncle gets these fully grown pigs and roasts them whole over a charcoal pit. That is the highlight of the reunion.

Counselor: Sounds like food plays a big role in your family.

Doris: Yeah, my mom always says, "You can never have too much food for company." We definitely don't have much money, but my mom will always put a big spread out. She'll clip coupons and buy things wholesale, like sides of beef. She and my aunts share this big freezer in our garage that they use to store food. We never suffered from a shortage of good food at my house growing up.

Counselor: What about exercise?

Doris: My mom always kids us about raising four kids being exercise enough. My brothers are very athletic. They play football and basketball in high school. My sister and I were never really very athletic. My mom was kind of old school about girls and sports. She didn't really encourage us to do that. She was always hustling us off to church to do community service stuff with the youth group. It was mostly singing in the choir and feeding the hungry. My sister and I still work one or two weekends a month with her in the church's soup kitchen.

Counselor: Sounds like you have a pretty full life that doesn't really involve too much physical activity.

Doris: Between school, my part-time job, and my responsibilities at church I have no time for myself.

Counselor: Doris, it looks like your mom is a big part of your life and you want to please her a lot.

Doris: Yes, I really love her and hate to see her with these health problems, but I don't think she'll ever change.

Counselor: Seems like you almost see yourself getting sucked into a pattern and you are worried about it.

Doris: Yeah, I'm not sure how to change this.

As a result of focusing the narrative, the client in this case study has now examined her problem from several different focal points. This exercise has enabled her to identify some factors that might be contributing to her problem as well as some of the strengths she has and the resources she can bring to bear in making positive changes. The information gained from refocusing is used by counselors to interpret clients' stories and reframe them, offering options for clients to explore.

Eliciting and Reflecting Meaning

Eliciting and reflecting meaning of clients' stories is concerned with helping clients uncover their most deeply held thoughts and feelings about their health problems. Eliciting and reflecting these thoughts and feelings is used to help clients interpret their stories and determine what they mean to them. It is very similar to the next microskill discussed in this chapter, interpretation of meaning and reframing. The major difference is that when reflecting meaning, clients are responsible for assigning meaning to their stories based on how they interpret them. In contrast, in interpretation of meaning and reframing, counselors draw not only from clients' stories but also from their own life experiences and theoretical frameworks to assign meaning to clients' stories and suggest alternative ways (reframing) for clients to view them (Ivey & Ivey, 2003).

Eliciting and reflecting meaning takes clients beyond the **explicit** (the concrete, observable facts of their stories) to the **implicit** (the hidden meanings of their stories). To elicit and reflect on the meaning of their health problems, counselors must help clients rethink their stories (restory) using information gleaned from the affective (attitudes and emotions), cognitive (thoughts, beliefs), and behavioral (actions) domains (Engen & Albert, 1995). **Figure 5.3** illustrates a three-part model of meaning that is useful in interpreting the meaning of clients' stories.

A major problem associated with use of this microskill is the developmental level of the client. Clients who are at the sensorimotor or concrete operational levels of the abstraction ladder (see Chapter 4) will have a difficult time or be unable to integrate the dimensions and reflect on the implicit meaning. Conversely, clients who are on the formal/operational or dialectic/systemic levels will readily be able to reflect on the underlying meanings.

Working with clients to elicit meaning is a lot like asking questions, reflecting feelings, and paraphrasing. The major difference lies in the determination of the meaning of the thoughts, feel-

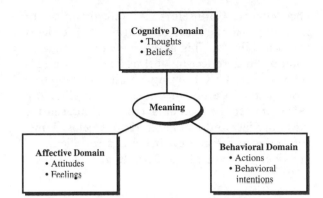

Figure 5.3 The meaning of a client's story is derived from the combined effects of information gained from the affective, cognitive, and behavioral domains.

ings, or behaviors compared to their mere acknowledgment. In a sense, reflecting meaning takes clients to the next level. It goes beyond having them concretely identify their thoughts, feelings, and behaviors and attempts to get them to uncover their deeper meaning (Ivey & Ivey, 2003).

Example: Eliciting and Reflecting Meaning

Counselor: Doris, it seems that you are very excited about the thought of changing your lifestyle but when you actually begin setting up a program of diet and exercise you don't follow through with it. What do you think that means?

Doris: I don't know. Maybe I am not really ready to make these changes yet.

Counselor: In what sense are you not ready?

Doris: I'm just too afraid that I will fail and that will set me back even further.

Counselor: So your way of dealing with this fear of failure is to stay the same?

Doris: Yes.

Interpretation and Reframing

Interpretation of meaning and reframing are separate skills but are used together during the third phase of microskills counseling to influence clients. Counselors use interpretation of meaning to make sense of what health problems mean to clients. This activity is very similar to eliciting and reflecting feelings but it is counselor directed. Reframing entails retelling the story with different meanings. Counselors use reframing to help clients consider alternative ways to view and manage their problems. Thus, reframing presents new meanings for clients to consider (Ivey et al., 1997a; Engen & Albert, 1995).

Interpretation of Meaning

Interpretation of meaning differs from eliciting and reflecting meaning in that it comes from counselors and includes their perspectives on the meaning of clients' stories. Counselors draw from their personal life experiences, their clinical experience, and their theoretical frameworks to develop their own meanings for clients' stories. To interpret the meaning of clients' health problems, counselors use the same model as clients (see Figure 5.3), drawing on information gleaned from the affective (attitudes and emotions), cognitive (thoughts, beliefs), and behavioral (actions) domains. This information, however, is filtered through the counselors' perspective and interpreted on four levels (see **Figure 5.4**): (1) what the story means to the individual client, (2) what similar stories have meant to other clients, (3) what the story means to the counselor, and (4) how the story meshes with the cumulative knowledge about similar problems expressed in professional training and literature. We have already discussed what the story means to the client. Identifying what the story has meant to other clients requires counselors to draw parallels to other clients with whom they have worked. Clients with similar stories and similar backgrounds may benefit from particular types of reframing. Determining what the story means to counselors draws on counselors' own life experiences with the problem. Counselors who have had problems with hypertension, maintaining a healthy body weight, or sticking to an exercise

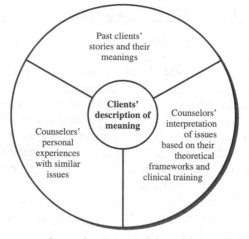

Figure 5.4 Counselors interpret the meaning of clients' stories based on the interaction of their interpretation and the clients' descriptions.

program, for instance, would have special insights into Doris's problem and what it means to her. Lastly, counselors' training and professionalism provide a broad background suggesting how to understand and interpret clients' problems. The various theoretical frameworks may explain clients' problems (and how to solve them) differently, but all generally provide a baseline to serve as a starting point in helping clients. Counselors draw from all four levels of information when interpreting the meaning of clients' stories.

Reframing

Once counselors interpret the meaning of health problems for clients, they can reframe the stories and present different versions for clients to ponder. These new stories offer alternative ways for clients to view their problems. They also provide new options to consider for dealing with their problems. In a sense, reframing takes the "blinders" off clients, allowing them to see their problems in new and different ways. It is critical that counselors use a nonjudgmental tone when using reframing so as not to threaten or alienate clients.

This is best accomplished by using nondirective, open-ended statements.

Example: Reframing
The counselor sets the reframe by putting Doris' story into context using confrontation.

Counselor: Doris, it seems that you are stuck. On the one hand, you want to change and feel that you have the ability to get your diet and exercise in order and control your hypertension. On the other hand, you seem afraid to take this step and seem hemmed in by your family and friends.

The counselor then moves into the reframe.

Counselor: Doris, did you ever think that maybe what is really going on is that you are holding back from making these changes because you know that once you succeed, there is no going back and that scares you?
Doris: I don't know what you mean.
Counselor: I see a strong, intelligent, capable young woman in front of me who is ready to break free from her past and move into the next phase of her life. Right now I think you are in a comfort zone as long as you stay where you are. I think you are ready to move on, take control of your health, and move in new directions. I think this health problem is just a metaphor for your whole life. I think you are afraid that if you really take control of your health, it will affect your entire life and change your relationship with your mother, friends, and living situation. What do you think about this?
Doris: I've never really thought about it this way, but maybe there is some truth to that. Part of me knows that the best way to take control of my lifestyle is to move out on my own and start to create a life that is more conducive to my health. I don't really think I can do this while living at home, and it kind of scares me.

The reframe in this example draws from the counselor's life experiences and clinical work with other clients. He helps Doris take the blinders off and look at her health problem as a metaphor for her entire life. Doris is at a crossroads in her life, and she is beginning to see how this ties uncertainty together with her health problem.

Counselors can go in many different directions with their reframing depending on their life experiences, work with former clients, theoretical framework, and a host of other variables. The purpose of reframing is to open clients up to different ways of viewing their problems. It also represents the next step in helping to narrow down the actual therapeutic plans. In the rest of this chapter, we will see how to tie together all of the skills learned so far to develop therapeutic regimens for clients that fit their needs, meet their goals, and are consistent with how they view their world.

Information, Directives, and Instructions

The final three influencing skills form the heart of health counseling and distinguish it from more generic counseling. Health counselors must teach clients how to manage, cure, or cope with their health problems. They also must teach clients how to prevent recurrences, reinfections, or reinjuries. In many cases, there is little room for interpretation. Medication is given according to established protocols, exercise prescriptions are performed according to exact instructions, and preventive methods are used in specific ways. This lack of leeway is why so much attention must be given to understanding clients' stories and the meaning of their health problems. Counselors can use their understanding of each individual client's health goals to tailor a therapeutic regimen to meet these goals.

Information

Health counselors often make two major mistakes when giving clients information: They give clients too much information and they give them the wrong type of information. In Chapter 2, we discussed adherence theory and some caveats for helping clients adhere to therapeutic regimens. In general, clients need to know the minimum information necessary to follow their therapeutic regimens. Less information is better than too much. What they need to know is information about how to adhere to their specific therapeutic regimen. What they do not need to know is biomedical information about their health problems. Adherence theory has revealed that no relationship exists between knowledge about a health problem and adherence with therapeutic regimens designed to manage that problem (Branon & Feist, 2000; Blonna, Legos, & Burlak, 1989).

Let's use cardiac rehabilitation as an example. Most clients who have suffered from heart attacks and participate in rehabilitation programs to get better are not fascinated by the anatomy and physiology of the heart and circulatory system. Unlike their counselors, they could not care less about how the heart, working in consort with the lungs, creates its own electrical charges to contract and relax cardiac muscle tissue so as to create a rhythmic intake and outflow of blood that exchanges waste products for oxygen and nutrients. What they *care about* (and need to know about) is what they must do to get this miracle organ back in proper working order. What they *really care about* is when they can go back to work, have sex again, and get on with their lives. Therefore, the information that cardiac rehabilitation patients need revolves around their prognosis, treatment, and schedule for returning to a normal life.

We like to use the analogy of a cake with extra frosting left over. The information clients need to know is the cake. Anything beyond it is extra icing on the cake. We don't want clients focusing on the icing before they eat the cake.

This limitation can be very difficult for health counselors to accept. People who are involved in health counseling (health educators, nurses, other healthcare providers, and generic counselors) are very interested in health. We are fascinated by the minutiae of the human body and could talk for hours about the miracles inherent in everything

from conception to immunity. We feel guilty if we don't share our enthusiasm and information with clients. It is as if we are doing them a disservice by not pouring the information on.

In actuality, we are doing them a disservice by giving them too much information. Learning theory shows that people can process only a limited number of instructions during any given educational experience (Branon & Feist, 2000). Health counselors need to ensure that they spend their limited time with clients giving them the information that is most central to their getting better.

Directives

Directives and **instructions** are very similar. Directives are broad, overall strategies or components in therapeutic regimens, whereas instructions are the specific details describing how to implement the directives. Directives are shaped by clients' stories, the meaning of health problems to them, and counselors' interpretations of what might or might not work for individual clients.

Let's use Doris's situation as an example for developing directives and focus on one component of her hypertension management—a regular exercise plan. Doris lives at home, goes to school full-time, works part-time, and is intelligent and motivated to start exercising. Because she is of modest means and has limited income and free time, we would propose different options for her than for someone with more free time and greater financial resources.

Example: Directives

Counselor: Doris, let's talk about some options for you to consider for starting a regular exercise plan. It is most important that you do aerobic exercise that will raise your heart rate and keep it elevated for 20–30 minutes. You need to repeat this every day or at least five days a week. Exercises such as walking or jogging, bicycling, swimming, rowing, and aerobic dancing are common activities people engage in. What do you think of these options?

Doris: I like to dance, but I have no time to go out and go dancing. I really don't have any time to go out anywhere and get any exercise.

Counselor: How do you feel about exercising at home or in your neighborhood?

Doris: I don't have any equipment.

Counselor: I'm not really talking about using equipment. Although a lot of people buy treadmills and exercise bicycles, you could just as easily walk in place or go outside and walk or jog around the block or at a nearby park or school.

Doris: I do live across the street from the high school. It has a quarter-mile track.

Counselor: Do you think this is something that might work for you?

Doris: Yes, at least in nice weather.

Counselor: What about when it is cold, snowy, or rainy outside? What do you see yourself doing then?

Doris: I guess I could walk inside. I also have an old bike that I could ride. I've seen these devices that attach to the wheels of a bike and raise it off the ground. I saw them for less than $20 at a local store.

Counselor: Is riding your bike inside something you think you could stick to?

Doris: I think so.

Counselor: Doris, you'll need to set your bike up somewhere comfortable, and out of the way of the normal household activity or it might get in the way of your family. Where do you see setting up your bike in the house?

Doris: My dad had his workshop area in the basement, which we've cleaned out since he died. It is about 10 feet by 10 feet and has a little old television set. I think that would be an ideal place.

Counselor: Sounds good to me. Let's go over this plan. You'll combine walking and jogging around the track at the school across the street with riding your bike in the basement on bad days and over the winter. Is that right?

Doris: Yes.

Counselor: I'd like you to buy that bike stand and set it up for next week. Can you do that?

Doris: Yes. I have a few bucks put aside as mad money, and this would be a good use of it.

You can see how the counselor used his understanding of Doris's unique situation to offer options for starting an exercise plan that might fit her needs and lifestyle. Once he put these ideas on the table, he and Doris negotiated the details. Notice how all of the attending, listening, and other influencing skills come into play when negotiating Doris's directives. Once the general directives are set up, the counselor can then proceed to the specific instructions.

Instructions

The quality of our instructions can mean the difference between clients getting better and gaining control over their health problems or clients getting worse (not getting cured, getting reinfected, or having a recurrence) and feeling out of control. Instructions are used by counselors in several ways:

- They are used in imagery activities to help clients visualize how things could be under different circumstances.
- They are used to teach relaxation exercises that are often employed to help clients relax while in counseling.
- They are used in role plays to help clients act out new ways of behaving (Ivey & Ivey, 2003).

In health counseling, counselors give instructions regarding taking medication, keeping logs and diaries, performing exercises and rehabilitative procedures, engaging in risk-reduction activities, and a host of other contexts.

Chapter 2 described key adherence strategies proven to be effective in increasing clients' compliance with instructions. Six specific educational strategies shown to be related to improved adherence are tailoring, written reinforcement, repetition, expectation citing, patient quizzes, and self-monitoring (Blonna et al., 1989; Davis, 1966). Let's quickly review them and then use Doris's case study to show how they can be applied to her exercise regimen.

Tailoring involves scheduling components of the therapeutic plan (e.g., medication taking, engaging in physical activity or exercise) at specific times during the day that best fit the patient's lifestyle rather than according to a predetermined schedule (Blackwell, 1978). *Written reinforcement* involves writing down each instruction that is specifically related to a desired patient behavior. It excludes all other general biomedical information about the health problem (Peck, Neville, & King, 1982). *Repetition* involves the planned verbal and written repeating of the specific instructions during the patient's visit (Blackwell, 1979). All instructions should be repeated at least three times during clients' visits. *Expectation citing* involves using the power differential in counselor–client or patient–provider relationships in a positive way by stating instructions as "expectations" (what counselors personally expect clients to do) (DiMatteo, 1994). *Patient quizzes* are verbal requests to repeat specific parts of the treatment plan. They are given both for individual segments of the plan and for the entire plan before the patient is allowed to leave (Blackwell, 1979). *Self-monitoring* involves the use of devices (e.g., medication packaging, logs) that allow patients to keep track of components of their therapeutic plan (Mahoney & Arkhoff, 1979).

Example: Giving Instructions

This example assumes that the counselor has already given Doris instructions on how to take her pulse and calculate her target rate for aerobic training and how to perform a few stretching exercises.

Counselor: Doris, let's put together a specific plan for how to walk or run so as to get the health benefits that you will need to manage your hypertension. I'm going to write this down on this instruction sheet for you (written reinforcement). Before I go over the instructions for how to walk or jog, we need to talk about when you will fit this in. Why don't you tell me a little about your daily schedule.

Doris: On Monday, Wednesday, and Friday, I get up at 6:00 A.M., get dressed, eat breakfast, help my mom clean up, and leave by 8:30 A.M. for school. I am in class all day from 9:30 until 3:15. I eat a quick sandwich in between classes. I drive home and get there about 4:00. I usually watch TV until dinner time, eat, and then do my homework until about 9:00 P.M. I watch more TV and go to sleep at 11:00 P.M. unless it is Friday night. That night I usually go out with friends or on a date.

On Tuesday, Thursday, and Saturday, I work at the mall from 10:00 A.M. to 3:00 P.M. I am home by 3:30. I watch TV until dinner time and then chill out after dinner until it is time to sleep. I go out with friends or on dates on Saturday nights.

On Sunday, I sleep until 8:00, get ready for church, and am there until 1:30 P.M. After that I just relax and see family and friends.

Counselor: Wow, Doris, you have a busy life. It looks like mornings are not too good for you to exercise unless you are willing to wake up early and go run before breakfast. That would mean getting up by 5:00 A.M. Otherwise, it looks like 4:00 P.M. instead of watching TV might be a good time. What do you think?

Doris: I think I could do it instead of watching TV at 4:00 P.M. It might help me unwind from school and work.

Counselor: Okay, how does trying to walk on Monday, Tuesday, Thursday, and Friday and one day on the weekend sound to start off?

Doris: I think I'd rather do it Monday through Friday at 4:00 P.M. and take the weekends off.

Counselor: Okay. Let's shoot for Monday through Friday from 4:00 to 5:00 P.M. (tailoring). If you miss a day, just work out on either Saturday or Sunday. Here, I'll write it down for you (Written reinforcement).

Doris: Okay, thanks.

Counselor: Let's talk about your actual jogging program. The first thing you need to do is warm up for 10 minutes or until you feel a light sheen of sweat on your forehead.

- Start by walking slowly around the track.
- Gradually pick up your pace a little just to get your blood flowing.
- When you feel a light sweat forming on your forehead or elsewhere, you are warm.

The counselor writes each step down and repeats them to Doris as he writes them (repetition and written reinforcement).

The next thing you do is complete the five stretching exercises we learned a little while ago.

- You can do the stretches in any order.
- Stretch to the point where you can feel a gentle pull on your muscles.
- When you feel that comfortable pull, stop and hold the stretch for 30 seconds.
- Do not stretch until you feel pain.
- If you feel pain, back off on your stretch a little.
- Do not lock your arms or legs when you stretch, and don't hold your breath.
- Do not bounce when you stretch.

The counselor writes each step down and repeats them (repetition and written reinforcement).

Counselor: Okay, Doris, I know this is all new to you and I probably made it harder than it needs to be. Before I continue, can you just tell me what you need to do as far as warm-up and stretching are concerned (patient quiz).

Doris: Okay. I'm going to go out to the track and walk around slowly for about 10 minutes or until I feel sweaty. Then I am going to do the stretches we discussed, in any order I want. I will stretch to the point just short of pain and hold the stretches for 30 seconds, being careful not to bounce.

Counselor: Very good. After you are warmed up and stretch, I want you to start jogging. After about five minutes, stop and take your pulse like we practiced.

- If your pulse is below 109 beats (55% of the maximum attainable heart rate [MHR] for a 22-year-old beginning jogger), try to jog a little faster.
- After another five minutes, stop and take your pulse again.
- Keep checking your pulse every five minutes to make sure it stays between 109 and 168 (55%–85% MHR).
- If your heart rate goes above that number, slow down or walk for a few minutes and recheck your heart rate.
- If at any time you feel faint, dizzy, or are in too much pain to keep jogging, slow down and walk.
- Keep this up for 20 minutes.
- After 20 minutes, walk slowly for another five minutes to cool down.
- When you are done cooling down, do your stretches again.

The counselor writes all of this information down and repeats each instruction (repetition and written reinforcement).

Counselor: Doris, I know that is a lot to remember. Why don't you just repeat those instructions to me so I know you understand them (patient quiz).

Doris: After I am all warmed up and stretched out, I start jogging around the track. After five minutes, I take my pulse to make sure it is over the 109 number. If it isn't, I pick up my pace and retake it after another five minutes. I basically keep this up and adjust my pace to make sure I don't go below 109 beats or above 168 beats per minute. When I am done, I cool off for five minutes and stretch again.

Counselor: Good, now how do you cool off (another quiz)?

Doris: I continue to walk slowly around the track.

Counselor: Okay, good. I want you to be sure to do this at least five times between now and when you come back to see me next week. I know you can do this and will talk to you about it next week (expectation citing).

Doris: Okay, I'll try.

Counselor: Oh, and don't forget to keep filling out the daily physical activity log we started two weeks ago. Make sure you write in all of your physical activity, including this new jogging/walking, just like we went over it two weeks ago (self-monitoring).

The counselor worked all of the adherence strategies into the specific set of instructions he wrote up for Doris. He used tailoring to assess Doris's schedule and help her find a good time to work out. He repeated and wrote down all of her instructions. Periodically he used patient quizzes to assess her level of understanding. He used expectation citing to let her know what he expected her to do. Lastly, he used self-monitoring (a log) to help her keep track of her workouts.

Logical Consequences

Logical consequences are the outcomes that occur as a result of following directives and instructions. There are two sets of logical consequences: (1) what counselors expect to happen if clients follow directives and instructions, and (2) what clients expect to occur if they follow directives and instructions. Ideally, counselors and clients will have similar expectations. This congruency is especially important in health counseling. Clients who have unrealistic expectations about the consequences of following their therapeutic regimens are more likely to be noncompliant (Basler, 1995). Counselors need to tell clients what to expect as a result of both following directives and not following them (Elder, Ayala, & Harris, 1999).

For example, if Doris continues to exercise for 30 minutes, five times a week, and everything else in her lifestyle stays constant, she can expect to feel initial fatigue and muscle aches and pains. She probably won't experience any dramatic weight loss. After a couple of weeks, however, she should begin to experience fewer aches and pains as her body adjusts to the exercise. After a month, she should start to feel slightly more energetic due to the effects of aerobic exercise. After three months, she should see noticeable weight loss and increases in endurance and energy levels.

If Doris's counselor informed her of these expected results, warning her about the initial pain and fatigue and encouraging her to stick it out for at least three months so she could experience the beneficial effects of the exercise, she would understand the logical consequences of the directives. If her counselor did not go over this and she had unrealistic expectations of the consequences of starting to exercise, she might be disappointed or upset and stop exercising. For instance, if Doris wasn't prepared for the aches and pains and initial fatigue, she might worry that the exercise is too much. If she expected to see dramatic results after two or three weeks, she also might be disappointed and stop exercising.

Similar mismatches in logical consequences can occur with expectations about the effects of medication or the healing process. For example, many antidepressant medications take several weeks to reach the concentrations within the bloodstream and tissues needed for clients to feel their effects. If clients are not told that they will not feel any different for two to three weeks, they may stop taking the medication after one or two weeks. Another example would be rehabilitation for athletic injuries. Often, it takes several months of physical therapy following surgery to regain enough strength and range of motion to allow clients to engage in any athletic activities. If clients go into rehabilitation expecting to be back on the playing field within six weeks, they might not follow through on the overall directives and specific instructions inherent in their therapeutic regimen. Counselors can assess clients' perception of logical consequences by using open-ended questions.

Example: Logical Consequences

Counselor: Doris, what are your expectations regarding the exercise program we mapped out for you?

Doris: What do you mean?

Counselor: You know, how do you see yourself in a couple of weeks, months, et cetera?

Doris: I guess I see myself losing about 20–30 pounds in a month or so and dropping a couple of dress sizes by then.

Counselor: Actually, Doris, the first couple of weeks are going to be rough. You'll be sore and tired a lot until your body adjusts. After a couple of weeks, that should go away. I'd give it a good three months before you will see any noticeable weight loss and changes in your dress size.

Doris: Really?

Counselor: Yes. You should really start to have more energy in a month or so, however. If you really watch your diet, you might lose weight more rapidly. I'd count on 1–2 pounds a week to be more realistic.

Even though the counselor disappointed Doris with this news, it was better to set things straight initially so she has more realistic expectations regarding the logical consequences of following the plan.

Summary

This chapter covered the influencing skills of confrontation, feedback, self-disclosure, eliciting meaning, interpretation of meaning, and reframing. All of these influencing skills work together when putting together a therapeutic plan for health counseling clients that will culminate with specific information, instructions, and directives.

Confrontation, also known as supportive challenge, is used to help clients identify and understand the discrepancies in their stories and lives. Working with them to minimize discrepant behavior and incongruencies in their lives helps them grow by becoming more genuine.

Feedback involves giving clients objective information about how they come across to others. As with confrontation, when feedback is presented in a caring, supportive fashion, clients can learn how the strengths and weaknesses in their words and actions affect their lives.

Self-disclosure is the sharing of counselors' personal information and experiences. When counselors share information about their own struggles and successes with problems that are similar to those of their clients, they demonstrate that everyone has issues in their lives that need to be worked through. Further, they show that the differences between counselors and clients are not as great as clients often think they are and empower clients in their efforts to get better.

Focusing the narrative is a microskill used to help clients see their stories from a variety of perspectives. Clients can then take a step back and think about their problems from new and different perspectives.

Eliciting and reflecting meaning is used to help clients understand the underlying significance of their problems. Counselors help clients move from the explicit (concrete aspects of their stories) to implicit (underlying meaning) aspects of their health problems. A similar skill, interpretation of meaning, is used by counselors to delve into the underlying meaning of clients' health problems. Counselors use their clinical training, theoretical frameworks, and life experiences to understand the true significance of clients' stories and then feed this information back to clients through the technique of reframing. Reframing involves retelling clients' stories to reflect counselors' interpretations of them. By reframing, counselors give clients different perspectives on their stories. Clients can then rethink their stories in different ways and see potential solutions of which they were previously unaware.

Study Questions

1. Define influencing skills, and explain how they are used to help clients change their personal constructs, behavior, coping skills, and decision making.
2. How can counselors influence clients without directly telling them how they "should" change?
3. How can counselors combine a nondirective approach with influencing?
4. What are the six major focal points used in exploring clients' stories?
5. How does changing focal points work in influencing clients to change?
6. What is confrontation, and when is it appropriate in counseling?
7. What does Ivey mean by calling confrontation a supportive challenge?
8. Give examples of three types of discrepancies that could be confronted.
9. What are appropriate and inappropriate uses of self-disclosure?
10. How does counselor self-disclosure influence client change?
11. How does reflection of meaning differ from paraphrasing?
12. How does understanding the meaning of a health problem for clients relate to helping them?
13. How does reflection of meaning differ from interpretation of meaning?
14. What is reframing?
15. How is reframing used to influence clients?

References

Allison DB, Edlen-Nezin L, Clay-Williams G (1997). Obesity among African American women: prevalence, consequences and developing research. *Women's Health* 3:243–274.

Banks-Wallace J (2000). Staggering under the weight of responsibility: the impact of culture on physical activity among African American women. *Journal of Transcultural Nursing and Health* 6:24–30.

Basler HD (1995). Patient education with reference to the process of behavioral change. *Patient Education and Counseling* 26:91–98.

Blackwell B (1978). Counseling and compliance. *Patient Counseling and Health Education* Fall:21–23.

Blackwell B (1979). The literature of delay in seeking medical care for chronic illness. In Haynes R, Taylor DW, Sacket DL (Eds.). *Compliance in Health Care*, pp. 1–15. Baltimore: Johns Hopkins Press.

Blonna R, Legos P, Burlak P (1989). The effects of an STD educational intervention on patient compliance. *Sexually Transmitted Diseases* 16:198–200.

Blonna R, Levitan J (2005). *Healthy Sexuality*. Pacific Grove, CA: Thomson Learning/Wadsworth.

Branon L, Feist J (2000). *Health Psychology: An Introduction to Behavior and Health*. Pacific Grove, CA: Wadsworth/Thomson Learning.

Davis DM (1966). Variations in patients' compliance with physicians' orders: analysis of congruence between survey responses and results of original investigations. *Journal of Medical Education* 41:1037–1048.

DiMatteo MR (1994). Enhancing patient adherence to medical recommendations. *Journal of the American Medical Association* 217:79–83.

Elder JP, Ayala GX, Harris S (1999). Theories and intervention approaches to health behavior change in primary care. *American Journal of Preventive Medicine* 17:275–284.

Engen H, Albert M (1995). *Microcounseling* (four-part videotape series). Iowa City, IA: University of Iowa.

Ivey AE, Gluckstern NB, Ivey MB (1997a). *Basic Influencing Skills,* 3rd ed. North Amherst, MA: Microtraining Associates.

Ivey AE, Gluckstern NB, Ivey MB (1997b). *Basic Influencing Skills,* 3rd ed. (videotape). North Amherst, MA: Microtraining Associates.

Ivey AE, Ivey MB (2003). *Intentional Interviewing and Counseling: Facilitating Client Development in a Multicultural Society.* Pacific Grove, CA: Brooks Cole.

Mahoney M, Arkoff D (1979). Self-management. In Pomerleau O (Ed.). *Behavioral Medicine Theory and Practice,* pp. 75–99. Baltimore: Williams and Wilkins.

Peck C, Neville J, King A (1982). Increasing patient compliance with prescriptions. *Journal of the American Medical Association* 248:743–757.

Rogers C (1965). *Client-Centered Therapy.* Boston: Houghton Mifflin.

United States Department of Health and Human Services (USDHHS), Office of Disease Prevention and Health Promotion (ODPHP) (2003). *Healthy People 2010: A Systematic Approach to Health Improvement.* www.healthypeople.gov/Document/html/uih/uih_bw/uih_2.htm#obj.

Walcott-McQuigg JA, Prohaska TR (2001). Factors influencing participation of African American elders in exercise behavior. *Public Health Nursing* 18:194–203.

Learning Objectives

By the end of the chapter students will:

1. Compare and contrast Blonna's definition with the four classic definitions of stress

2. Describe the three types of stress arousal

3. Understand how stress arousal is associated with a variety of health problems

4. Compare and contrast stress and challenge

5. Understand the relationship between perception and stress

6. Describe the goals of stress counseling

7. Describe the five R's of coping with stress model

8. Describe the role of introductory skills in assessing clients' perceptions of the role of stress in their lives

9. Explain how body language is related to assessing stress in clients

10. Discuss the importance of language when discussing stress with clients

11. Describe how to use self-disclosure effectively

12. Discuss how changing the focal point can help clients appraise stressors differently

13. Describe the key directives for each of the five R's of coping

Health Counseling for Primary Prevention

Chapters 6 and 7 focus on health counseling for primary prevention. As discussed in Chapter 1, health counseling, like health promotion and health education, can target any of the three levels of prevention: primary, secondary, or tertiary. Health counseling for primary prevention focuses on helping clients who are at risk reduce those risks. For example, this chapter focuses on stress counseling. Clients who seek stress counseling have risk factors for stress. They might think illogically or have trouble managing their use of time, or they might not know how to relax and unwind. These "risk factors" for the stress response are areas that can be modified. Counselors can teach stress clients how to think more logically and rationally, manage their time more efficiently, and build relaxation activities into their lifestyles that help them unwind from their hectic lives. Similarly, most clients coming in for birth control counseling (Chapter 7) are sexually active and not currently using contraception consistently and correctly. This behavior puts them at risk for an unintended pregnancy. Birth control counselors can help them reduce this risk by assisting them in finding birth control methods that are a good fit for their sexual lifestyles and moral/ethical positions.

In both chapters, the starting point is dealing with clients who are well, but at risk. The entire focus of primary prevention counseling is helping clients reduce their risks and remain well.

What Is Stress?

Blonna (2005) defines **stress** as "a holistic transaction between the individual and a stressor resulting in the body's mobilization of a stress response." A **holistic transaction** is an appraisal process involving a potential stressor, the individual, and the environment. A **stressor** is any stimulus appraised by the individual as being threatening or capable of causing harm or loss. The **stress response** is a set of physiological adaptations made by the body to maintain homeostasis in the face of threat, harm, or loss. This definition of stress recognizes the importance of perception in the appraisal of potential stressors. Perception of potential stressors is influenced by the individual's overall level of well-being and incorporates environmental factors into a model of personal stress. This holistic model emphasizes that stress doesn't occur in a vacuum **(Figure 6.1)**.

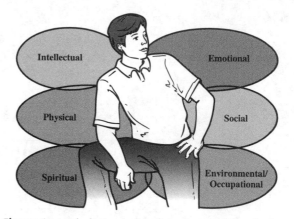

Figure 6.1 A holistic model of stress recognizes the importance of the dimensions of health and wellness in understanding stress.

Blonna's (2005) definition is derived from the four classic ways of viewing stress: (1) as a stimulus, (2) as a response, (3) as a transaction, and (4) as a holistic phenomenon.

Stress as stimulus conceptualizes stress as being an outside force that puts demands on people. This perspective really makes it synonymous with the presence of "stressors" such as work, taxes, and traffic. This way of viewing stress was popularized by Holmes and Rahe (1967), who developed a point system based on life events to quantify the level of stress experienced by people in the previous year. They coined the term "life events" to characterize everyday situations that place demands on people and force them to adapt. Holmes and Rahe then quantified the effects of life events and their relationships to the stress response. Life event scales, while seriously flawed, remain popular today and are used by many stress counselors to help clients quantify their stress levels.

Stress as response defines stress as a physical response going on within people. It is viewed as a migraine, lower back pain, a knot in the stomach, and so on. This way of viewing stress grew out of the pioneering work of Hans Selye (1956), who is generally considered the father of modern stress research. He was the first to document the physiological effects of stress on the body. Selye's research grew out of the work of Walter Cannon (1932), which qualified and quantified the effects of various stressful stimuli on the body.

Selye (1956) created a model, called the general adaptation syndrome (GAS), to qualify and quantify the stress response (see **Figure 6.2**). He believed that the GAS was temporal in nature and consisted of three parts: (1) alarm (initial mobilization of energy for "fight or flight"); (2) resistance (lower level, but more complex and more dangerous response to chronic stressors); and (3) exhaustion (burnout of "weak link" due to chronic stressors). If stressors were not removed or handled effectively, the response would progress from one stage to another.

Selye based GAS on the premise that all stressors throw the body out of balance. Like Cannon, he believed that the human body normally attempts to maintain a balance, or homeostasis. When exposed to noxious stimuli that put demands on it, the body mobilizes energy and attempts to maintain homeostasis through a complex physiological response involving many different body parts and systems. This response changes over time. If the source of stress is not removed, resistance is lowered, and the body can become exhausted and break down. To get back into balance and maintain homeostasis, the body must adapt to the stressor by mobilizing energy. Selye called this energy *adaptation energy,* and he believed all living things have a finite supply of it.

Selye was less concerned about perception and other psychological aspects of stress than its physiological effects on the body. A key component of his conceptualization of stress is the distinction drawn between **eustress** (good stress) and **distress** (bad stress). He believed that stress could be either a positive or a negative phenomenon.

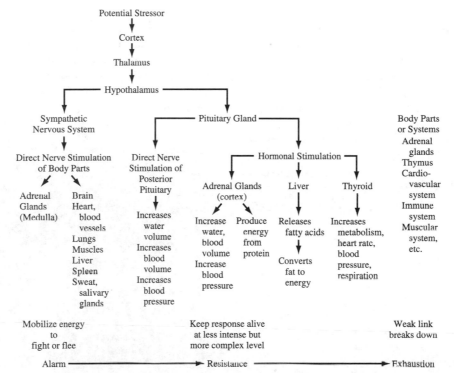

Figure 6.2 During the general adaptation syndrome (GAS), the body mobilizes energy to maintain homeostasis in the face of stressors.

Selye felt that both good and bad stress affect the body in the same way—that is, both use adaptation energy.

Stress as transaction views stress as an exchange between a stimulus, the perception of it, and the response it causes. For example, stress might be the composite of the muscle tension one gets when thinking about giving a speech in front of a class. Lazarus and Folkman (1984) integrated stimulus and response by creating a transactional model of viewing stress. They described various factors involving both the stimulus and the personality of the individual and identified their roles in the assessment of potential stressors as threatening or not (see **Figure 6.3**). Their pioneering work showed that stress was more than just a simple stimulus or response and broke ground for future research into the key aspect of stress, the role of perception. Lazarus (1966) showed that stimuli are neutral (as far as stress is concerned) until they are perceived as stressful. For someone or something to trigger a stress response, it must first be perceived as threatening (meaning one cannot cope with it). Once someone or something is perceived as threatening, the brain triggers the stress response.

Lazarus and Folkman's (1984) way of viewing stress takes issue with the notion of eustress and distress. Their transactional model of stress supports the idea that people and things are stressors only if they are capable of initiating a stress response—that is, only if they are perceived as threatening. In other words, eustress is not stress at all because it is associated with good feelings.

Instead, eustress is a totally different phenomenon called **challenge** by Lazarus and Folkman (1984). When we are challenged, the body mobilizes energy similarly to the way it does during the beginning of the stress response (see **Figure 6.4**). However, this energy is accompanied by positive thoughts and emotions and a feeling of being in control (not threatened). This positive, short-term phenomenon dissipates after whatever sparked the challenge is removed. An example is the "psyching" that goes on with athletes prior to a competition. They mobilize energy and get energized in a positive way because of being challenged by their competition, but they are not stressed (Lazarus, 1999).

The final way of defining stress, as a holistic phenomenon, views it as part of a larger whole. That is, stress is a part of an individual's physical, social, spiritual, emotional, and intellectual well-being. It is "being a student" or "feeling helpless in trying to control one's life." This perspective grew out of the wellness movement and takes into account lifestyles and circumstances beyond single events that may trigger stress responses. The stress response, according to adherents of holistic health, is viewed as a process mediated by a person's level of functioning across the physical, emotional, intellectual, spiritual, social, environ-

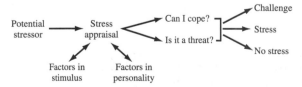

Figure 6.3 The stress transaction is based on appraising whether a potential stressor is a threat and if one can cope with it.

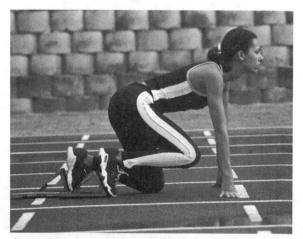

Figure 6.4 Being challenged summons the energy and focus in a way that is similar to being alarmed. (© Photos.com)

mental, and occupational dimensions of health. People who are more whole—that is, functioning at high levels in each dimension—are better able to minimize their stressors and effectively cope with the stress in their lives.

This chapter will adhere to Blonna's (2005) conceptualization of stress, which is based on the four classic definitions and recognizes the importance of perception in the stress response.

Personality and Stress

Albert Ellis (1997, 1991a, 1991b), the founder of a type of psychotherapy called rational emotive behavior therapy (REBT), identified a core group of **illogical beliefs** that are common in stressful personalities and form the basis for his theory on stress and neurotic behavior. Ellis's theory proposes that people and things don't make clients feel bad and behave neurotically. Rather, their negative thoughts and illogical beliefs about these people and things are the basis of clients' stress and neuroses. Ellis, like Lazarus and Folkman, believes that perception of situations determines whether these situations become stressors.

In their clinical work with patients, Ellis and Harper (1998) found that clients' illogical beliefs about life form the basis of an irrational belief system. Such a belief system creates a distorted perspective for appraising potentially stressful situations. Walen, DiGuiseppi, and Wessler (1980)—colleagues of Ellis—identified four categories of illogical/irrational beliefs:

1. *Awfulizing statements*. These statements "awfulize," or exaggerate the negative effects of, a situation, especially ones that don't warrant such treatment. Clients who tend to react to potentially stressful situations in this way could be referred to as "awfulizers" or "catastrophizers." The least little stressor is a catastrophy for them.
2. *Should, must, ought statements*. These advice-giving statements are based on a one-dimensional view of situations. People who are advice givers think that their way of

viewing the world is the correct and only way. They are referred to as "musterbators" because everyone must see things their way.
3. *Evaluation of worth statements*. These statements imply that some people or things are worthless or a complete waste of time. People who make such judgments could be called "evaluators."
4. *Unrealistic need statements*. These statements set unrealistic, unattainable requirements for happiness. People who view the world in this way are "needy" people. They are constantly finding fault with everything and are never happy because nothing is ever good enough for them.

Millon (1996) proposes a biosocial learning theory model of stress and personality. According to his theory, humans develop, as a result of an interaction of genetic/biological factors and learned experiences, a "personologic style" that can predispose them to stress. Each individual has idiosyncratic vulnerabilities that contribute to development of a stress-prone personality style. Millon identified eight specific stress-prone personality styles: aggressive, narcissistic, histrionic, dependent, passive-aggressive, compulsive, avoidant, and schizoid. Everly and Lating (2002) provide an excellent overview of these styles and summary of how they contribute to increased vulnerability to stress.

People who are exceptionally aggressive are more stressed because they mistrust others and are always on the defensive. They fear loss of control and use anger, intimidation, and dominance to try to retain control at all costs. This creates heightened susceptibility to stress (Millon, 1996; Everly & Lating, 2002).

Narcissistic people are preoccupied with themselves and being perceived by others as unique and special. They are self-absorbed to the point of being incapable of seeing any other point of view but their own, and they lack empathy for others. Their stress comes from their fear of not being viewed as special, their inability to postpone gratification, and their inability to communicate with others (Millon, 1996; Everly & Lating, 2002).

Histrionic personalities crave affection, support, constant stimulation, and interpersonal approval. These needs are accompanied by an exaggerated outpouring of affect and flair for the dramatic. The histrionic personality is more stress-prone because of excessive fear of rejection, fear of loss of approval and affection, and the constant need for stimulation and change (Millon, 1996; Everly & Lating, 2002).

Dependent personalities require unusually high levels of support from others. To gain this support, they will be passive and submissive. Their increased susceptibility comes from their inability to view themselves as competent and their fear of loss of support or outright rejection (Millon, 1996; Everly & Lating, 2002).

Passive-aggressive personalities are ambivalent, chronically negative, and pessimistic. They desire independence but lack the skills to achieve it. This conflict causes dependency and a resultant passivity. Their proneness to stress comes from their struggle between the aggressive pursuit of independence and the passive dependence on others for approval (Millon, 1996; Everly & Lating, 2002).

Compulsive personalities are rigid, inflexible, and driven by the need to behave in proscribed, socially approved ways. They also need to maintain rigid self-control. Their increased susceptibility to stress comes from their lack of flexibility and their inability to deal with ambiguity and abstraction (Millon, 1996; Everly & Lating, 2002).

Avoidant personalities desire social support and affiliation but fear rejection so much that social avoidance becomes their way of life. They are highly sensitive to interpersonal situations and relationships. Their vulnerability to stress comes from the combination of their lack of social support and their fear of interpersonal rejection (Millon, 1996; Everly & Lating, 2002).

Schizoid personalities are placid and bland, and lack virtually all desire for interpersonal contact. They might be viewed as the polar opposites of histrionic personalities. Schizoid personalities are more prone to stress because of their hyper-sensitivity to social stimuli and fear of interpersonal intrusion. They also lack social supports (Millon, 1996; Everly & Lating, 2002).

Psychosomatic Disease and Stress

Philip Deutsch (1959) is credited with inventing the term **psychosomatic** to explain the interaction between the mind and the body in the disease process. Diseases associated with stress have often been trivialized as being psychosomatic or "all in one's head." **Psychogenic** disease and **somatogenic** disease are two categories of psychosomatic disease.

Psychogenic disease refers to psychosomatic illnesses that lack a causative organism, or germ. These diseases, such as chronic backache, migraine headaches, peptic ulcers, and colitis, are conditions that arise when the structure and function of body parts and tissues are altered by a chronic stress response.

Chronic stress is a risk factor that contributes to the development of some psychogenic diseases. Cardiovascular disease presents an interesting example. The degenerative process of atherosclerosis is worsened by the physiological changes in the body caused by the ongoing stress response. No causative germ is involved, however.

With somatogenic disease, a causative organism does exist. The long-term effects of the stress response weaken the body's defenses, rendering a person more susceptible to infection and the development of disease. For example, college students may be susceptible to mononucleosis, for instance, due in part to the effects of chronic college stressors on their immune systems. The link between somatogenic disease and stress is less direct and more difficult to prove, however, because many other factors—ranging from a person's behavior to the **virulence** of the invading organism—must be taken into consideration.

Everly and Benson's Disorders of Arousal

Everly and Benson's (1989) disorders of arousal model provides the most comprehensive analysis of the mechanisms by which the stress response manifests itself in disease (see **Figure 6.5**). The model starts with a potential stressor, which can be cognitive, affective, environmental, or personality type (i.e., personologic predisposition). The leap from potential stressor to stress arousal, however, is mediated by the **limbic system**. Everly and Benson (1989) found that people with stress-related diseases were highly susceptible to limbic system arousal. They called this relationship the **limbic hypersensitivity phenomenon (LHP)**. LHP, it is believed, develops as a result of either acutely traumatic or repeated extraordinary limbic system excitation due to stress. Once limbic arousal occurs, it triggers the stress response described by Selye (1956). If the stress response is evoked too often or sustained for too long, it produces overstimulation that leads to wear and tear and eventual breakdown of target organs and systems. This breakdown can be the result of biochemi-cally induced trauma or toxicity or actual overwork. The ensuing "disorders of arousal" include all of the classic stress-related physical disorders as well as most anxiety and adjustment disorders and some forms of depression (Everly & Lating, 2002).

The Effects of Stress on Disease

The effects of acute, or alarm-phase, stress responses are usually not harmful. The rapid mobilization of energy created to assist people in confronting threats to their well-being originated as a positive, life-saving adaptive mechanism. Although the effects are intense, they are short-lived and begin to reverse once the source of stress is removed or handled effectively. The result of this type of stress response on the body is fatigue. With a lifestyle that is balanced and includes proper nutrition, exercise, and adequate rest, the body can rejuvenate itself and not suffer any harm from acute stress. The greater the frequency of events that provoke alarm reactions, the greater the need for rest to help the body regenerate the energy that was used up in coping with the stressor. The effects of a moderate amount of short-term stress on psychogenic and somatogenic disease are negligible.

Unfortunately, we are often stressed by situations and people that we cannot fight or run away from—stressors that will persist for some time. When we do not act and use the energy that has been mobilized to either eliminate or cope with the source of stress, our bodies cannot remain in this state of activation for long periods. Our bodies subsequently shift into a lower-level, resistance-phase response, and we begin to suffer the effects of dealing with a long-term, chronic stressor (see **Table 6.1**).

The effects of chronic low-level stress on disease are most clear with psychogenic diseases. Over time, the stress response leads to generalized wear and tear on the body. When body parts and systems are forced to work overtime for long periods without rest and rejuvenation, they begin to malfunction and eventually break down. The re-

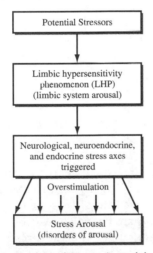

Figure 6.5 In Everly and Benson's model, a potential stressor arouses the limbic system and triggers a stress response along the neurological, neuroendocrine, and endocrine stress axes. If the stress response is evoked too often or sustained for too long, it will result in overstimulation, leading to breakdown of target organs and systems and "disorders of arousal." (*Source:* Blonna R (2005). *Coping with Stress in a Changing World,* 3rd ed. New York: McGraw-Hill. Reproduced with permission of The McGraw-Hill Companies.)

The Acute and Chronic Effects of Stress

Short-Term (Mobilizes Energy)	Long-Term (Wears Body and Mind Down)	
	Physiological	**Psychological**
Increased:	Cardiovascular system	Post-traumatic stress
Blood sugar	(atherosclerosis, high	disorder (PTSD)
Fats/cholesterol	blood pressure, heart	
Hormones (adrenaline)	attack, stroke)	Anxiety disorders
Blood pressure		(panic attack, mania,
Heart rate	Muscular system	generalized anxiety
Breathing rate	(increased tension,	disorder, insomnia)
Muscle tension	tension headaches,	
	TMJ, backaches, low	Depressive disorders
	back pain)	(dysthymic disorder,
		major depression)
	Immune system	
	(greater susceptibility to	
	illness, reduced ability to	
	fight infection and disease,	
	allergies)	
	Digestive system	
	(esophageal reflux, ulcerative	
	colitis, irritable bowel	
	syndrome, peptic ulcers)	

Source: Everly & Lating, 2002.

lationship between stress and psychogenic disease is most direct with five body systems: the endocrine, muscular, digestive, cardiovascular, and immune systems. Excess strain on these systems results in inefficiency and a gradual breakdown in their performance, followed by increased susceptibility to a host of illnesses (Everly & Lating, 2002).

The Goals of Stress Management Counseling

Everly and Lating (2002) use their disorders of arousal model to identify three key elements of arousal that characterize the stress response and are precursors to the development of stress-related

diseases: (1) increased neurotransmitter arousal and activity, (2) increased neuromuscular arousal, and (3) increased negative cognitive arousal. All three elements are linked and work together in initiating and sustaining the stress response. A comprehensive model for coping with stress should incorporate strategies designed to break this chain, stop the stress response, and initiate a relaxation response.

Blonna's five R's of coping is such a model (see **Figure 6.6**). The five R's—Rethink, Reduce, Relax, Release, and Reorganize—represent a multilevel, wellness-based approach to stress management. The stress management strategies incorporated into this model are designed to combat one or

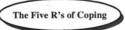

The Five R's of Coping

Rethink: Change the way you think about potential stressors

Reduce: Cut back on the overall number of stressors

Relax: Put your body into a relaxed state

Release: Purge the by-products of stress through physical activity

Reorganize: Increase your overall level of health (physical, social, spiritual, mental, emotional, occupational/environmental)

Figure 6.6 Coping strategies from the five R's can be used individually or collectively to build a personal stress management plan.

more of the three levels of arousal identified by Everly and Lating (2002). The five levels of coping and the strategies contained within each level work both independently and collaboratively to reduce arousal and the stress associated with it. A synergistic effect occurs when all of the levels of coping are working together simultaneously.

Rethink strategies work by minimizing cognitive (and subsequent neurotransmitter and neuromuscular) arousal and by decreasing repetitive negative self-talk. The strategies help clients examine their thoughts and illogical beliefs about life and potential stressors and replace the illogical, irrational beliefs with more logical, rational ones. In this way, people can defuse potential stressors by changing the way they view them.

Most rethink strategies are drawn from cognitive-behavioral therapy techniques.

Reduce strategies minimize all three levels of arousal by focusing on reducing the overall volume of stressors in clients' lives. When clients are involved in too many activities and demands (pleasurable as well as unenjoyable), they reach a point of physical, intellectual, and emotional overload, and feel that they can no longer cope with these demands. These demands then become stressors (see **Figure 6.7**). One of the overall goals of stress counseling is to help clients find an optimal level of demand in their lives. Reduce strategies diminish arousal by reducing the number of stressors. Assertiveness training and time management are two common types of reduce strategies.

Relax strategies work by inducing a relaxation response. Relaxation is incompatible with stress and decreases neurotransmitter, neuromuscular, and cognitive arousal. Many types of relaxation techniques exist, ranging from diaphragmatic breathing to biofeedback. They work in a variety of ways to reduce arousal.

Release strategies provide a positive, vigorous, physical outlet for the energy produced by the stress response created to maintain homeostasis in the face of threat. These strategies help reduce all three levels of arousal by inducing a relaxing state of fatigue associated with physical activity. The fatigued, relaxed state that follows the activ-

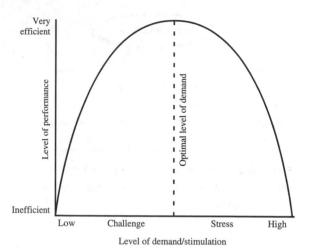

Figure 6.7 Our level of performance is related to our level of demand. As our level of demand/stimulation increases, we are challenged and our performance increases. When we reach our optimal level of demand, we reach peak performance. If we exceed our optimal level of stimulation, the same demands that challenged us become stressors. (*Source:* Blonna R (2005). *Coping with Stress in a Changing World,* 3rd ed. New York: McGraw-Hill. Reproduced with permission of The McGraw-Hill Companies.)

ity is incompatible with the stress response. Two popular release strategies are kickboxing and karate, both of which employ vigorous kicks and punches that release stress tension.

Reorganize strategies work by integrating healthy behaviors into daily living so as to provide a more stress-resistant lifestyle. Daily practice of these techniques creates a hardier, more stress-resistant lifestyle by increasing clients' levels of wellness across all six dimensions (physical, social, spiritual, emotional, intellectual, occupational and environmental). Such a lifestyle is designed to reduce the frequency and intensity of clients' stress arousal.

The five R's of coping model provides a variety of strategies and levels of coping that can work independently or together. A key to effective stress management is realizing that different techniques and stressors are influenced by space and time. What worked for clients in coping with spe-

cific stressors under past circumstances may not be effective the next time they confront similar stressors under different circumstances. Having a stress management plan that incorporates several kinds of strategies and levels of coping will enable clients to meet the challenge of coping with stress in an ever-changing world. For a comprehensive discussion of the various stress management techniques utilized under each of the five R's, consult Blonna (2005).

Counseling Someone with Stress Using Microskills

As a stress counselor, you have three primary goals for your clients: (1) assessment of personal stressors, (2) finding the client's optimal level of stimulation, and (3) development of a personal stress management plan based on the five R's model (Blonna, 2005). In addition to these primary goals, counselors must assess clients' goals regarding their stress. The best way to do so is to describe your goals and assess clients' needs.

Case Study 6.1
John

John is 27 years old, is married, and identifies as Italian American.

John was a returning student in one of Dr. Blonna's Stress Management evening classes. This very mature student was a member of the National Guard who had served in post–World Trade Center bombing security activities. John had been married for six years and was the proud father of a newborn son, Ricky. He worked in the telecommunications industry installing high-end telephone and data systems for medium-size and large corporations. He had a very secure job with a good salary, benefits, and seniority. After Ricky was born, John and his wife Kathy bought a modest house in a northeastern New Jersey suburb. John's work often took him into New York City.

John took the class because he was suffering from tension headaches and low back pain and frequently had trouble sleeping because of excessive worrying over financial concerns. Even though things in John's life were moving according to his plans, he still felt stressed by the pressures of fatherhood, home ownership, and everyday concerns in the modern world such as taxes, war, and terrorism.

Introductory Skills

As discussed in Chapter 3, a good introduction is essential to establishing trust and building the foundation necessary to help clients manage their stress. Many issues in clients' lives contribute to their stress, and a solid introduction sets the stage for exploring these issues.

Identify Yourself and Explain Your Role

Try writing a script for this part of the introduction and practice it until it becomes second nature to you. When introducing yourself, it is very important to make a concerted effort to establish a skin-to-skin human connection with the client. A firm handshake is a good way to do so. Extend your hand, make eye contact, and smile as you give the client a firm (but not crushing) handshake.

Example

Counselor: (Extending hand, smiling) Hi, I'm . . . . I'm one of the counselors here. My job is to help you understand what stress is all about and to work with you in developing a personal stress management plan based on your needs and lifestyle. Many different things and situations are capable of causing stress, ranging from sexual problems to the economy. I'd like you to feel free to discuss these and any other issues you believe are related to the stress in your life. I'm going to have to ask you to discuss some very personal issues so that I can better understand your stress. I am not here to judge you. My job is

to help you make the best decisions for yourself about how to manage your stress. Together we will work out a plan for helping you manage your stress. I want you to understand that everything we say is confidential and that your name and anything we talk about cannot be shared with anyone else.

Clarify Client's Name

A simple way to verify the client's name is to use an open-ended statement following your introduction. Do this while you are still standing and immediately following your handshake and self-identification.

Example

Counselor: (Before sitting and explaining his role) And your name is . . . ?

John: My name is John.

Counselor: Nice to meet you, John.

Explain the Client's Role

After exchanging names and describing your role, explain the client's role. A simple explanation should include the three key elements of the client's role discussed in Chapter 3: (1) active participation, (2) self-responsibility, and (3) honesty.

Example

Counselor: John, your role in this process is to be as open and honest as possible when talking to me. The only way I can help you is if you tell me exactly what is going on with your stress. You'll have to take an active role in this process and take responsibility for getting better. Together, we can work out a stress management plan that will work best for you in managing your life and your stress.

Set Goals for the Session(s)

As mentioned earlier in this chapter, the three primary goals of stress counseling are (1) assessment of personal stressors, (2) finding one's optimal level of stimulation and demand, and (3) development of a personal stress management plan based on the five R's of coping model (Blonna, 2005). In addition to these primary goals, counselors must assess clients' goals regarding their stress. The best way to do so is to describe your goals and assess clients' needs.

Example

Counselor: John, my work with you will revolve around three goals: (1) helping you assess the stress in your life, (2) helping you find an optimal level of stimulation and demand in your life, and (3) working with you to develop a personal stress management plan. These are the things I must discuss with you. What other goals do you have for our time together?

It is important for counselors to give clients adequate time to think this question through before moving into the next part of the session.

Transition to the Client's Story

A good way to make the transition from the introduction to getting clients to tell their stories is to use open-ended statements regarding what happened. The goal in making these open-ended statements is to get clients talking about their current stress and how it manifests itself in their lifestyles and relationships.

Example

Counselor: John, why don't you tell me what led to you being here today.

Counselor: John, tell me a little bit about what you know about stress.

Counselor: John, tell me a little bit about your stress for the past month.

Counselor: John, tell me what are the three greatest sources of stress in your life.

John: I came in because of something you said in class the other night about how the symptoms of the stress response are warnings about what is going on in people's bodies. You know, that things like low back pain, tension headaches, and other types of muscle tension could mean that the person is in the resistance phase of the stress response.

Counselor: Um, hum.

John: Well, I have all three of those symptoms and am worried about it. I want to get con-

trol of my stress before it leads to other symptoms or a real problem.

Attending Skills

One of the most interesting things about stress management counseling is the diversity in how people define stress and stressors. Counselors must be very careful to not get caught in the "universal stressors" trap. Most people (counselors as

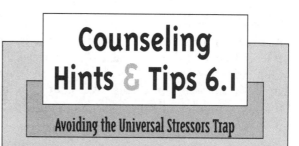

Counseling Hints & Tips 6.1

Avoiding the Universal Stressors Trap

Counselors must be vigilant in taking a neutral stance toward the notion of "universal stressors," such as death and divorce. These and other life events are always viewed initially as "potential stressors." Here are some tips to help counselors avoid this trap:

1. Remind yourself that there is no such thing as a universal stressor.
2. Relabel all previously described universal stressors as "potential stressors."
3. Remember that potential stressors become stressors only when clients perceive them to be something they cannot handle.
4. Do not assume that the counselor's personal stressors are stressful for all clients.
5. Keep an open mind regarding the range of possible ways clients will perceive potential stressors.
6. Do not prejudge potential stressors; let clients describe their significance.

Listening to clients' stories without prejudging how they perceive potential stressors will give you insights into the nature of their stress in general as well as their tendency to perceive things either logically and rationally or illogically and irrationally. The way clients think about potential stressors is a major factor in becoming able to manage their stress.

well as clients) believe in the "stress as stimulus" way of defining stress. They assume that certain people/events/situations are inherently stressful for all people under all circumstances. These "stressors"—for example, death, taxes, divorce, or loss of a job—are just assumed to be stressful for everyone, all of the time. The authors of this textbook do not believe this to be true. For example, even events such as death and divorce are not always perceived as stressors. The death of someone who has suffered for months or years might be perceived by a loved one as a blessing, not a stressor. Divorcing someone who has been abusive or hurtful can be perceived as liberating, not necessarily stressful. In both cases, clients do not feel that they cannot cope with the event. Rather, the event liberates them from a sense of hopelessness and inability to cope.

Nonverbal Attending Skills

The way clients appraise potentially stressful situations and events will often differ markedly from the way counselors perceive them. It is important to remember that clients create much of their own stress because of their illogical/irrational way of viewing the world. Counselors must remain neutral in their nonverbal behavior and body language when listening to clients describe their stress for this reason.

Often, when confronted by clients' illogical thinking, counselors want to intervene and help clients think more clearly about their potential stressors. It is important for counselors to avoid becoming impatient at this point in the interview and to allow clients to freely discuss their lives and stress before helping them.

Verbal Following

A key aspect of verbally following stress-related stories is paying particular attention to logical versus illogical thinking. This endeavor is crucial in helping clients later in counseling. Illogical thinking plays a major role in determining whether potential stressors become actual stressors. Because all stimuli are merely "potential stressors" until clients decide that they can't cope

with them, the way clients view these stimuli (logically or illogically) is the determining (and most important) factor in the creation of stress in their lives. Clients will give counselors clues about their ability to think logically or illogically by using "red flag" words and phrases. As mentioned previously in this chapter, these words and phrases serve as clues to categories of illogical thinking.

A big part of helping clients manage their stress is assisting them in avoiding illogical thinking and the use of broad generalizations and **global words**. During verbal following, it is important to listen for global words such as "total," "complete," "should," "must," and "ought," as well as phrases such as "what a complete waste of . . ." and "what a totally useless . . . ." These words and phrases are evidence of illogical thinking and need to be followed up on later in the interview.

Example

John: (Continuing with his story) I am very busy lately. Between work, the new house, the new baby, and school, it seems that I have *absolutely no* free time anymore. I get so aggravated with anything that wastes my time. To tell you the truth, lately it seems that school is a *total* waste of my time. I haven't learned *anything* there in the two years I've been trying to finish my four-year degree. It's not like my two-year degree. That was fun because most of the coursework was related to my job in telecommunications. The liberal arts and general education courses I have to take now are a *complete* waste of time. I'm running up to school after work or after playing with my son and wasting my time and money on some stupid philosophy class. I don't get *any* satisfaction from this at all.

The temptation for John's counselor is to get sucked into agreeing with John about the uselessness of his schoolwork, which doesn't seem to be meeting his needs. In actuality, John just gave several clues about his own illogical thinking about school. While John may be bored by school and hemmed in by other responsibilities, the logical reality is that he has learned *something* at school and it hasn't been a *total* waste of his time. His time may have been better spent elsewhere, but it hasn't been a *total* loss. John fails to realize that all educational experiences and required courses compromise individual wants and needs to some extent as part of a plan to meet degree requirements. Therefore, these courses haven't been a *complete* waste of his time. Such subtle nuances in illogical thinking are picked up only if counselors pay close attention to the nature of their clients' thinking as well as their actual stories.

Vocal Tone

Try to match the pace and tone of clients' stories. Stress counseling clients experience a range of emotions regarding their situations and express them in the way they tell their stories. Some will be very animated, almost manic in their descriptions of stress and stressors. Their stories will burst forth in a stream of consciousness accompanied by many emotional highs and lows. Other clients will appear overwhelmed by the magnitude of stress in their lives. They will be quiet and appear overburdened by the task of putting their stress into words. Often these clients will need more time to formulate their thoughts and organize their stories in their own heads before sharing their tales with counselors. Don't respond to clients' stories with your own tone and pace. Let their emotions and style dictate yours.

Responding Skills

Nonverbal Minimal Encouragers

Use nonverbal encouragers liberally to keep clients talking. Remember, stress appraisal is highly personalized and clients must be given the maximum opportunity to describe the situations and people that are the basis for the stress in their lives. The less talking counselors do initially, the better. Use encouraging body language to keep clients talking. Be sure that your body language and nonverbal

feedback come across as nonjudgmental. Discomfort about being judged is a major barrier with working with stress patients. In many cases, they will feel guilty about being stressed by interpersonal issues and thoughts and feelings directed toward others and are on the lookout for any signs of disapproval from counselors. Try to maintain a relaxed posture, and periodically scan your own body for signs of any tension that might be transmitted to clients. Chapter 3 described open and closed body language. Try especially hard to avoid judgmental poses such as folding your arms over your chest or looking "down" at clients.

Verbal Minimal Encouragers

Simple acknowledgments such as "uh huh," key words, and mirroring are very important tools that can be used to encourage clients to continue their stories. They are especially helpful in getting clients to explain how they appraise potential stressors. We will continue with John's story to illustrate this point.

Example

John: Anyway, I'm just annoyed at wasting my time and money on things that don't seem to be worth it.

Counselor: Um, huh. (Simple acknowledgment)

John: You know, especially with the new baby, I want to spend more time home with him, not taking some stupid philosophy class.

Counselor: Stupid? (Key word)

John: Maybe "stupid" isn't the best word to use. It just doesn't seem that important to me now. I guess I have so little free time to spend with my family and since I am working so much overtime now I really don't want to be in school right now.

Counselor: Really don't want to be in school? (Mirroring)

John: Finishing my four-year degree just doesn't seem to be as important as it was last year. I really was motivated last year, because I realized I needed it to move up in my job. Lately, however, I am even questioning that. Sometimes I like being where I am. I can work all the overtime I want to make extra money and not have the hassles of management.

Counselor: Hassles? (Key word)

John: You know, playing the game, dealing with all the company bullshit. It's like I'd have to turn my back on all of the things I see that are wrong with the job. Right now, I can see all the day-to-day issues that can be improved. If I get into management, I really can't speak out against them like I do now.

Open Invitation to Talk
Careful use of questioning to clarify how clients perceive potentially stressful situations is very important because of the diversity in the ways people appraise stressors. Because the stress appraisal process is very complicated, clients' stories are often quite confusing. A skillful, nonjudgmental use of questions will help counselors clarify how clients view their world and their stress.

Open-Ended Statements and Questions
Using open-ended statements liberally can create a more relaxed, conversational tone. Making a couple of open-ended statements and then sitting back and listening to clients' stories is much less threatening than asking clients a string of closed questions. Use closed questions to tease out information not covered by clients' answers to open-ended queries.

Example
Instead of asking multiple questions like

- "John, is working so much overtime a source of stress for you?"
- "John, do you work a lot of overtime hours?"
- "John, is playing games the only thing you dislike about management?"
- "John, are your working conditions stressful?"

ask

- "John, how does working so much overtime factor into your stress?"

- "John, what is your work schedule like?"
- "John, tell me a little more about what you dislike about management."
- "John, tell me what about the working conditions in your job that you find stressful."

Instead of asking

- "John, do you dislike your philosophy class?"
- "John, do you dislike your philosophy professor?"

ask

- "John, could you tell me a little more about this philosophy class?"
- "John, what about your philosophy class is stressful?"
- "John, tell me about your philosophy professor."

You'll notice that many of the open-ended statements seem to make assumptions that certain issues related to work, management, his class, and his professor are related to John's stress. Don't worry about these assumptions. Clients will let counselors know if such assumptions are valid or off base. Counselors can always use additional open-ended statements or closed questions to go back and clarify information.

Example: Overtime
John: I really don't find overtime stressful at all. I look at it as a great opportunity to make extra money to do things around the house and fix up the baby's room. I also enjoy the work I am doing on some high-end communications projects that are really interesting and state-of-the-art.

Example: Management
John: I guess I just feel that there are certain things about management in my company that are dishonest. All of our managers came from the field, so they know how the working conditions are. As soon as they get into management, it seems that they forget the very concerns that they spoke out against six

months ago. I think I'd have a hard time do-ing that.

Example: Philosophy Class

John: It really isn't anything going on in class. The professor is pretty interesting, and the subjects we discuss are really very interesting. I guess it just doesn't seem that important given the fact that I have a new son and house and I'd rather be there.

Paraphrasing

As described in Chapter 4, effective paraphrases have three elements: (1) a short restatement of the client's story in your own words, (2) use of a key word or phrase, and (3) a checkout phrase. It is important to use paraphrasing extensively with stress clients, because their appraisals of events are the determining factors in their stress. Counselors must not assume that their interpretation of stress is the same as that of their clients. It is important to use paraphrasing to clarify clients' stress appraisals.

Example: Overtime

Counselor: John, it seems that you have mixed feelings about overtime. You really enjoy the work, and the money is good, but it seems to cut into the time you want to spend at home and the time you need to spend at school. Is that right?

John: Yeah, that about sums it up.

Example: Management

Counselor: John, it seems that you don't find moving into a management job as appealing as you did last year because of the games you'll be forced to play. Is that accurate?

John: Yeah, I'm not sure if I am ready to do that anymore.

Example: Philosophy Class

Counselor: John, it seems that while your philosophy class and professor are interesting, it doesn't seem like it is the right time to be in school. Is that correct?

John: I'm not sure. I guess that is part of my feeling stressed about it.

Reflection of Feelings

Accurate reflection of feelings and emotions is crucial when counseling clients about stress because of the strong link between key emotions and stress. Lazarus (1999) believes that appraising potential stressors as being actually stressful is directly linked to specific "stress emotions." When key emotions are associated with potential stressors, they are much more likely to be appraised as stressors. Lazarus (1999) identifies several key emotions that are linked to stressful appraisals:

- Anger, hostility, envy, and jealousy (the nasty emotions)
- Anxiety-fright, guilt, and shame (the existential emotions)
- Relief, hope, and sadness-depression (emotions provoked by unfavorable life conditions)
- Gratitude and compassion (empathic emotions)
- Happiness-joy, pride, and love (emotions provoked by favorable life conditions)

Accompanying each of these emotions are what Lazarus terms "core relational themes," which are linked to emotional narratives or scripts that accompany the emotions for the person. These emotional narratives are similar to Ellis's (1997, 1991a, 1991b) illogical beliefs and link the emotions to stressful appraisals (Lazarus, 1999).

Most people can readily understand how negatively toned feelings—anger and hostility, for example—can result in stress by linking these powerful negative emotions to people and situations that are appraised as threatening or harmful. It is more difficult to understand how positively toned emotions—happiness-joy, pride, and love, for instance—can be linked to stress. The best way to understand how emotions linked to favorable life conditions can result in stress is to examine them within the framework of the entire stress appraisal model. One's perception of love, for instance, isn't always completely accompanied by altruistic feelings and logical thinking. Often loves comes with emotional strings and historical baggage from previous relationships and interactions with significant others. Because of this past history, we may have illogical expectations of love and potential loved ones. For instance, we may put loved ones on a pedestal and fail to see their flaws. We may expect too much from them. We all know of people who fall madly in love with someone, rush head-long into a relationship, and refuse to recognize obvious cues that the loved one is not the picture of perfection who will provide 24/7 bliss and happiness. When the reality of the loved one sets in (he or she isn't as beautiful, sexy, intelligent, kind, and patient as expected), the appraisal changes. Love can also create stress when it steers us into directions that compromise our goals, values, morals, and ethics. Lovers often make demands on us that put us in positions where we are forced to choose between them and family friends, career, freedom, and so on.

The key to understanding how these emotions play out and whether they will result in a stress transaction is recognizing how well (if at all) we cope with them. Lazarus (1999) is quite clear, in his most recent synthesis, that stress appraisals and reappraisals revolve around our ability to cope with potential stressors. If we feel we can't cope (or can't cope well), the aforementioned emotions will be aroused, the core relational themes will play out in our heads, and we will experience stress. If we feel that we can cope effectively, the emotions, although strongly felt, won't result in a stressful appraisal.

Example

Counselor: John, it seems that you have mixed feelings about the things that seem to be causing you the most stress right now. You seem to be grateful for being able to work overtime and earn money, but this also seems to make you angry because it makes it hard to be home and go to school. Is that right?

John: Yeah. I almost feel guilty because I really have such a good life and am lucky, but I just feel hemmed in right now.

Summarizing

Once clients' thoughts and feelings about specific stressful situations are expressed, summarization helps clarify them and put them into context. This summary offers an opportunity for clients to hear the story again and decide if anything needs to be added, deleted, or clarified. It also shows them how well counselors are following the story. Remember, summaries include both cognitive (thoughts, facts) and affective (feelings, emotions) dimensions of clients' stories.

Example

Counselor: John, before we move on, let me see if I understand what is going on with your stress. The three things that seem to be coming to a head here are overtime, school, and the joys and responsibilities of being a homeowner and new father. While you seemed grateful and happy with your life and blessings, you are beginning to feel pressured by your commitments, and it makes you angry. I get the impression that you are not doing anything to relieve this pressure. Is this accurate?

John: Yeah, especially the last part. In the past I used exercise and sports to get rid of stress, but over the past six months I haven't really done anything at all. I bought some fitness equipment for the house but haven't even had a chance to unpack it yet. I have put on about 15 pounds over the past year and I'm really not happy about it.

Counselor: Okay, that's something we'll talk about when we start to set up your stress management plan.

Influencing Skills

As mentioned earlier in this chapter, the three primary goals of stress counseling are (1) assessment of personal stressors, (2) finding one's optimal level of stimulation and demand, and (3) development of a personal stress management plan based on the five R's of coping model (Blonna, 2005). Many of the influencing skills can be used to achieve these goals. It is important to remember that clients and counselors often have cultural differences that come into play when using influencing skills (see Diverse Perspectives 6.1).

Self-disclosure

As mentioned in Chapter 5, self-disclosure is an excellent technique for building confidence in clients regarding their perceived ability to change. Self-disclosing to clients that you, the counselor, know what they are going through because you also struggle with balancing the needs of family, children, work, and self-development and advancement can help instill confidence in clients. You do not need to go into great detail regarding your stress. The important thing is to establish a real connection with clients, based on shared experience. Clients need to see that even mental health professionals struggle with stress. The goal

of stress management isn't eliminating stress from one's life, but rather learning how to manage a tolerable level of stress. Even counselors have stress and have to cope with it.

Example

Counselor: John, I know what you are experiencing. This is something I have struggled with my entire life—cramming all of the things in life that I enjoy into 24 hours. It's not that I feel oppressed by these demands; I relish them and they add meaning to my life. It's just that sometimes, to use an old adage, too much of even a good thing can be stressful.

John: Yeah, that is it exactly. On the one hand, I want to pinch myself because things are going so great, yet on the other hand, I get angry because sometimes it seems like I am too busy to enjoy it all.

diverse perspectives 6.1

Susie Chen

Susie Chen was a senior marketing major and the youngest daughter of a first-generation Chinese American family. Susie's two sisters were married and worked with their husbands in the family business, which included three laundries. Susie, the first of the family to attend college, managed one of the three laundries.

Susie enrolled in a stress management class because she needed help in managing her time more efficiently. She attended college during the day and worked at the family business more than 40 hours per week and on weekends. She also lived at home with her mom, dad, and grandparents.

After a few weeks of class, it became apparent that time management was not Susie's problem; she had excellent time-management skills. Rather, Susie's real problem was that she was feeling extremely anxious and stressed anticipating her impending graduation. Upon graduation, her family expected her to become more involved in the family business, perhaps opening a fourth outlet, and to continue to live at home. The issue was never discussed—they just assumed that Susie would obey their wishes.

Susie, however, had no desire either to remain in the family business or to continue to live at home. She longed to join a multinational company and see the world as an international marketing representative. She also wanted her own apartment. When she was asked by her professor whether she had explained these desires to her family, she exclaimed, "Oh no! I couldn't do that. They would never understand or accept it. Plus, it would be considered impolite." When her professor probed further concerning how she expected to pursue her plans, Susie explained that they would have to wait either her parents died or else she did something shameful like run away and leave them a letter, praying for their future forgiveness. The professor was dumbfounded. He really did not know what to do. It was obvious that cultural reasons were keeping Susie, an excellent student with great communication skills, from using the assertiveness techniques that her professor recommended. They decided that she was better off learning how to live with this stressor and cope with it using other techniques rather than to try to eliminate it through the use of assertiveness.

Counselors need to be careful to not allow clients to use counselor self-disclosure as an opportunity to shift the discussion away from themselves. By self-disclosing, counselors are trying to establish an empowering connection with their clients. Only immature counselors waste this opportunity by talking too much about themselves and their stressors.

Confrontation

Confrontation will come into play extensively, especially when responding to incongruities related to the stress in their lives. Chapter 5 noted that confrontation is a skill that respectfully and gently makes clients aware of discrepancies in their lives and their stories. Like John, most clients have conflicting stories or send mixed messages about their stress and how they appraise potential stressors. These discrepancies occur for a variety of reasons. Sometimes people just behave in discrepant ways. They get into ruts and don't even realize it. A big part of stress counseling is helping clients see these discrepancies and devise strategies for overcoming or coping with them.

Sometimes clients honestly cannot recall details about prior stressful situations, so their stories come out as disjointed or with pieces missing. Other times clients will intentionally tell discrepant stories. Many clients who have discrepancies in their stories try to hide parts of their stories either that are too difficult for them to deal with or that they feel will lead to too many problems if discussed. These issues range from ethical issues to involvement in illegal activities. Clients who are embarrassed about their stress will sometimes discuss only parts of their stories and withhold other parts, especially if they sense that they are being judged by counselors.

Confronting discrepancies is essential to meet the goals of the counseling session. Using Ivey and Ivey's (2002) one hand, other hand approach is most helpful when employing this skill.

Example

Counselor: John, on the one hand, you just mentioned how important exercise is to you as a way to stay in shape and deal with stress. On the other hand, you say that you haven't exercised in more than six months. Can you explain that to me, please?

John: I guess with the new house, the baby, school, and working overtime so much, I just let it slip.

Example

Counselor: John, on the one hand, it seems that you know how to use exercise as a way to deal with your stress and feel good about yourself. On the other hand, you haven't done this in six months. What happened?

John: I guess I just haven't made it as big a priority as other things in my life over the past six months.

Changing the Focal Point

Changing the focal point is an excellent way to help clients gain a new perspective on their problem. In viewing their problem through the eyes of another person involved in their story, they often gain insights that change the way they view their situation and influence their future behavior.

Example

Counselor: John, let's step back from the problem for a minute and try to look at what is going on from your wife's perspective. Take a couple of minutes and try to think about how your wife views what is going on with your stress. When you can visualize this, share your thoughts with me.

John: (A couple of minutes later) It's funny you should mention this, because lately she has been trying to get me out of the house to go for a run or go to the gym.

Counselor: So how do you think she views the situation?

John: I think she basically feels that she has things under control and I am actually being a bit intrusive.

Counselor: Intrusive?

John: Yeah. She would actually like to work on Ricky's room herself. She wants to paint and organize his closet, stuff like that. She has actually told me to take more time for myself.

She really seems to want me to go back to what our schedule was like before we had the baby.

Counselor: What was that like?

John: We both worked until about 5:00. I used to stop by the gym or dojo after work and come home for dinner at around 7:00. She usually got home about 5:30 and had more than an hour to herself to unwind, read the paper, talk to her friends and family on the phone.

Counselor: And now?

John: She swings by her mom's house at about 5:15 to pick up Ricky after work and comes home to play with him and prepare dinner. I usually work a little overtime two nights a week and finish up at around 6:30 P.M. On one of those nights, I swing by the house for about 15 minutes on my way to school for my night class. On the other night, I go straight home. The other three nights I come right home after work and am there by 5:30 P.M.

Counselor: So it seems that you are home a lot more right after work than you used to be. How do you think your wife feels about this?

John: I never really thought about it, but now that you mention it she seems a little bitchy about me being there. It's almost like I am intruding on her time to be with Ricky.

Counselor: So, rather than this being a time for you to help out or relax with your son and wife, it almost seems tense and stressful.

John: Yeah, I guess so. It's not like my wife is mad at me. I think she knows I want to be there to help out with Ricky, but it is a real change for her. She's not used to sharing that time with me. If Ricky wasn't around, that would be her time to unwind after work. I guess she is also still trying to adjust to all the changes in her life over the past six months.

Counselor: Well, John, how can we use this information to help with your stress?

John: Maybe I should try to get back into the habit of stopping off at the gym or dojo on my way home to get a workout in and burn off some stress. It would give Kathy some time alone to be with Ricky and unwind from work. I could still have about an hour with him before he goes to sleep.

Counselor: It seems like everybody wins in this situation. Both you and Kathy return to some semblance of the schedule you had before Ricky was born. She has her time to unwind and you have your time to release some of your stress. What do you think?

John: I guess so. It made me feel a little guilty to take this time for myself. I felt kind of selfish and thought I should be home with my wife and kid, but I think it is something Kathy really needs and wants.

Counselor: Why don't you talk it over with her?

John: Okay, I'll do that.

As a result of changing the focal point and looking at the situation through the eyes of his wife, John was able to gain new insight into the way he was viewing this stressful situation. This changed his perception, and hence his appraisal of the potential stressor was changed. The new perspective led to his willingness to change his actual behavior.

Another interesting focal point to explore with John would be his Italian American cultural heritage. Cultural expectations often set up expectancies regarding family roles that can be stressful if they are not embraced by individuals.

Example

Counselor: John, tell me a little bit about how people of your culture would view your situation.

John: This is something I struggle with. There are a lot of things I embrace as an Italian American, but I also have some major problems with many of the cultural expectations of my father, family, and culture in general regarding being a man and a father.

Counselor: Go on.

John: I have these vivid memories of growing up and attending or hosting holiday get-togethers. My family was pretty clannish.

They never socialized with "outsiders." I can never remember my parents hosting a dinner party for friends or relatives. It was always family. Even friends were somehow related to somebody in the family. There was this loosely used term "paisanos" to refer to friends who were somehow linked to the villages of our family's origins in Italy.

Anyway, these family get-togethers always seemed to segregate the men from the women and children. I can recall always playing in the kitchen where the women spent the entire day preparing, serving, and cleaning up the meal. The men, meanwhile, were catered to and never had to help prepare, serve, or clean up. They were always ensconced in the living room smoking cigars, drinking wine, and talking about "important" things. I really couldn't stand this and promised myself that when I grew up and got married I would have a more egalitarian relationship.

Counselor: So how does this relate to what you are going through now?

John: I'm not sure. I feel pulled in different directions. I guess I feel that Kathy needs a break from working all day and having to care for Ricky and prepare dinner. I don't want to fall into this separation of roles like I experienced with my family. I really want to be an active participant in my family and our household. I don't want her to have to shoulder all of this responsibility herself.

Counselor: It seems that she wants to do this. Her wanting to do these "motherly" things seems to evoke a kind of fear in you of returning to the past. It seems to rekindle some of these cultural dislikes you had growing up.

John: Yeah, I think so. Even though she tells me she wants to have these responsibilities, I have a hard time accepting this. I'm worried that she'll start to embrace a more traditional role, the kind that I grew up with.

Counselor: So what you are saying is that you are worried that Kathy, now that she is a mother, will change and be more like the women in your culture that you grew up with. You're afraid that the kind of life you've had together with her will change and become more like the one you grew up in?

John: I guess so. What is really weird is that another part of me wants to be like the men in my history. My father always told me to be the "man of the house" or the protector, as he put it. I guess I embrace this part of my cultural upbringing. I really like feeling responsible for everyone's security and happiness. I believe that as the husband, and now father, it is my job to put my family's needs ahead of mine. I guess I want to be the patriarch without any of the sexist implications that go along with it.

Counselor: Seems like an awesome responsibility, feeling responsible for everyone's happiness.

John: Yeah, maybe. I'm always thinking about their happiness. Are you saying I need to focus more on my own?

Counselor: I just want you to think about how things were up to now and how they are changing.

John: Maybe I need to just relax and trust Kathy more. She's always been very open and honest with me regarding how she feels about our relationship. She is very different from my mom and the other women in my family. I know she wouldn't want to have the kind of traditional family life they had.

As a result of changing the focal point and looking at the situation as another man from his culture would, John was able to gain new insight into his conflicting feelings about his roles as husband and father. This new perspective changed his appraisal of the situation and his willingness to reexamine these roles and how taking more time for himself might affect them.

Eliciting and Reflecting Meaning
Chapter 5 described how eliciting and reflecting meaning helps influence clients by giving them insights into the meaning of aspects of their stories.

Before counselors move on to giving directives and instructions for changing behavior, they need to be sure that they understand the meaning of clients' stories. A good way to elicit meaning is to ask clients to make sense of the meaning of their stories.

Example

Counselor: John, we've been talking a lot about your life and the things in it that seem to be the root of your stress. Why don't you take a moment and see if you can make sense of it by telling me what all of this means to you.

John: All right, I'll try. I guess I am feeling pulled in many different directions. Part of me wants to work overtime to earn extra money to do more around the house, make Kathy happy, and plan for my son's future. Another part of me wants to cut back on overtime so I can spend more time around the house helping out and being with Ricky. Part of me wants to get my degree so I can earn more money and advance in my job, but another part really likes what I am doing as a craftsman and is turned off by moving to the next level. I guess I am also having a harder time adjusting to fatherhood than I thought I would. I always thought I could just merge the man I am with the responsibilities of being a father. I never realized this would resurrect all the emotions I had about my childhood and the father roles I grew up with in my culture.

Interpretation of Meaning and Reframing

Counselors use interpretation of meaning to make sense of what health problems mean to clients. This process is very similar to eliciting and reflecting feelings but is counselor directed. Interpretation of meaning differs from eliciting and reflecting meaning in that it comes from counselors and includes their perspectives on the meaning of clients' stories.

Example

Counselor: John, this is a very exciting time in your life. You have a lot on your plate: a good job that you find personally and professionally rewarding, a new house, a healthy new son, a solid marriage, your college coursework. It seems that all of these challenges are starting to turn into stressors because they are evoking contradictions and mixed feelings. It seems like this build-up is beginning to tax your abilities to cope with these demands. Remember, your perception of these things determines whether they actually become stressors. Work, school, being a husband and father—these things are merely potential stressors until you feel that you can't cope with them. It seems that you are feeling as if you are at a crossroads. You need to make some decisions about changes you have to make in your life, and change is stressful.

John: I guess so. I feel like there isn't enough time to do all of the things that I need to do, or even think them through. I know something's got to give, but I'm not sure what.

Reframing

After interpreting the meaning of clients' stories, counselors can reframe those stories and present different versions for clients to ponder. As mentioned in Chapter 5, these new, alternative ways of viewing their problems provide new options to consider for dealing with the problems and allow clients to see their problems in new and different ways.

Example

Counselor: John, I understand that you are feeling pretty confused and stressed out about work, school, and your home life. Have you considered that this might be a normal part of adjusting to the new demands of being a homeowner and father?

John: You mean that I am blowing this out of proportion?

Counselor: No, I think it is very real for you. I just mean that maybe your expectations for adjusting to these new challenges were a little off. Maybe adding just two new things to your life—a baby and a house—created more change than you imagined?

John: I never looked at it this way, but there are just so many more things to think about than before. I get exhausted just thinking about what I should be doing for Ricky's future and for the house.

Counselor: You might want to share some of this confusion with Kathy to see how and where she can help.

John: Yeah, I have been keeping this all to myself.

Counselor: I think it might not be a bad idea to take a closer look at the demands of work and school combined with these two new additions (house and Ricky) to your life. Most of your plans about work and school were made before you had Ricky and bought the house. It might not be a bad idea to revisit them. What do you think?

John: I think that would be a good idea. I'm having lots of second thoughts about some of my past plans related to work and school.

Reframing John's story sets the stage for developing a stress management plan based on directives that fit his unique needs. A key component will be helping him examine the way he views work, school, and his roles as husband and father to help him think more logically about these parts of his life.

Directives and Logical Consequences

Several potential directives, instructions, and logical consequences are associated with each of the four goals of stress counseling: (1) assessment of personal stressors, (2) finding one's optimal level of stimulation and demand, and (3) development of a personal stress management plan based on the five R's of coping model (Blonna, 2005). The specific directives and instructions used will vary depending on the stress management model employed by counselors. This book will use Blonna's five R's model of stress management. As described earlier in the chapter, this model provides several different strategies for each level of coping.

Directives Associated with Assessment of Personal Stressors and Use of Time

Counselors should not assume that all clients have the same stressors. For this reason, the logical starting point in helping clients manage the stress is having them assess their stressors. There are many different ways to do this. We recommend use of two simple logs: one that keeps track of a variety of stressor-related variables (see **Figure 6.8**) and another that monitors time management (see **Figure 6.9**).

1. Fill out the stressor and time logs for the next four weeks.
2. Bring the logs in each week for analysis and discussion.
3. Use the logs to help develop personal stress management plans.

Logical Consequences of Assessment of Personal Stressors and Use of Time

1. Keeping the stress and time logs will provide information about the nature of your personal stress profile.
2. You can use the information in the stress log to plan a stress management program (which includes time management plans).
3. You can use the stress log to monitor the success of your stress management program.

Specific Instructions for Assessment of Personal Stressors

1. List all of your stressors every day. Make sure to include all stressors, even the most trivial (such as the morning paper being late).
2. You can make multiple days' entries on one assessment sheet.
3. Describe how you perceived the stressor (exactly what you told yourself about it).
4. Describe how your body and mind reacted to the stressor. This is your stress response (*not* your appraisal).
5. Rate each stressor on a scale of 1 to 10 (with 10 being the most stressful).
6. Describe what you did (if anything) to cope with the stressor.

Day/Date	Stressor	Response	Intensity	Coping	Specific Details That Bothered You

EXAMPLE

Day/Date	Stressor	Response	Intensity	Coping	Specific Details That Bothered You
Monday, Sept. 1	Stuck in traffic	Muscle tension in neck; anger	8	Yelled at other drivers	Felt trapped, like there was nothing I could do
Tuesday, Sept. 2	Fight with girlfriend	Anger; stomach churning	9	Stormed out of the room; avoided her	Fought over silly comment made by a TV talk-show host

EXAMPLE

Figure 6.8 Stressor assessment log

Day/Time	Activity
5:00 A.M.	
5:30 A.M.	
6:00 A.M.	
6:30 A.M.	
7:00 A.M.	
7:30 A.M.	
8:00 A.M.	
8:30 A.M.	
9:00 A.M.	
9:30 A.M.	
10:00 A.M.	
10:30 A.M.	
11:00 A.M.	
11:30 A.M.	
12:00 P.M.	
12:30 P.M.	
1:00 P.M.	
1:30 P.M.	
2:00 P.M.	
2:30 P.M.	
3:00 P.M.	
3:30 P.M.	
4:00 P.M.	
4:30 P.M.	
5:00 P.M.	
5:30 P.M.	
6:00 P.M.	
6:30 P.M.	
7:00 P.M.	
7:30 P.M.	
8:00 P.M.	
8:30 P.M.	
9:00 P.M.	

Figure 6.9 Time assessment log

7. At the end of a week, look for patterns or trends in what causes you stress, how you perceive potential stressors, how you respond to stressors, what the overall volume and intensity of your stressors are, what you do to cope, and whether it works.

8. Write a summary of the items contained in step 7 and bring the log with you every week when you meet with your counselor.

Example

Counselor: John, before you start keeping this log, make a few copies of the blank sheet so you have enough copies to fill in.

In the first column, list all of your stressors every day. I want you to keep track of even the smallest annoyances, such as the weather or the morning paper being late.

In the second column, write down exactly what you told yourself about the stressor. Don't worry about your language. Be as expressive as you want.

In the next column, describe how you felt. Things like muscle tension, worry, and so on go in this column.

In the next column, you must give each stressor a point value from 1 to 10. Use 10 to denote the biggest stressors.

In the next column, put down anything you did to cope. Be sure to include even negative things like screaming or yelling.

Every Sunday night, write up an analysis of any patterns or trends you find for each of the columns.

I expect you to bring this in every week for our appointment together so we can look it over and talk about it.

Specific Instructions for Assessment of Time

1. Use a new time log sheet for each day.
2. Each day fill in how each 30-minute block of time throughout the 24-hour period was used.
3. Use ditto marks for several lines if you repeat the same activity, such as sleeping.
4. At the end of a week, look for patterns or trends in the following types of time: paid work time, unpaid work time, fun/play time, commuting time, sleep time.
5. Write a summary of the items contained in step 4 and bring the log with you every week when you meet with your counselor.

Example

Counselor: John, instructions for filling out the time log are similar to those for keeping the stressor log. Once again, you should make

extra copies of these sheets. Unlike the stressor logs, where you can log in multiple days on one sheet, you will use a new time log sheet for each day.

You will have to log in everything you do during each 24-hour period. I will leave it up to your discretion how to log in activities like making love.

You can use single words or phrases to fill in how you used each 30-minute block of time throughout the 24-hour period. You can use ditto marks or slashes for several lines if you repeat the same activity (like sleeping) through multiple time periods.

Once again, every Sunday night write up an analysis of any patterns or trends you find in your use of time.

As with your stressor log, I expect you to bring this in every week for our appointment together so we can look it over and talk about it.

Directives Associated with Finding One's Optimal Level of Demand

Unfortunately, finding one's optimal level of demand (see Figure 6.7)—that point beyond which even pleasurable activities become stressors—isn't easy to do. There is no chart, based on height and weight, that tells you how much stimulation you need to reach optimal functioning. Finding one's optimal level is derived through trial and error and is somewhat subjective. It starts with assessment of stressors and the consequences of stress and involves a willingness to adapt to the changing demands of life.

Directives

1. Assess your current level of functioning and position on the stress curve.
2. Identify your optimal level of demand.

Logical Consequences Associated with Finding One's Optimal Level of Demand

1. Assessing their optimal level of demand will provide clients with additional information (it builds on the information gleaned from assessing stressors and use of time) about the level of demand in their lives.

2. Comparing this information to their subjective assessment of where they are on the stress curve (Figure 6.7) gives clients a visual picture of the level of demand in their lives and the results of this stimulation.

3. Only clients know how they feel about their current level of demand and what their optimal level of demand is.

4. Completing this work prepares clients for taking action (part of their plan based on the five R's) to cut back on unwanted demands.

Specific Instructions for Finding One's Optimal Level of Demand

1. Look at Figure 6.7 (the inverted stress curve) and describe where you think you are on the curve at this time in your life.

2. Describe where you would prefer to be on the curve.

3. Describe three major demands/stimuli that you think are responsible for putting you in your present position on the stress curve.

Example

Counselor: John, I want you to pick where you think you are on this stress curve at this time in your life. Where would you prefer to be on the curve? What are the two or three major demands on your time that you think are responsible for keeping you where you are on the stress curve? What do you think you can do to change your position on the curve?

Directives Associated with Developing a Personal Stress Management Plan Based on the Five R's of Coping

More than 25 different stress management strategies are associated with the five R's of coping model. Counselors need to help clients choose those strategies that are most likely to work for them. Counselors should use their knowledge of clients' stories to help them pick strategies that most closely fit their personalities and lifestyles. In this way, clients can tailor a personal stress management plan geared toward their needs and wants.

Directives

1. Develop a personal stress management plan based on the five R's model.

2. Pick one strategy from each of the five R's to build your plan.

Logical Consequences of Developing a Personal Stress Management Plan Based on the Five R's of Coping

1. Clients will tailor a stress management plan to their needs.

2. Clients should choose strategies that interest them and are consistent with their personalities and lifestyles.

3. Clients are more likely to comply with plans they develop personally.

Specific Instructions for Developing a Personal Stress Management Plan Based on the Five R's of Coping

1. Have clients review **Table 6.2** and give them information about the various coping strategies available.

2. Tell clients to take the materials home, read them, and think about how the strategies mesh with their personalities, needs, and lifestyles.

3. Tell clients to come back the next week prepared to choose at least one strategy for each of the five R's.

4. Work with clients in developing their personal plans.

Example

Counselor: John, the first step in developing a personal stress management plan for you is to go back and look at all of the strategies available using the five R's of coping model. Here is a copy of the chart I gave you to take home that describes these strategies associated with the five R's model [hands John the chart to look at]. We talked a little about these and I gave you some material to read last week regarding how they work. Take a minute to look at this material again and try to decide which ones do you think you'd be interested in trying.

Table 6.2

Strategies for Reducing Stress Arousal

Relaxation Strategy	Arousal Reduction
Diaphragmatic breathing	Reduces neurotransmitter arousal (Everly & Lating, 2002; Zhang, Harper, & Ni, 1986)
	Reduces neuromuscular arousal (Everly & Lating, 2002; Van Peski-Oosterbaan et al., 1997)
	Reduces cognitive arousal (Everly & Lating, 2002; DeFilippo & Overholser, 1999)
Meditation and relaxation response	Reduces neurotransmitter arousal (Everly & Lating, 2002; Benson & Friedman, 1985)
	Reduces neuromuscular arousal (Everly & Lating, 2002; Jeving, Wallace, & Biedebach, 1992)
	Reduces cognitive arousal (Everly & Lating, 2002; Kabat-Zinn et al., 1992)
Quieting reflex/calming response	Reduces neuromuscular arousal (Stroebel, 1979)
Autogenics and visual imagery	Reduces neurotransmitter arousal (Everly & Lating, 2002; Linden, 1994; Lusk, 1992)
	Reduces neuromuscular arousal (Everly & Lating, 2002; Linden, 1994, 1999; Lusk, 1992)
	Reduces cognitive arousal (Everly & Lating, 2002; Linden, 1994, 1999; Lusk, 1992)
Biofeedback	Reduces neurotransmitter arousal (EMG and EEG techniques) (Everly & Lating, 2002; Schwartz, 1995)
	Reduces neuromuscular arousal (EMG and EDR techniques) (Everly & Lating, 2002; Rokicki et al., 1997)
	Reduces cognitive arousal (EEG technique) (Everly & Lating, 2002; Schwartz, 1995)
Systematic muscle relaxation	Reduces neurotransmitter arousal (Everly & Lating, 2002; McGuigan, 1991, 1993; Jacobsen, 1970, 1978)
	Reduces neuromuscular arousal (Everly & Lating, 2002; McGuigan, 1991, 1993; Jacobsen, 1970, 1978)
	Reduces cognitive arousal (Everly & Lating, 2002; McGuigan, 1991, 1993; Jacobsen, 1970, 1978)
Hatha yoga and stretching	Reduces neuromuscular arousal (Seward, 2002; Birkel & Edgren, 2000)
Tai chi	Reduces neuromuscular arousal (Seward, 2002; Jacobsen, 1970; Koh, 1981)
Massage	Reduces neuromuscular arousal (Seward, 2002; Naliboff & Tachiki, 1991)

John: I looked at these over the week and I've picked these five strategies: Seligman's ABCDE model [Rethink], the triple A's of coping [Reduce], diaphragmatic breathing [Relax], punching the heavy bag [Release], and exercise [Reorganize]. I think these might work for me.

Counselor: Excellent choices, John. I think all of these are consistent with what you've told me about your stressors and your lifestyle. I notice that physical activity plays a big part in your coping style.

John: Yes, I agree. I've come to realize how important this really is in keeping me sane.

Counselor: Let's go over each of these to make sure you know how to do them.

Readers are directed to Blonna (2005) for a comprehensive explanation of the theory behind each of these strategies.

Specific Instructions for Seligman's Model (Rethink Strategy)

Whenever you are confronted by stressors or potential stressors that are based on illogical, pessimistic thinking, you should *analyze them in writing,* using Seligman's (1998) ABCDE model (see **Figure 6.10**).

A: Identify the adversity in the potential stressor.

A	(Adversity) Stressful situation, person, event, etc.
B	(Beliefs) Your illogical beliefs about **A** (pessimistic beliefs about permanence, pervasiveness, and personalization)
C	(Consequences) Your feelings and actions resulting from your beliefs about **A**
D	(Distraction) Divert your attention away from your beliefs or (Dispute) Substitute more optimistic beliefs for each **B**
E	(Energization) Your new feelings and actions resulting from **D**

Figure 6.10 Seligman's (1998) ABCDE model for coping with stress and emotional problems is similar to Ellis and Harper's model but focuses on potential stressors that are related to optimism and pessimism.

B: List each illogical belief about the potential stressor, paying particular attention to statements regarding permanence, pervasiveness, and/or personalization.

C: List all of the stressful consequences you are experiencing as a result of your beliefs about A.

D: Describe the distractions (divert your attention away from) or disputes (substitution of more optimistic beliefs) you can use to change your perception of each B.

E: List your new feelings based on your more optimistic thinking.

Specific Instructions for the Triple A's of Coping (Reduce Strategy)

1. Examine one week's worth of stressor logs.
2. Organize stressors into groups that can be (1) abolished, (2) avoided, or (3) altered.
3. Take each stressor (or category of stressors) and describe how to abolish, avoid, or alter it.
4. Describe, in writing, how this reduces the overall level of demand in your life.
5. Describe, in writing, how these actions will affect your position on the inverted stress curve (Figure 6.7).

Example

Counselor: John, I want you to go through your stressor logs and identify stressors you think you can abolish (get rid of), avoid (be exposed to less often), or alter (change somehow to destress them).

Write down what you think will happen to your life and stress when you abolish stressors. Do this for each stressor you think you can abolish.

Describe exactly how you will be exposed to the avoidable stressors. Once again, describe how you think this will affect your life.

Describe exactly how you will change those stressors you can alter. Once again, describe how you think this will affect your life.

Bring this material with you next week, and we'll go over it to see how this works out.

Specific Instructions for Diaphragmatic Breathing (Relax Strategy)

1. Find a quiet place away from others to practice.
2. Minimize distractions by closing doors and turning off the radio, television, and phone.
3. Practice this activity a few times a day.

In time, with regular practice, you will automatically shift into a deeper, more even breathing pattern whenever you feel stressed. Deep breathing is an excellent first choice for reducing stress.

Example

Counselor: John, I'd like you to relax and follow these simple instructions for practicing this breathing technique.

Pick a comfortable chair. Sit on the chair with your back straight, head up.

Visualize a picture of your lungs. Picture all of the smallest branches of your lungs where the oxygen actually enters your bloodstream.

Inhale slowly through your nose.

As you breathe in, push your stomach forward and let your ribs expand and your shoulders rise as the air fills your lungs completely from the bottom up.

Once your lungs feel full, slowly exhale through your mouth, letting your shoulders fall and your ribs shrink back as the air slowly passes through your mouth.

Gently pull your stomach back in with your stomach muscles, fully draining all of the air from the lower portion of your lungs.

Keep this up for five minutes.

Specific Instructions for Punching a Heavy Bag (Release Strategy)

1. Warm up properly.
2. Assume the ready position.
3. Assume a forward stance.
4. Measure your punch against the bag.
5. Bring your hands up.
6. Hit with the knuckles first.
7. Practice throwing a few easy punches.
8. Increase your punching power.

Example

Counselor: John, there are a few things we need to go over just to ensure that you are using proper technique when punching a heavy bag.

Make sure that before you hit the bag you warm up properly by jogging in place, walking on a treadmill, or gently riding an exercise bike for five to ten minutes.

Make sure your feet are shoulder width apart, your knees slightly bent, and your hands closed lightly. Your eyes should be focused straight ahead and your shoulders square with your body.

John, are you right- or left-handed?

John: I'm right-handed.

Counselor: You'll need to assume a left forward stance. Move your left leg straight forward the distance of two shoulder widths. Your right leg should be straight, your feet pointed forward with the left knee bent and directly over the heel. Your hips and shoulders should be square with one another, while the back is straight.

Measure your punch against the bag by rotating your hips forward and extending your punching arm as if you were throwing a punch so that the distance between yourself and the bag allows you to hit the bag solidly without your elbow locking.

Bring your hands up and hold your left fist just below your eyes, parallel to the left shoulder, with the back of your forearm and fist facing forward. Hold your right arm horizontally across your body, with your right fist held at shoulder height.

Make sure you use a proper fist, with your thumb wrapped around and across the rest of your fingers. Always keep your fist in a straight line with your wrist and arm. Bending at the wrist can cause pain and injury.

When throwing a punch, you want to make sure the first two knuckles of the hand connect with the bag first. These are the knuckles above the index and middle fingers. You also want to hit squarely on these knuckles, and not with a combination of knuckle and first section of your fingers. It is easy to sprain or dislocate a finger if they hit first.

Throw a few easy punches. Do not hold your breath when you connect with your punch. Breathe out, grunt, or yell as you throw the punch. This will help you prevent holding your breath and aid in releasing stress.

After throwing several easy punches, increase the force of your punching. Follow through by imagining that you are throwing your punches through the bag.

Specific Instructions for Overall Increasing of Physical Activity Levels (Reorganize)

1. Try to incorporate 30 minutes of moderate physical activity into each day (see **Table 6.3**).
2. Pick activities that are enjoyable.
3. Develop a "four-season approach" to physical activity and fitness by picking at least one activity that can be performed every season, regardless of the weather.
4. Choose some activities that include family members to incorporate them into your reorganizing plan.
5. Do not let physical activity become a source of stress.

Example

Counselor: John, there are countless things you can do to reorganize your life to make it healthier and therefore stress resistant. You've mentioned that in the past you worked out at the gym and dojo to deal with stress. What do you think about focusing on these activities once again?

John: I think that is a good idea.

Counselor: The first thing I'd like you to do is to go back over the stress curve and triple A's activities we worked on to see how they freed up some additional personal time for you. I'd like you to reexamine two blocks of time: your after-work time and weekends.

I'd like you dedicate the after-work time to your personal physical activities and the weekend time to physical activities you can engage in with Kathy and Ricky. This way

---

Table 6.3

Moderate Physical Activity

The *Surgeon General's Report on Physical Activity and Health* (1999) recommends getting a moderate amount of physical activity each day. A moderate amount of physical activity is roughly equivalent to physical activity that uses approximately 150 calories (kcal) of energy per day, or 1000 calories per week.

This table lists a variety of ways to obtain a moderate amount of physical activity. Because amount of activity is a function of duration, intensity, and frequency, the same amount of activity can be obtained in longer sessions of moderately intense activities (such as brisk walking) as in shorter sessions of more strenuous activities (such as running).

Less Vigorous, Requires More Time

Washing and waxing a car for 45–60 minutes

Washing windows or floors for 45–60 minutes

Playing volleyball for 45 minutes

Playing touch football for 30–45 minutes

Gardening for 30–45 minutes

Wheeling self in wheelchair for 30–40 minutes

Walking 1.75 miles in 35 minutes (20 minutes/mile)

Basketball (shooting baskets) for 30 minutes

Bicycling 5 miles in 30 minutes

Dancing fast (social) for 30 minutes

Pushing a stroller 1.5 miles in 30 minutes

Raking leaves for 30 minutes

Walking 2 miles in 30 minutes (15 minutes/mile)

Water aerobics for 30 minutes

Swimming laps for 20 minutes

Wheelchair basketball for 20 minutes

Basketball (playing a game) for 15–20 minutes

Bicycling 4 miles in 15 minutes

Jumping rope for 15 minutes

Running 1.5 miles in 15 minutes (10 minutes/mile)

Shoveling snow for 15 minutes

Stairwalking for 15 minutes

More Vigorous, Requires Less Time

Source: Surgeon General's Report on Physical Activity and Health. www.cdc.gov/nccdphp/sgr/ataglan.htm.

you can get the benefits of physical release, which seem to work for you, while not feeling that you are sacrificing time with your wife and son. How does that sound?

John: It sounds like a good idea.

Counselor: Good. Lastly, I want you to identify two kinds of physical activities: one for your after-work workouts and one for your weekend activities with your family. By next week I want you to pick four activities (one for each season) that you can fit into each slot (personal and family).

You can see that comprehensive stress counseling using the five R's of coping model (Blonna, 2005) is time-consuming but tailors activities to the needs of clients. Tailoring of stress management activities results in greater compliance with stress management plans.

Summary

Stress is defined as "a holistic transaction between the individual and a stressor resulting in the body's mobilization of a stress response." This eclectic definition of stress emphasizes the importance of the stress appraisal process involving a potential stressor, the individual, and the environment. In this appraisal process, any stimulus appraised by the individual as threatening or capable of causing harm or loss is considered to be a stressor. These stimuli remain "potential stressors" until they are actually appraised as threatening.

The stress response is a potentially harmful set of physiological adaptations by the body to maintain homeostasis in the face of threat, harm, or loss. Eustress is an outdated concept, having been replaced by the notion of challenge, a positive mobilization of energy that is accompanied by the perception of being in control and able to cope. Stress transactions are influenced by the individual's overall level of well-being and incorporate environmental factors into a model of personal stress.

Various models have been developed to explain how stress is related to illness. Stress disorders are characterized as "disorders of arousal,"

and the mechanisms of arousal were described in detail in this chapter. Different types of coping strategies can be used to combat stress arousal. Blonna's five R's of coping model is a comprehensive model that uses different levels and techniques of coping to help clients develop personalized individual stress management plans. This holistic model emphasizes that stress doesn't occur in a vacuum.

The last part of the chapter demonstrates the application of the microskills model to counseling clients with stress. Using John as a case study, the counselor worked through the application of introductory, attending, responding, and listening skills to someone with stress.

Study Questions

1. Describe the major differences in the five ways of defining stress.
2. Compare the authors' definition of stress with the four classical definitions.
3. Explain what a holistic transaction is by using a personal example.
4. What are life events, and how do they relate to stress?
5. What is homeostasis, and how does it relate to the stress response?
6. What is the role of threat perception in the stress response?
7. What is psychosomatic illness?
8. List and describe the two types of psychosomatic diseases.
9. Compare and contrast Everly and Benson's disorders of arousal model with Selye's GAS.
10. Describe the role of chronic stress in the weakening and eventual breakdown of various body parts and systems.

References

Benson H, Friedman R (1985). A rebuttal to the conclusions of David S. Holmes article: meditation and somatic arousal reduction. *American Psychologist* 40:725–728.

Birkel DA, Edgren L (2000). Hatha yoga: improved vital capacity of college students. *Alternative Therapies* 6:55–63.

Blonna R (2005). *Coping with Stress in a Changing World,* 3rd ed. Dubuque, IA: McGraw-Hill.

Canon W (1932). *The Wisdom of the Body.* New York: W. W. Norton.

DeFilippo JM, Overholser JC (1999). Cognitive behavioral treatment of panic disorder: confronting situational precipitants. *Journal of Contemporary Psychotherapy* 29:99–113.

Deutsch P (1959). *On the Mysterious Leap from Mind to Body.* New York: International Universities Press.

Ellis A (1991a). The philosophical basis of rational emotive therapy. *Psychotherapy in Private Practice* 8:97–106.

Ellis A (1991b). The revised ABC's of rational-emotive therapy (RET). *Journal of Rational-Emotive Therapy* 9:139–167.

Ellis A, Gordon J, Neenan M, Palmer S (1997). *Stress Counseling: A Rational Emotive Approach.* New York: Springer.

Ellis A, Harper R (1998). *A New Guide to Rational Living* North Hollywood, CA: Wilshire Books.

Everly GS, Benson H (1989). Disorders of arousal and the relaxation response. *International Journal of Psychosomatics* 36:15–21.

Everly GS, Lating JM (2002). *A Clinical Guide to the Treatment of the Human Stress Response.* New York: Kluwer Academic Plenum Publishers.

Holmes HT, Rahe HR (1967). The social readjustment rating scale. *Journal of Psychosomatic Research* 11:213.

Ivey A, Ivey M (2002). *Intentional Interviewing and Counseling: Facilitating Client Development in a Multicultural Society,* 5th ed. Pacific Grove, CA: Thomson/Brooks Cole.

Jacobsen E (1970). *Modern Treatment of Tense Patients.* Springfield, IL: Charles C. Thomas.

Jacobsen E (1978). *You Must Relax.* New York: McGraw-Hill.

Jeving R, Wallace RK, Biedebach M (1992). The physiology of meditation: a review. A wakeful hypometabolic wakeful exposure. *Neuroscience and Biobehavioral Reviews* 16:415–424.

Kabat-Zinn J, Massion AD, Kristeller J, et al. (1992). Effectiveness of a meditation based stress reduction program in the treatment of anxiety disorders. *American Journal of Psychiatry* 149:936–943.

Koh TC (1981). Tai chi chuan. *American Journal of Chinese Medicine* 8:15–22.

Lazarus RS (1966). *Psychological Stress and the Coping Process.* New York: McGraw-Hill.

Lazarus RS (1999). *Stress and Emotion: A New Synthesis.* New York: Springer.

Lazarus RS, Folkman S (1984). *Stress Appraisal and Coping.* New York: Springer.

Linden W (1994). Autogenic training: a narrative and quantitative review of clinical outcomes. *Biofeedback and Self-regulation* 19:227.

Lusk JT (1992). *Relaxation, Imagery, and Inner Healing.* New York: Whole Person.

McGuigan FJ (1991). *Calm Down: A Guide for Stress and Tension Control.* Dubuque, IA: Kendall-Hunt.

McGuigan FJ (1993). Progressive relaxation: origins, principles and clinical applications. In PM Leher, Woolfolk TL (Eds.). *Principles and Practices of Stress Management,* 2nd ed. (pp. 17–52). New York: Guilford.

Millon T (1996). *Disorders of Personality,* 2nd ed. New York: Wiley.

Naliboff BD, Tachiki KH (1991). Autonomic and skeletal muscle response to non-electrical cutaneous stimulation. *Perceptual and Motor Skills* 72:575–584.

Rokicki LA, Holroyd KA, France CR, et al. (1997). Change mechanisms associated with combined relaxation/EMG biofeedback training for chronic tension headache. *Applied Psychophysiology and Biofeedback* 22:21–41.

Schwartz MS (1995). *Biofeedback: A Practitioner's Guide,* 2nd ed. New York: Guilford.

Seligman MEP (1998). *Learned Optimism: How to Change Your Mind and Your Life.* New York: Free Press.

Selye H (1956). *The Stress of Life.* New York: McGraw-Hill.

Seward BL (2002). *Managing Stress,* 3rd ed. Boston: Jones and Bartlett.

Stroebel CF (1979). Non-specific effects and psychodynamic issues in self-regulatory techniques. Paper presented at the Johns Hopkins Conference in Clinical Biofeedback, Baltimore, MD.

Surgeon General of the United States (1999). *Surgeon General's Report on Physical Activity and Health. www.cdc.gov/nccdphp/sgr/atagan/htm.*

United States Department of Health and Human Services (USDHHS), Office of Disease Prevention and Health Promotion (ODPHP) (2003). *Healthy People 2010: A Systematic Approach to Health Improvement.* www.healthypeople.gov/Document/html/uih/uih_bw/uih_2.htm#obj.

Van Peski-Oosterbaan AS, et al. (1997). Cognitive behavioral therapy for unexplained noncardiac chest pain: a pilot study. *Behavioral and Cognitive Psychotherapy* 25:339–350.

Walen S, DiGuiseppi R, Wessler R (1980). *A Practitioner's Guide to RET.* New York: Oxford University Press.

Zhang J, Harper R, Ni H (1986). Cryogenic blockade of the central nucleus of the amygdala attenuates aversely conditioned blood pressure and respiratory response. *Brain Research* 386:136–145.

Chapter 7

Birth Control Counseling

Learning Objectives

By the end of the chapter students will:

1. Differentiate between the following terms: fertility control, contraception, birth control, and family planning

2. Compare the meanings of theoretical and actual use effectiveness

3. Explain the different mechanisms of fertility control

4. Evaluate a variety of fertility control methods

5. Understand how fertility control needs change over the life cycle

6. Identify which methods work best for clients in reducing the risks for unintended pregnancy and sexually transmitted diseases

7. Describe the goals of birth control counseling

8. Describe the role of introductory skills in assessing clients' sexuality and perceptions of birth control

9. Explain how body language and other nonverbal messages are related to assessing sexuality concerns in clients

10. Describe how to use sexual self-disclosure effectively

11. Discuss how changing the focal point can help clients appraise their birth control needs differently

12. Describe the key directives for each of the goals of birth control counseling

Introduction

People use the terms "birth control," "contraception," and "family planning" interchangeably when referring to controlling fertility. Al-

though the three terms are similar in that they all refer to strategies for preventing unintended pregnancy, they are vastly different in terms of their implications for counseling. It is important for counselors to understand the subtleties in these terms and their implications when working with clients.

Family planning implies the desire to have children at some planned point in time. Counseling clients about family planning involves helping them postpone childbearing until it is desired, spacing subsequent births, and avoiding pregnancy at other times. Besides discussing how to prevent getting pregnant, counseling clients about family planning may include discussing how to facilitate a pregnancy as well as adoption when these issues seem desirable. It is important for counselors to remember that not all clients who want to prevent getting pregnant ever want to plan or have families.

Contraception refers to all methods designed to prevent conception or fertilization. As we will discuss in detail in this chapter, contraceptive methods work by preventing the sperm and egg from uniting to cause fertilization. They include non-penetrative sexual activity, barrier methods, hormonal contraception, withdrawal, fertility awareness, and sterilization. These methods vary in their effectiveness and appropriateness for clients at different points in their reproductive lives. Because contraception works by preventing conception, it may be the more appropriate term to use with clients whose religious or cultural beliefs condemn the use of abortion. Counselors should also be aware that more conservative clients might be uncomfortable discussing some of these methods, especially the noninsertive sexual behaviors.

Birth control is a broad term encompassing all methods designed to prevent pregnancy and birth. It includes all contraceptive methods, emergency contraception, and abortion, which is designed to interrupt an established pregnancy. The term "birth control" is perceived negatively by many people because of its association with abortion, one of many birth control methods. Many clients mistakenly refer to oral contraceptives and birth control as being synonymous.

Fertility control is a neutral term that can be used by counselors to alleviate many of these concerns. It is self-explanatory and refers to all attempts by women to control their own fertility.

Effectiveness: Theoretical and Actual Use

Fertility control methods vary in their effectiveness. Two measures of effectiveness are used to evaluate fertility control methods: theoretical use and actual use (see **Table 7.1**).

Theoretical Effectiveness

The **theoretical effectiveness** of any fertility control method is the estimate of how well it should work if it is used consistently and correctly. It is the ideal effectiveness of the method, determined through laboratory research and experimental studies. Theoretical effectiveness research designs attempt to control for as many variables as possible that could potentially interfere with correct and consistent use. Failure of the method accounts for most of the ineffectiveness. Theoretical effectiveness is the lowest expected percentage of women who will get pregnant while using the method. For instance, a method might be said to have a 99% theoretical use effectiveness, meaning that there is a 1% theoretical risk of getting pregnant while using it (Hatcher, Trussel, Stewart, et al., 1998).

Actual Use Effectiveness

The **actual use effectiveness** of any fertility control method is how well it actually works when real people use it under normal circumstances. That is, it is the observed effectiveness of the method, determined by following a group of actual users for one year to see how many get pregnant. Actual use effectiveness studies are not subject to the same rigorous controls as most theoretical effectiveness studies are. For this reason, user failure (failure to use the method consistently and correctly each time a couple has intercourse) largely accounts for the lack of effectiveness. Actual use effectiveness estimates combine the effectiveness of the actual method with user failure rates. The effectiveness is expressed as the percentage of women who get pregnant after one year of using the method. For instance, a method might be said

Table 7.1

Theoretical Versus Actual Use Effectiveness

The Actual Use Effectiveness Represents the Typical Failure Rate, While the Theoretical Effectiveness Is the Lowest Observed Failure Rate

Method	Typical Failure Rate (%)	Lowest Observed Failure Rate (%)
No method (chance)	85	85
Withdrawal	19	4
Combination birth control pill	5	0.1
Progestin-only pill	5	0.5
Depo-Provera	0.3	0.3
Norplant	0.09	0.09
Copper T IUD	0.8	0.6
Male latex condom	14	3
Female latex condom	21	5
Diaphragm	20	6
Cervical cap	20	9
Spermicide alone	26	6
Fertility awareness	25	1–9
Female sterilization	0.5	0.5
Male sterilization	0.5	0.5

Data are percentage of women becoming pregnant using a method for one year. Typical failure rate means that the method was not always used correctly and with every act of sexual intercourse. Lowest observed failure rate means the method was used correctly and with every act of sexual intercourse.

Source: U.S. Food and Drug Administration, 1998.

counseling and to be able to separate their own risk tolerance from that of their clients. This consideration is essential when helping clients choose methods that fit *their* needs and wants. Counselors are cautioned against accepting catchy phrases such as "zero risk tolerance" when counseling clients. Such phrases are great for marketing and public relations campaigns but might create more harm for clients by setting unrealistic expectations for success.

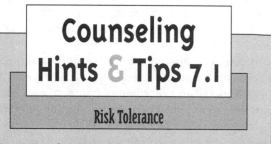

Counseling Hints & Tips 7.1

Risk Tolerance

Here are a few tips to help you remember how to communicate risk to clients:
1. Tell clients that all birth control methods involving penetration carry some risk of pregnancy. *None* is 100% effective in preventing pregnancy.
2. Ask clients what an acceptable percentage of risk for pregnancy is *for them,* at this stage of their lives.
3. *Never* assume that your tolerance for risk is the same (or should be the same) as that of your clients.
4. Explain to clients that risk tolerance varies over the course of one's sexual life cycle.

to have an 85% actual use effectiveness, meaning that 15% of the people who used it for one full year got pregnant while relying on it (Hatcher et al., 1998).

Pregnancy Risk

It is important for counselors to understand the concept of risk in the context of birth control

In essence, to live is to be at risk of injury, illness, and death. Every day we engage in activities associated with risk, from driving a car to engaging in recreational pursuits and hobbies. **Table 7.2** describes the risk of dying associated with some common activities. Even mundane things such as taking a shower involve some level of risk. Indeed, the risk of slipping in the tub or shower, falling, hitting one's head, and dying increases as we age. Risk of death is a reality of life. Our risk of dying naturally increases with our age. Most

Table 7.2

Relative Risks for Death from Various Activities Including Preventing Pregnancy

Risks Per Year for Men and Women of All Ages Who Participate in the Activities

Activity	Chance of Death in a Year
Motorcycling	1 in 1000
Automobile driving	1 in 5900
Power boating	1 in 5900
Rock climbing	1 in 7200
Playing football	1 in 25,000
Canoeing	1 in 100,000
Health Risks for Women	
Using tampons	1 in 350,000
Hysterectomy	1 in 1600
Risks for Women from Preventing Pregnancy	
Using oral contraceptives (nonsmoker)	1 in 66,700
Using oral contraceptives (<35 years old)	1 in 200,000
Using oral contraceptives (35–44 years old)	1 in 28,600
Using oral contraceptives (heavy smoker)	1 in 1700
Using IUDs	1 in 10,000,000
Using diaphragm, condom, or spermicides	None
Using fertility awareness methods	None
Undergoing sterilization (tubal ligation)	1 in 38,500
Risk from Terminating Pregnancy	
Legal abortion (<9 weeks)	1 in 262,800
Legal abortion (9–12 weeks)	1 in 100,100
Legal abortion (13–15 weeks)	1 in 34,400
Legal abortion (>15 weeks)	1 in 10,200
Risk of Continuing Pregnancy	1 in 10,000

Source: Adapted from Hatcher R, Guest F, Stewart G, et al. (1998). *Contraceptive Technology*, 17th ed., p. 230. New York: Ardent.

commonly accepted medical procedures—from having x-rays to undergoing local and general anesthesia—carry health risks that clients are willing to assume. They realize that the benefits associated with complying with these procedures outweigh the risks associated with not having them done.

When discussing the risks associated with birth control methods and preventing pregnancy, it is important to remember that being pregnant is also risky. In fact, carrying a pregnancy to term is associated with a greater risk of dying than any individual birth control method. No birth control method is 100% perfect and without risk. Two types of risks need to be discussed with clients: health risks and pregnancy risks. *Health risks* are associated with health problems that can arise as a result of combining clients' preexisting health status and medical history with the use of a specific contraceptive method. For example, the risk of acquiring pelvic inflammatory disease (PID), an infection of the upper reproductive tract, is greater for women who use intrauterine devices (IUDs) than for women who use other forms of birth control. *Pregnancy risk* is the risk associated with the method's theoretical and actual use effectiveness. In essence, it is the risk of getting pregnant while relying on the method.

Risk tolerance (and consequently the appeal of certain methods) changes over time. An acceptable level of risk for a single, 19-year-old woman just entering her second year of college might be very different from that for her married, 27-year-old sister who is well established in her career and at a different point in her life. The needs of their 47-year-old mother are even more different. Yet all of these women share one thing in common—the desire to prevent an unintended pregnancy.

Clients should review their fertility control needs periodically and make changes in their methods as necessary. It is not unusual for clients to try several different methods over the course of their reproductive lives.

Mechanisms of Action

Blonna and Levitan (2005) propose an interesting yet simple way to group fertility control methods according to how they work in preventing unintended pregnancy. They identify seven mechanisms of action:

1. *Provide nonpenetrative sexual pleasure.* This group of methods, sometimes called *outercourse,* provides options for the satis-

faction of sexual desire and orgasm that do not involve the penis penetrating the vagina. Methods in this category include kissing, hugging/rubbing, massage, masturbation, use of sex toys, and oral-genital sexual contact.

2. *Prevent sperm from meeting egg.* These methods work either by withdrawing the penis prior to ejaculation or by predicting ovulation and avoiding unprotected intercourse during fertile times.

3. *Provide barrier between sperm and egg.* This group of methods works by putting a mechanical or chemical barrier between the sperm and the egg. These barriers prevent the sperm and egg from uniting in the fertilization process. Such methods include male condoms, female condoms, diaphragms, contraceptive sponges, cervical caps, and various types of chemical spermicides.

4. *Prevent implantation.* Methods in this group work by preventing the implantation of a possibly fertilized egg in the uterine lining. They encompass intrauterine devices (IUDs) and emergency contraceptives.

5. *Prevent release of egg.* This group of methods works by suppressing ovulation through alteration of the hormonal balance in the body. Changing the hormonal balance in the bloodstream prevents the pituitary gland from chemically triggering the release of an egg from the ovary. Methods in this group include oral contraceptives (birth control pills), hormonal injections (Depo Provera shot), hormonal cervical rings (NuvaRing), and hormonal release patches (Evra patch).

6. *Surgically block passage of sperm or egg.* Methods in this category work by sealing off the main egg and sperm transport routes (fallopian tubes and vas deferens, respectively). Female (tubal ligation) and male (vasectomy) sterilization procedures belong in this group.

7. *Terminate an established pregnancy.* This group consists of methods that end an es-

tablished pregnancy. Methods include medical and surgical abortion.

The fertility control options available under each mechanism of action present distinct advantages to clients depending on a host of factors ranging from level of effectiveness to cost. The relative attractiveness of one method over another will also vary according to where clients are in their reproductive life cycle. We will discuss these issues later in this chapter.

Methods Associated with Each Mechanism of Action

Nonpenetrative Behaviors

Nonpenetrative sexual behaviors that can be used to control fertility include massage, masturbation, outercourse, and anything else that doesn't involve vaginal penetration (McDonough, 1995). It is important for clients (especially sexually inexperienced ones) to understand that there are many ways to enjoy sexual pleasure without risking pregnancy. The actual use effectiveness of sexual activities that do not involve vaginal penetration has not been established. Their effectiveness lies in their theoretical attributes. If vaginal penetration doesn't occur, no mechanism is available for live sperm to reach a mature ovum. Theoretical effectiveness, therefore, should approach 100%.

Unprotected anal intercourse is not included in this group because, although it doesn't involve vaginal penetration, the close proximity of the anus could permit migration of fluids across the perineum and into the vagina. Ejaculating near the vagina is discouraged for this reason.

Celibacy/Abstinence

The first category of nonpenetrative methods comprises celibacy and abstinence. Blonna and Levitan (2005) point out that while these two terms are often used interchangeably, their meanings are distinctly different. Although the literal definition of **celibacy** is avoidance of sexual relations, the term is usually associated with a religious decision not to marry. **Abstinence** refers to practicing self-restraint. It is often taken to mean not having sexual intercourse. Although clients often assume that celibacy and abstinence mean total avoidance of all forms of sexual release, in fact people can be celibate or abstain from sexual intercourse but still masturbate or use other forms of nonpenetrative behaviors to release sexual tension (Norris, 1996).

Case Study 7.1
Susan: Choosing to Be Celibate

Susan, 31, is a divorced white female who identifies as a bisexual. Here is her story.

I've been celibate for the past year and a half. I'm 31 years old, have a 5-year-old daughter, work full-time, and go to school full-time. Things just never worked out with my daughter's father and ever since I've been back to school, I haven't had the energy to even think about sex. My schedule is crazy and I don't have much free time. When I have time off, I prefer to spend it with my daughter. I don't have the time to spend on cultivating a relationship. I really want to finish school and get good enough grades to get into graduate school someday.

I don't miss intercourse. It's not that I don't like sex. Before I got married, I used to really get off on sex with both men and women. My sex life with my daughter's father was really great, and eventually I stopped having sex with anyone else but him and got pregnant. Things between us were never the same after that. Since we split up, I've just been burned out on the idea of starting a new relationship. I masturbate a couple of times a week and prefer to deal with my sexual needs that way. I can see this changing someday and hope to meet a woman who can love and satisfy me and love my daughter. For now, though, I'm not looking for a relationship.

Kissing/Hugging/Massage

Kissing can provide intense sensual and sexual delight while imposing no risk for pregnancy. Kissing is often associated with hugging, rubbing, and massage. Once commonly referred to as petting, these activities can be carried to the point of orgasm with no risk of pregnancy. With a little imagination, these safe sex activities can be erotic and provide a satisfying outlet for sexual desire by themselves or when other fertility control methods are unavailable.

Masturbation

Although masturbation is usually associated with solo sexual activity, it is an excellent way to share an orgasm with a partner without worrying about conception. Masturbation can offer a break from having to worry about who is supplying the contraception.

Sex Toys

Sex toys such as vibrators and dildos come in a variety of shapes and sizes. They offer a safe, low pregnancy risk, sexual option (Davis et al., 1996).

Oral-Genital Sexual Behavior

The various forms of oral-genital sexual contact (**fellatio, cunnilingus, anilingus**) offer a sexual option with low risk for pregnancy. Unlike abstinence and nonpenetrative sexual behavior, however, oral-genital sexual contact can pose risks of disease transmission. These activities should never be practiced without barrier protection if engaged in with anyone except a disease-free partner.

Methods That Prevent Sperm from Reaching Eggs

There are two nonsurgical methods that work by preventing sperm from reaching eggs: coitus interruptus and fertility awareness (Blonna & Levitan, 2005).

Coitus Interruptus (Withdrawal, Pulling Out)

Coitus interruptus, also known as withdrawal or pulling out, is one of the most commonly used and least understood of all fertility control strategies. The actual use effectiveness of coitus interruptus ranges from 65% to 70%. Three factors seem to contribute to the relatively low actual use effectiveness: human error (not withdrawing the penis in time), method failure (sperm present in pre-ejaculatory fluid), and using the method during peak fertility (mid-cycle versus other times during a woman's menstrual cycle) (Blonna & Levitan, 2005; Hatcher et al., 1998). More than half of all couples around the world use coitus interruptus as their primary method of fertility control (Hatcher et al., 1998). Although most counselors would consider 65%–70% actual use effectiveness to be unacceptably low, clients must understand that this is significantly better than the 5% level of effectiveness associated with chance.

Fertility Awareness

Fertility awareness is also known as natural family planning and the rhythm method. This strategy relies on avoiding unprotected intercourse during days of peak fertility. Peak fertility can be estimated by combining knowledge about an individual woman's menstrual cycle with the latest scientific findings about egg and sperm viability. The four fertility awareness methods are calendar, basal body temperature, cervical mucus, and combined. Actual and theoretical use effectiveness data are available for both individual fertility awareness methods and the combined method.

Methods That Provide Barriers Between Sperm and Egg

Barrier methods are among the oldest and most well-known methods used to control fertility. They derive their names from their mechanism of action: They work by literally placing a mechanical, chemical, or combination-type barrier between the sperm and the egg. Mechanical devices use latex and polyurethane barriers to cover the penis (male condom), line the vagina (female condom), or protect the cervix (diaphragm, cervical cap). Chemical devices provide a spermicidal barrier that covers the cervix (foam, suppositories, film) or are used in combination with a mechanical device (gel/diaphragm or cap, spermicide impregnated in sponge, or spermicidal lubricant for condoms).

Male Condom

The male condom is one of the oldest known fertility devices. Three types of condoms are currently available in the United States: latex, polyurethane, and natural lamb membrane (Nelson, Hatcher, Zieman, et al., 2000). Condoms are available in different colors, sizes, shapes, and flavors. Each type is manufactured under stringent quality controls and regularly inspected for leaks and other damage. For a batch of condoms to be legally sold, only four defects in 1000 condoms are allowed. If more than one defective condom is found, the entire batch is destroyed (*Consumer Reports*, 1995).

Putting on a Condom
For pleasure, ease, and effectiveness, both partners should know how to put on and use a condom. To learn without feeling pressured or embarrassed, practice on your penis or a penis-shaped object, such as a ketchup bottle, banana, cucumber, or squash.

Remember: Practice Makes Perfect
- Put the condom on before the penis touches the vulva. Men leak fluids from their penises before and after ejaculation. Pre-ejaculate ("pre-cum") can carry enough sperm to cause pregnancy and enough germs to cause STDs.
- Use a condom only once. Use a fresh one for each erection ("hard-on"). Have a good supply on hand.
- Condoms usually come rolled into a ring shape. They are individually sealed in aluminum foil or plastic. Be careful—don't tear the condom while unwrapping it. If it is brittle, stiff, or sticky, throw it away and use another.
- Put a drop or two of lubricant inside the condom.
- Place the rolled condom over the tip of the hard penis.
- Leave one-half inch of space at the tip to collect semen.
- If the penis is not circumcised, pull back the foreskin before rolling on the condom.
- Pinch the air out of the tip with one hand. (Friction against air bubbles causes most condom breaks.)
- Unroll the condom over the penis with the other hand.
- Roll it all the way down to the base of the penis.
- Smooth out any air bubbles.
- Lubricate the outside of the condom.

Taking off a Condom
- Pull out before the penis softens.
- Don't spill the semen—hold the condom against the base of the penis while you pull out.
- Throw the condom away.
- Wash the penis with soap and water before embracing again.

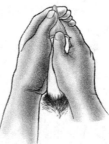

(a)

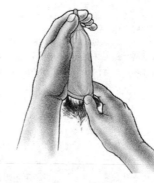

(b)

Figure 7.1 How to put on a male condom. (*Source:* Planned Parenthood Federation of America, Inc. http://www.plannedparenthood.org/.)

The theoretical effectiveness of condoms is 97%, as the stringent manufacturing standards ensure uniformly high quality. Actual use effectiveness is 88%. The disparity between actual use and theoretical effectiveness is attributed mostly to human error regarding storage and application. Counseling Hints 7.2 provides some ideas regarding how to make condom use more attractive to clients.

Female Condom

The female condom is a loose-fitting pouch that is inserted into the vagina, covering its walls and protruding over the vulva (see **Figure 7.2**). Female condoms are made from a polyurethane material that is similar to latex but less penetrable and are lubricated with a spermicide. The female condom works by containing a man's semen after he ejaculates into his partner's vagina. It also offers protection against sexually transmitted disease (STD) infectious agents that might be in the man's semen or emanate from penile lesions (Hatcher et al., 1998)

Female condoms are uniform in size and have a ring at both ends that helps with insertion and ensures a proper fit. The theoretical effectiveness of female condoms is 95%; actual use effectiveness is 79% (Hatcher et al., 1998).

Communicating about condoms is essential to their effective use. Often, sexual communication is more of a challenge because of the way men

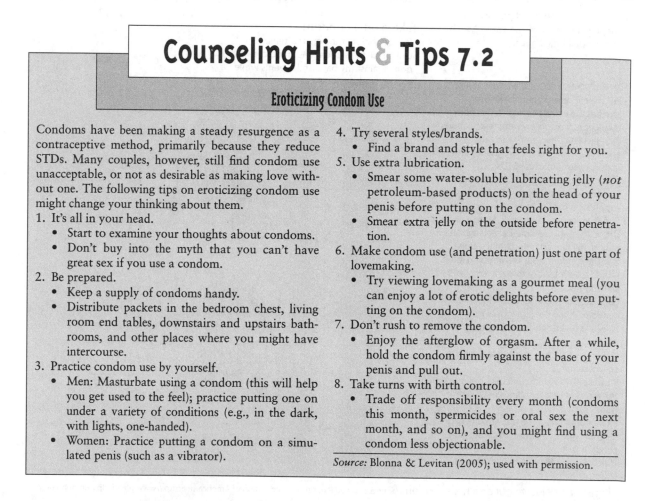

Counseling Hints & Tips 7.2

Eroticizing Condom Use

Condoms have been making a steady resurgence as a contraceptive method, primarily because they reduce STDs. Many couples, however, still find condom use unacceptable, or not as desirable as making love without one. The following tips on eroticizing condom use might change your thinking about them.

1. It's all in your head.
   - Start to examine your thoughts about condoms.
   - Don't buy into the myth that you can't have great sex if you use a condom.
2. Be prepared.
   - Keep a supply of condoms handy.
   - Distribute packets in the bedroom chest, living room end tables, downstairs and upstairs bathrooms, and other places where you might have intercourse.
3. Practice condom use by yourself.
   - Men: Masturbate using a condom (this will help you get used to the feel); practice putting one on under a variety of conditions (e.g., in the dark, with lights, one-handed).
   - Women: Practice putting a condom on a simulated penis (such as a vibrator).
4. Try several styles/brands.
   - Find a brand and style that feels right for you.
5. Use extra lubrication.
   - Smear some water-soluble lubricating jelly (*not* petroleum-based products) on the head of your penis before putting on the condom.
   - Smear extra jelly on the outside before penetration.
6. Make condom use (and penetration) just one part of lovemaking.
   - Try viewing lovemaking as a gourmet meal (you can enjoy a lot of erotic delights before even putting on the condom).
7. Don't rush to remove the condom.
   - Enjoy the afterglow of orgasm. After a while, hold the condom firmly against the base of your penis and pull out.
8. Take turns with birth control.
   - Trade off responsibility every month (condoms this month, spermicides or oral sex the next month, and so on), and you might find using a condom less objectionable.

Source: Blonna & Levitan (2005); used with permission.

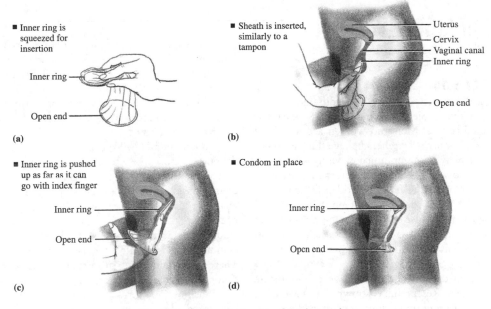

- Inner ring is squeezed for insertion
  - Inner ring
  - Open end

(a)

- Sheath is inserted, similarly to a tampon
  - Uterus
  - Cervix
  - Vaginal canal
  - Inner ring
  - Open end

(b)

- Inner ring is pushed up as far as it can go with index finger
  - Inner ring
  - Open end

(c)

- Condom in place
  - Inner ring
  - Open end

(d)

Figure 7.2 How to insert a female condom.

and women communicate. Diverse Perspectives 7.1 describes some of these differences.

Diaphragm

The diaphragm is a spring-loaded, rubber or plastic, nonlubricated dome that is inserted into the vagina and is anchored between the wall of the vagina and the cervix. Prior to insertion, spermicidal jelly must be placed around the rim and on the inside of the dome for it to work properly. The diaphragm is not designed to form an impenetrable barrier against the cervix. It works by covering the cervix, thereby blocking sperm's access to the egg. Any sperm that are able to get around the edge of the diaphragm are immobilized by the spermicide contained in the dome (Hatcher et al., 1998). Diaphragms are available by prescription only and must be fitted by an experienced healthcare professional. Their theoretical effectiveness is 97%. Their actual use effectiveness is 82%—slightly lower than that of the male condom. As with condoms, the dropoff in effectiveness primarily results from human error associated with incorrect and inconsistent use (Hatcher et al., 1998).

Cervical Cap

The cervical cap is a small, thimble-shaped plastic or rubber cap that fits snugly against the cervix through suction. It is available in four sizes and must be prescribed and fitted by a healthcare professional. It works in a fashion similar to the diaphragm, blocking the passage of sperm while utilizing spermicidal jelly as a backup to immobilize sperm that may enter around its rim. The theoretical effectiveness of the cervical cap is comparable to that of other vaginal barrier methods—namely, the female condom, diaphragm, and sponge (Hatcher et al., 1998).

Vaginal Contraceptive Sponge

The vaginal sponge is a soft, white, polyurethane sponge impregnated with spermicide. It works the same way as the diaphragm and cervical cap: It creates a double barrier (absorbent polyurethane sponge and spermicide) that blocks and absorbs

He Said/She Said

Do men and women communicate differently? Research about this subject over the past 20 years has yielded mixed results. Men and women are socialized differently, and many researchers believe this difference emerges in the way we communicate. Many women are socialized to show their feelings, whereas men are typically taught to keep their feelings hidden (Machaud & Warner, 1997). Men are taught to keep their fears and doubts disguised, because showing these vulnerabilities is considered a sign of weakness. Men are also socialized to believe that admitting weakness is unmanly (Tannen, 1990).

These beliefs can affect the way we communicate with our partners. Research has shown that wives send clearer and more emotional messages than their husbands (Noller & Fitzpatrick, 1991). Wives tend to frame their message in an emotional context, whereas husbands deemphasize affect and focus instead on issues and facts. Husbands send more neutral, less expressive messages that are more difficult to interpret (Tannen, 1990). Machaud and Warner (1997) found that men and women communicate differently when dealing with problems. When dealing with "troubles talk," these researchers found that women were much more likely to offer sympathy than men. Men were much more likely to tell a joke. Women were typically supportive, while men sought to avoid the trouble. Lastly, Tannen (1990) found that women were much more likely to listen as a way to offer support, while men were much more likely to try to "solve" the problem by offering advice.

McGinty et al. (2003) found that female college students were more likely to engage in nonverbal feedback and were more proficient at using it than their male counterparts. Female college students in their study were also more proficient at decoding nonverbal feedback than the males who participated. In the same study, males and females also differed in how they communicated based on the nature of the relationship. There were significant differences in the communication patterns of students in "involved" versus "casual" relationships. The former group was significantly more concerned about nonverbal communication than the latter group. The involved students also demonstrated greater skill in communicating nonverbally with their partners than the casual daters (McGinty, Knox, & Zusman, 2003). Involved daters were also "less confused" about their communications than the casual daters and reported "working harder" on communicating (both verbally and nonverbally) clearly.

Source: Blonna & Levitan (2005); used with permission.

---

sperm while chemically deactivating them. Like the diaphragm and cervical cap, the sponge can be inserted as long as 6 hours before intercourse. Unlike the other methods, the sponge can be left in place for 24 hours and used more than once without any need for additional applications of spermicide. The vaginal contraceptive sponge is similar in effectiveness to the diaphragm and the cervical cap. Its theoretical effectiveness is 96%, and actual use effectiveness is 84% (Hatcher et al., 1998).

Chemical Spermicides

A wide variety of chemical spermicides are available as stand-alone fertility control methods or for use in conjunction with mechanical barriers as previously discussed. They all work by immobilizing and killing sperm, though they vary in form and method of application. Spermicides are available as nonprescription fertility control devices at most drug stores. The best-known forms are films, foams, gels, and creams. They work by creating a chemical barrier suspended in either a shaving-cream-like foam, clear gel, or smooth cream. All are inserted deep into the vagina, near the cervix (see **Figure 7.3**). They create an immediate, effective chemical barrier against sperm. These spermicides may be inserted no more than 30 minutes prior to intercourse (Hatcher et al., 1998).

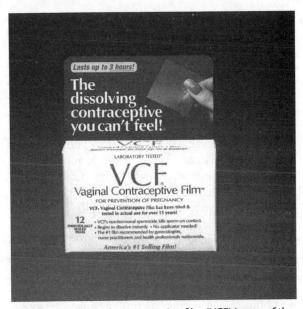

Figure 7.3 Vaginal contraceptive film (VCF) is one of the least messy types of chemical spermicides available for use. (*Source:* VCF Vaginal Contraceptive Film. Courtesy of Apothecus Pharmaceutical Corp. Reprinted with permission.)

Methods That Prevent Implantation of a Fertilized Egg

Intrauterine Devices

The IUD is designed to prevent implantation of a fertilized egg. Recent studies show that IUDs also work by slowing sperm down and keeping them from reaching viable ova (Hatcher et al., 1998).

IUDs are available only by prescription. These pieces of plastic are inserted into the uterus by a gynecologist or other trained reproductive health-care professional. The three models currently available for use in the United States are T-shaped and covered with a layer of either synthetic progesterone or copper.

The presence of the IUD within the uterus triggers the inflammatory response, and the synthetic progesterone or copper produces biochemical changes within the uterus and fallopian tubes. Theoretical effectiveness and actual use effectiveness of IUDs are similar: Theoretical use effectiveness is approximately 99%; actual use effectiveness is 97%.

Most of the failure associated with IUD use has to do with the body's attempt to reject the device through uterine contractions.

The IUD is best suited for a woman who already has given birth to at least one child. Women who have never been pregnant tend to experience more severe cramping, as the uterus becomes accustomed to the presence of this device. Many IUD users report heavier than normal menstrual flow. The IUD is not recommended for women with a history of **pelvic inflammatory disease (PID)**, as they are eight times more likely than women who have never had PID to experience a second episode if they use an IUD (Hatcher et al., 1998).

Methods That Prevent the Release of Ova

The methods that prevent the release of an egg comprise hormonal contraceptives. Oral hormonal contraceptives, also known as birth control pills, come in two types: **combination pills** and **minipills.** Combination pills combine synthetic estrogen and progesterone. Minipills contain progesterone only (Hatcher et al., 1998).

Combination pills are the most commonly used oral contraceptives. They work in several ways, though their main action is to suppress ovulation by elevating estrogen levels within the bloodstream. An abnormally high level of estrogen inhibits the secretion of follicle-stimulating hormone (FSH), which is necessary for the release of a mature ovum. Progestin, the artificial progesterone in combination pills, provides additional protection by keeping the cervical mucus thick. This makes it harder for sperm to penetrate the cervix. Oral contraceptives are highly effective in controlling fertility. Their theoretical effectiveness is greater than 99%; their actual use effectiveness is 97%. The dropoff is associated with human error—that is, failing to take pills consistently and correctly (Hatcher et al., 1998).

Progesterone-only minipills are meant to be taken every day. The same precautions and instructions for missed combination pills apply to minipills. Progestin, the same artificial progesterone used in combination pills, is taken by itself. Its action in minipills is identical to the way it works in combination pills: It keeps cervical mucus thick and alters the composition of the endometrium, reducing the likelihood of fertilization and implantation (Hatcher et al., 1998).

The **hormonal contraceptive patch** administers hormones through the skin, and is reported to be as effective as birth control pills. The patch is thin, is beige in color, and measures 1.75 inches on each side (see **Figure 7.4**). A woman wears a patch for one week, replaces it on the same day for three consecutive weeks, and goes "patch free" during the fourth week (Ortho-McNeil Pharmaceutical, 2003). The patch is contraindicated for the same women who are at risk for using birth control pills. Its effectiveness for pregnancy prevention is high (99% theoretical effectiveness), but it offers no protection against STDs (Ortho-McNeil Pharmaceutical, 2003).

The **hormonal contraceptive ring**, like all hormonal contraceptives, works on the principle of a woman having a 28-day menstrual cycle: three weeks of hormonal control followed by one week where the reduced endometrium is shed. The hormonal contraceptive ring appears similar to the plastic ring at the end of the female condom, and is inserted by the woman deep into the vagina, where it remains for three weeks. At the

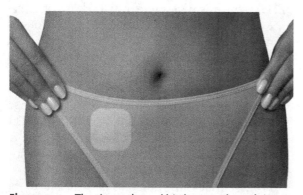

Figure 7.4 The time-released birth control patch is an innovative way to deliver hormonal contraception. (*Source:* Courtesy of Ortho-McNeil Pharmaceutical, Inc.)

end of the three-week period, it is removed by hooking the index finger under the ring and pulling it out.

The **hormonal contraceptive shot** is a progestin-only hormonal contraceptive. Its action is the same as that of the minipill. A major advantage of the shot over the other hormonal methods is the way in which it is administered. An injection is given every three months. The injections can be administered in either the arm or the buttocks. A single injection provides three months' worth of protection (Hatcher et al., 1998).

The **emergency contraception pill,** commonly called the "morning-after pill," is a combination of synthetic estrogen and progestin. It is designed to be administered under medical supervision within 72 hours after unprotected intercourse. The early administration of the pills works to prevent the release of an ovum, or slow the movement of the ovum, or prevent implantation (Hatcher et al., 1998).

Methods That Prevent Sperm from Reaching Egg (Surgical)

The surgical **sterilization** methods that prevent sperm from reaching the ova consist of **vasectomy** and **tubal ligation.** Sterilization does not prevent sperm and ova from being released. Rather, it blocks the path of either the sperm or the egg as a result of surgical removal of a small section of the vas deferens (vasectomy) in the male or fallopian tubes (minilaparotomy and tubal ligation) in the female (see **Figure 7.5**). The ends of the vas deferens and fallopian tubes are either folded back and sewn shut or cauterized.

Ova or sperm that are produced after sterilization cannot continue their journey, so they die, break down, and are excreted from the body as waste products. Both male and female sterilization have theoretical and actual use effectiveness rates exceeding 99%. Once the surgery has been performed, the user has to do nothing more to ensure safe, effective fertility control. All sterilization procedures should be viewed as permanent,

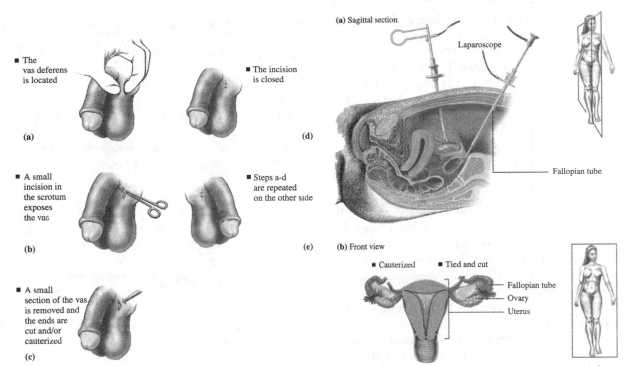

The vas deferens is located

(a)

A small incision in the scrotum exposes the vas

(b)

A small section of the vas is removed and the ends are cut and/or cauterized

(c)

The incision is closed

(d)

Steps a-d are repeated on the other side

(e)

(a) Sagittal section

Laparoscope

Fallopian tube

(b) Front view

Cauterized   Tied and cut

Fallopian tube
Ovary
Uterus

Figure 7.5 Of the two procedures, male vasectomy is cheaper, is easier to perform, and does not require an overnight hospital stay.

because once these structures have been surgically altered, there is no guarantee that they can be rejoined (Hatcher et al., 1998).

Methods That Terminate an Established Pregnancy

This group consists of methods that end an established pregnancy. It includes both medical and surgical abortion.

Abortion is defined as the termination, either spontaneous or induced, of an established pregnancy.

About one-third of all abortions are spontaneous abortions, also known as miscarriages. They result from a variety of conditions, ranging from physical trauma to a breakdown of the uterine lining. Induced abortions account for the remaining two-thirds of abortions. They involve re-

moving the lining of the uterus after pregnancy has been established. This procedure removes not only the endometrium but also the placenta and embryo or fetus. Abortion procedures are of several types, with their distinctions being related to the length of the pregnancy and other extenuating circumstances (Blonna & Levitan, 2005).

Surgical Abortion Methods

There are four major types of surgical abortions: (1) vacuum aspiration, (2) dilation and curettage (D&C), (3) dilation and evacuation (D&E), and (4) hysterotomy.

Vacuum aspiration is the most widely used procedure for early abortions. It can be performed in a medical office or clinic for pregnancies less than 14 weeks' gestation (Hatcher et al., 1998). It can be carried out as outpatient surgery under local anesthesia and does not require an overnight stay in a hospital. The cost for the procedure varies between $225 and $575.

A vacuum aspiration abortion usually takes approximately 10 minutes. It is safe and usually causes few side effects. The cervix is dilated, and a vacuum tube is inserted into the cervix. At the end of the tube is a **cannula,** which is attached to a vacuum pump (aspirator). This pump is used to suction off the contents of the wall of the uterus (endometrium, fetus/embryo, and placenta).

Dilation and curettage (D&C) is performed from the end of the first month of pregnancy throughout the first trimester and is similar to vacuum aspiration. Instead of using a cannula, however, it relies on both suction and the use of a curette—a narrow metal loop—to clean the walls of the uterus (Planned Parenthood Federation of America, 2002).

Dilation and evacuation (D&E) combines the two previously described techniques and can be used in abortions up to the fifth month of gestation. The cervix is dilated and most of the contents of the uterus are removed through suction. In preparation for the procedure, practitioners may insert a laminaria 6–24 hours prior to the D&E; the laminaria is made of dried seaweed, which expands and gently dilates the woman's cervix. Two other synthetic dilators, Lamicel and Dilapan, have also been used. They have the advantage of producing faster cervical dilation (Hatcher et al., 1998).

Because of the more advanced stage of fetal development at this point in gestation, not all of the uterine contents can be removed through aspiration alone. A curette is inserted, and the remaining uterine contents are scraped out. General anesthesia or a paracervical block is required for the procedure (Blonna & Levitan, 2005).

Hysterotomy is a major surgical procedure used in second-trimester pregnancies. It is similar to a cesarean section. An incision is made through the abdomen and uterus, and the fetus is removed and destroyed. This surgery requires general anesthesia and a hospital stay of several days. It is not used very often (Planned Parenthood, 2002).

Healthy People 2010 Leading Health Indicators

Responsible Sexual Behavior (Unintended Pregnancy)

Health Implications of Irresponsible Sexual Behavior: Unintended Pregnancy

Unintended pregnancies and **sexually transmitted diseases (STDs),** including infection with the human immunodeficiency virus (HIV) that causes AIDS, can result from unprotected sexual behaviors. Abstinence is the only method of complete protection. Condoms, if used correctly and consistently, can help prevent both unintended pregnancy and STDs. In 1999, 85% of adolescents abstained from sexual intercourse or used condoms if they were sexually active. In 1995, 23% of sexually active women reported that their partners used condoms (USDHHS, 2003).

While unintended pregnancy rates in the United States have been declining for the past two decades, nearly half of all pregnancies in the country are unintended; that is, at the time of conception the pregnancy was not planned or not wanted. The highest rates of unintended pregnancy occur among teenagers, women aged 40 years or older, and low-income African American women. Approximately 1 million teenage girls each year in the United States have unintended pregnancies. The economic costs associated with unintended adolescent pregnancy are estimated to be between $7 billion and $15 billion per year (USDHHS, 2003).

Objectives for the Nation

- Increase the proportion of adolescents who abstain from sexual intercourse or use condoms if currently sexually active
- Increase the proportion of sexually active persons who use condoms

Medical Abortion

Medical abortions do not involve surgical intervention but rather the use of medications to terminate a pregnancy. These nonsurgical abortions can be induced by administering agents that work in one of two ways: (1) by causing the uterus to contract and expel its contents, or (2) by initiating the breakdown of the endometrium, making it impossible to sustain the pregnancy.

RU-486 is the drug mifepristone, which was introduced in the United States in 2000 with the brand name Mifeprex. This antiprogesterone agent works by blocking the absorption of progesterone, the hormone necessary for continued viability of the endometrium. If progesterone is blocked, the uterine lining will no longer support fetal development. A second drug, misoprostol (a type of prostaglandin), is administered 3–7 days later and produces uterine contractions. These contractions cause the uterine lining and products of conception to be sloughed off within 24 hours (Nelson et al., 2000).

Case Study 7.2
Luz

Luz is a 23-year-old single heterosexual who identifies as Latina. Luz is a first-semester senior in a New York City metropolitan-area public college. She was referred for birth control counseling from her college health center after a recent pregnancy scare. Luz works 25 hours per week as a music production assistant for a major record label based in New York. She is on schedule to graduate from college in the spring with a bachelor's degree in music management. Her ultimate goal is to own her own record company specializing in Latina music.

Communicating About Sexuality and Birth Control

Communication encompasses a whole range of issues, from emotional comfort and security, to cultural considerations, to discrete behavioral skills. Sexual communication poses unique challenges because the difficulty of communicating in general is compounded by the personal nature of sexuality. Communicating effectively requires skill, patience, and commitment as well as an understanding and mastery of sexual information. Honest and accurate sexual communication is essential in developing and maintaining good relationships and in fostering consistent and correct use of birth control (Blonna & Levitan, 2005).

Sexual Vocabulary

One thing that makes sexual communication difficult is the lack of a common sexual vocabulary in our culture. The United States has no uniform set of agreed-upon words, phrases, and sexual language level. Often we are unsure of the proper terminology for sexual topics such as anatomy and physiology and sexual behaviors. Insecurity about sexual terminology, coupled with emotional discomfort, makes talking about sex difficult.

Language level plays a part in effective sexual communication. Mandel (1981) identified four levels of language that make influence sexual communication:

1. *Childhood language* is simple, cute, and fun to use when discussing sex. It can also be used to hide embarrassment about addressing sexual issues. Clients have their own pet names and phrases for sexual body parts and behaviors. Couples often communicate sexually using childhood language, especially when they are being playful with each other.
2. *Street language* is tough, expressive, and emotional. It can be disarming and often is used to level the playing field between counselors and clients who do not share equal power or prestige. Tough talk can bestow power and superiority. Street language also serves to create bonds between members of subcultures who share a language that members of mainstream society do not understand. Rap music incorporates the power and raw sensuality of street language into a unique art form.

3. *Common discourse* is the language level of mainstream society. It is the generally accepted form of language with which most people in a society communicate. It is taught in schools and runs through all subject matter. Unfortunately, because sex education is not taught in most public schools across the United States, students don't develop common discourse in sexuality.

4. *Scientific/professional language* is the discourse of the work world and professional community. It is the language that professional peers use as they communicate about the subtleties of their chosen professions. Like street language, it is usually understood only by those who share its culture.

When we communicate with clients about birth control and sexuality, we must use the level of language with which they are most comfortable. Miscommunication can occur when the language levels of the two parties are not the same. A common language level is a good starting point for effective sexual communication.

Counseling Clients About Birth Control Using Microskills

The overall goal of counseling clients about birth control is to help them pick methods that they will use consistently and correctly every time they have sexual intercourse (Hatcher et al., 1998). To achieve this goal, clients must choose methods that meet the following criteria:

1. The method is safe for them to use based on their personal health risks.
2. The method meets their criteria for an acceptable level of effectiveness and risk.
3. The method is a good fit for their sexual lifestyles.
4. They can afford to use the method.
5. The method is culturally acceptable to them.

Counselors must assess all of these issues before helping clients choose specific birth control methods. Counselors must avoid applying their own

standards for safety, effectiveness, and cultural acceptance when working with clients.

Introductory Skills

It is essential that counselors pay particular attention to their introductions when working with birth control clients, because this step is critical in establishing trust and setting a nonjudgmental tone that is essential to success in any form of counseling but particularly with any form of sex counseling.

Identify Yourself and Explain Your Role

Counseling birth control clients requires that counselors explore clients' sexual/medical histories in great detail. It is critical that counselors have a full understanding of clients' prior success and failures with birth control methods. This point needs to be explained to clients up front, so they have no misconceptions about what will be brought up and why it needs to be discussed. Counselors should be prepared to justify asking any sexual questions that clients might find objectionable. Try writing a script for this part of the introduction, then practice it until it becomes second nature to you. When introducing yourself, remember to extend your hand, make eye contact, and smile as you give the client a firm (but not crushing) handshake.

Example

Counselor: (Extending hand, smiling) Hi, I'm [name]. I'm one of the birth control counselors at the clinic. My job is to make sure you understand how all of the available methods work and how they fit your particular birth control needs. I also need to make sure you leave here with the ability to pick a method that you will use consistently and correctly, every time you have sex.

To do this, I must talk to you about some very personal issues related to your sex life. I am going to ask you about your current and past sexual relationships. I'm also going to ask you about the kinds of sexual activities you engage in, and the successes and failures you've had with birth control over the years. I am not asking about these issues to judge you. I need to know this information so I can help you pick the best method for you. Together we will work out a plan for helping you prevent unwanted pregnancy. I want you to understand that everything we say is confidential and will not be shared with anyone else.

Clarify the Client's Name

A simple way to verify the client's name is to use an open-ended statement before you sit down and begin your introduction.

Example

Counselor: (Before sitting and continuing the counselor says) And your name is . . . ?

Luz: My name is Luz.

Explain the Client's Role

After exchanging names and describing the counselor's role, explain the client's role. A simple explanation should include the three key elements of the client role discussed in Chapter 3: (1) active participation, (2) self-responsibility, and (3) honesty.

Example

Counselor: Luz, we just talked a little bit about my role in this process. Equally important is your role in this process. You need to be as open and honest as possible when talking with me. The only way I can help you find a birth control method that will work for you is if you are honest with me about your sex life. You'll have to take an active role in this process and take responsibility for choosing a method that best suits your needs. Together, we can find a method that will work best for you and prevent you from getting pregnant in the future.

Luz: Okay, I'll do my best.

Set Goals for the Session(s)

As mentioned earlier, the overall goal of counseling clients about birth control is to help them pick methods that they will use consistently and correctly every time they have sexual intercourse (Hatcher et al., 1998). To meet this goal, clients must choose methods that meet the following criteria:

1. The method is safe for them to use based on their personal health risks.
2. The method meets their criteria for an acceptable level of effectiveness and risk.
3. The method is a good fit for their sexual lifestyles.
4. They can afford to use the method.
5. The method is culturally acceptable to them.

In addition to this primary goal, counselors must assess clients' goals regarding birth control. The best way to deal with this issue is to describe your goals and assess your clients' needs.

Example

Counselor: Luz, there is one main goal that I have for our sessions together—helping you pick a birth control method that you will use consistently and correctly every time you have sexual intercourse. To meet this goal, I must make sure that you understand how several issues affect your ultimate choice. First, is the method safe for you to use based on your personal health risks? Second, does the method meet your criteria for effectiveness and risk? Third, is the method a good fit for your sexual lifestyle? Fourth, can you afford the method? Fifth, is the method culturally acceptable to you? What goals do you have for our sessions?

Give the client time to think this through before moving into the next part of the session.

Luz: I guess my main concern is making sure I don't get pregnant. What happened last month really scared me. It made me realize how close I came to getting pregnant. I couldn't stand to go through such uncertainty again.

Counselor: I can appreciate that. I'll do the best I can to help you find a method that gives you some peace of mind.

Transition to the Client's Story

A good way to make the transition from the introduction to getting clients to tell their stories is to use open-ended statements regarding what happened. Here are a few examples:

"Luz, why don't you tell me what led to you coming in to see me today."

"Luz, tell me a little bit about your experience with using birth control."

"Luz, tell me a little bit about your sex life for the past couple of years."

"Luz, tell me what you think your birth control needs will be over the next couple of years."

The idea in using these open-ended statements is to get clients talking about their knowledge of birth control as well as their sexual lifestyles. You can start with either, but understanding both of these components of the overall story is essential to meeting your goal for birth control counseling.

Example

Luz: I'm here today because I missed my period last month and thought I was pregnant. I'm very regular and when I missed my period I was really scared. I didn't know what to do and was afraid to talk to anyone about it, so I just kind of waited it out to see if it would come. I let four weeks go by before I actually went into the health center and had a test. I actually felt like I was gaining weight and had morning sickness. It was very freaky. When my test came back negative, the nurse at the health center referred me to you to be sure I got on some kind of birth control before I started having sex again.

Counseling Hints & Tips 7.3

Guidelines for Talking About Birth Control

Clients are often very apprehensive about discussing their sexual histories. Counselors must take extra care in providing a safe environment for clients to do so. The following general tips will help you create such an environment.

1. *Never assume anything.* Try not to stereotype clients based on physical appearance. Sexual interests, activity level, past experience, and a host of other relevant issues have little to do with external appearance. Don't even assume that your clients are heterosexual simply because they are coming to you for birth control advice.

2. *Ensure confidentiality.* Tell clients that everything you will discuss with them will be kept in the strictest confidence, even from their husbands, wives, and lovers. Demonstrate confidentiality by not talking to other clients on the telephone, discussing previous clients in the presence of your current one, or keeping existing clients' records on your desk for new clients to see.

3. *Be able to justify any question.* If you don't have a good reason to delve into certain sexual issues, don't go there. The purpose of asking about sexual stories is to help clients find methods that match their sexual lifestyle needs.

4. *Be nonjudgmental.* Birth control clients will often have sexual values, morals, and lifestyles that are different from those of their counselors. The counselor's job is to help clients by working within their personal sexual constructs to help them see and understand how their sexual lifestyle relates to their risk.

5. *Use the appropriate language level.* Try to use sexual terms that clients understand. Using a word like "coitus" instead of the more commonplace "intercourse," for instance, can create distance between you and the client.

Attending Skills

One of the most interesting (and challenging) things when counseling clients about birth control is the diversity of their birth control experiences. Listening to their stories will give you insights into the nature of their sexual/medical histories and how these relate to their current birth control needs. Central to these stories are sexual themes involving various combinations of settings, partners, and behaviors. It is essential that you set a nonjudgmental tone from the start while attending. Counseling Hints 7.3 describes a few key points to consider when eliciting clients' birth control stories.

Nonverbal Skills

As mentioned in Chapter 3, positive (open) body language is demonstrated by a relaxed posture, steady eye contact, nods of the head, and an occasional smile or happy expression. These cues signal that you are an approachable sender or a receptive receiver (McGinty et al., 2003).

Negative (closed) body language shows visible signs of tension, such as clenched fists or tight jaw muscles, a closed posture (arms folded, body shifted sideways), and facial expressions ranging from anger to disbelief. Negative body language can indicate a variety of things, from apathy or disturbance about something to something as simple as having to go to the bathroom.

When counseling clients about sex-related issues, it is very important that counselors pay particular attention to their own body language in addition to that of their clients. Clients' sexual knowledge, attitudes, values, and behaviors will often differ from those of counselors and might make them feel uncomfortable. It is important not to show this discomfort through nonverbal cues related to body language and eye contact.

Verbal Following Skills

A key aspect of verbally following birth control clients' stories is paying particular attention to sexual lifestyle issues. To help clients choose those birth control methods that best meet their sexual lifestyle needs, it is crucial to understand their sexual histories. It is important to pick up on clients' subtle nuances in language, such as the use of the plural form when discussing sex partners. Whether clients refer to one partner or to multiple partners will create an entirely different scenario for choosing an appropriate method of birth control. For example, clients with one monogamous partner have different contraceptive needs and options than clients with multiple, nonmonogamous partners.

Examples

Counselor: Luz, tell me a little about your sex life so I can understand your birth control needs.

Luz: Like what do you mean?

Counselor: You know, things like how long you have been having intercourse, your partners, birth control you've used in the past. Those kinds of things.

Luz: Well, the guys I have been having sex with really don't use birth control.

Counselor: Guys?

Luz: Whoa, it's not like I am some kind of a slut or anything.

Counselor: I didn't mean to imply that. I'm just trying to clarify that there is more than one guy we are talking about.

In this instance the client got a little defensive, so the counselor just reassured her about the purpose of the question. By closely verbally following Luz's own words, the counselor, at this early stage in hearing the story, was just picking up where Luz left off. The next logical step is to get Luz to continue her story by resuming her story where she stopped.

Example

Counselor: Luz, tell me more about these guys.

Luz: Right now, there are two guys I am involved with: this boy Raul from school, who I have been going with for about a year, and Randi (pause . . .), one of my managers from work.

Luz: (Continues in a lower, softer volume) Randi is married (pause . . .) but he's getting a divorce from his wife.

Vocal Tone

Try to match the tone and pace of clients' stories. Birth control clients experience a range of emotions regarding their infections, and they express these emotions in the way they tell their stories.

At this point Luz's tone is somewhat cautious. The pause in her speech indicates that she is testing the counselor regarding her relationship with Randi, a married man. Her pace is conversational and her vocal tone is even. While she is not rushing through her story or drawing it out with overly long pauses, her pace is guarded.

Luz's emotions regarding her story begin to show in her pace and volume. Clients who are emotionally upset might pause more frequently to compose themselves, get the courage to discuss painful issues, or assess how counselors react to what they are saying. For this reason, it is important to respond in a nonjudgmental way. The volume of clients' speech also tells counselors something about their stories. Luz's speaking more softly and at a lower volume imply that she might be feeling some embarrassment, guilt, or shame regarding her story. It is worth noting for later follow-up.

Example

Counselor: (In an even, moderate-volume, nonjudgmental tone) Tell me more about Raul and Randi.

Luz: I've known Raul since high school. He also goes to my college but we only started dating last year. We've been friends for a while. Last year when I broke up with Tommy, my long-term boyfriend from high school, Raul kind of stepped in.

Responding Skills

Nonverbal Minimal Encouragers

As mentioned in Chapter 4, nonverbal minimal encouragers include the following: (1) overall re- laxed open body posture; (2) facial expressions (e.g., nods, eyes, smile, eyebrows); and (3) hand gestures (roll hands to indicate "continue") (Engen & Albert, 1995; Ivey, Gluckstern, & Ivey, 1997a, 1997b). Liberal use of these nonverbal gestures indicate that you are listening, hear what clients are saying, and want them to continue. A client like Luz, who talks freely and easily, will often respond to these minimal efforts to get her to continue to tell her story

Verbal Minimal Encouragers

Combine the nonverbal minimal encouragers with verbal ones such as "ummm" or "uh huh," key words, and mirroring to show clients you are paying attention and understand their stories. Key words and mirroring are excellent techniques for getting clients to expand on sexual information. Their simplicity and absence of interpretation allow clients the opportunity to fully explain their situations without fear of being judged.

Example

Counselor: (In response to Luz's last statement, ". . . Raul kind of stepped in"). Stepped in. (Key words)

Luz: Yeah, I think he had been looking for an opportunity to hook up with me.

Counselor: Hook up.

Luz: Yeah, you know, have sex. I was feeling kind of lonely after my Tommy dumped me for some Anglo sorority girl Jessica. Raul, being Puerto Rican, like me, made me feel beautiful and wanted again. I slept with him on our first date.

Counselor: You slept with him on your first date. (Mirroring)

Luz: (Slightly blushing and turning her head a little) Yeah. It had been about two weeks since my boyfriend dumped me, and I was really missing him and the sex we had been having. When Tommy and I were together, we'd do it like four or five times a week. I was really missing this. Raul was real sweet and not pushy at all on our date, but I know he wanted me. We went to a party at his friend's fraternity and danced a little. When he held me, I could tell he was excited. I couldn't wait to take him back to my dorm room and get him in bed.

Counselor: Uh humm.

Luz: Yeah, he got so excited the first time, he pulled out after about 30 seconds and shot all over my leg.

Open Invitation to Talk

As mentioned in Chapter 4, using questions carefully is an excellent way to clarify clients' stories as well as keep them talking. From the case study, it is obvious that Luz is not having any major problems talking about her sexual history. A few well-placed questions at this point of the interview would be all that is necessary to get her to clarify ambiguous issues and to continue with her story.

Open-Ended Statements and Questions

Open-ended statements can be used to maintain a relaxed, conversational tone such as the one established with Luz. While there are lots of missing pieces to her story so far and much more to be told, it is better to proceed by asking the client one or two well-crafted open-ended statements than a series of yes/no direct questions.

Examples

The counselor might ask these questions

"Luz, tell me about your sex life with Raul."

"Luz, tell me about your relationship with Randi."

"Luz, tell me about your sexual relationship with your long-term boyfriend Tommy."

compared to these questions:

"Luz, when you have sex with Raul, do you have vaginal intercourse?"

"Luz, when you have sex with Raul, do you use birth control?"

"Luz, how often do you have sex with Raul?"

"Luz, when was the last time you had sex with Raul?"

"Luz, how many times have you had sex with Raul?"

"Luz, when you have sex with Randi, do you have vaginal intercourse?"

"Luz, when you have sex with Randi, do you use birth control?"

"Luz, how often do you have sex with Randi?"

"Luz, when was the last time you had sex with Randi?"

"Luz, how many times have you had sex with Randi?"

You can get the answers to these questions by asking each question directly, or you can ask one or two indirect, open-ended questions, listen to Luz describe her sexual behavior, and then follow this up with closed questions.

Example

Counselor: Luz, tell me a little more about your use of birth control with Raul.

Luz: We have mostly used rubbers and pulling out. When he has a condom, we'll use it. If not, he pulls out when he is about to come. He doesn't like to use condoms, but I usually insist.

Counselor: What do you mean "usually"?

Luz: When I remember to and when I haven't been drinking or doing weed.

Counselor: Tell me more about this.

Luz: Raul is kind of a street guy. He deals pot sometimes and usually has some. We like to get high together and have sex. The only problem is that it makes me very horny and I don't think so clearly. We also like to drink when we are partying. When I am drinking or smoking weed, I usually don't remember to bug him about using rubbers.

Counselor: About how often do you get high when you have sex?

Luz: Usually only on weekends. Monday through Thursday we have to be straight to get up for class and go to work. Neither of us works on the weekends, so we usually get high then.

Counselor: So how long has this been going on?

Luz: I guess for about six months.

Counselor: Tell me more about Randi.

Luz: Wow, I don't know, he is married and has a kid.

Counselor: Luz, I told you, everything we talk about is confidential. I am legally bound to protect your privacy.

Luz: Well, okay. Randi is a former pro football player who got into the music business about 10 years ago. He owns a small record label that specializes in mostly hip hop music, but he wants to expand into the Latin market. I met him doing an internship there for my college last semester. He is a really great guy. I've learned a lot from him about the business. He's going to help me launch my Latina record company some day.

Counselor: Tell me about your sexual relationship with him.

Luz: It started innocently enough. I must admit that I've always found him attractive but I didn't want to get involved with him because he was my internship supervisor and he's married. All last semester, everything was cool between us. We'd work late and talk and get to know each other. He's like 15 years older than me but really understands me.

   As the semester went along, I saw that things between him and his wife were not going so good. She is a West Coast lady. He met her when he played football in California, and she's from that area. She's a typical California beach bunny and hates the cold weather in New Jersey. She also doesn't dig the music scene and really hates all of his industry friends.

Counselor: Go on.

Luz: This semester he asked me to stay on and work there. This has nothing to do with school, he said, just business. He pays me really good money and I'm learning the business. So over the break we were working late and doing a little blow.

Counselor: Blow?

Luz: Cocaine. We were high and he came on to me big time, telling me how he loves my ass and I'm so sexy. He calls me his little JaLo. So I was kind of telling him to shut up and stop screwing around, when he stopped me, looked me in the eyes, and said he's stone-cold serious. He then said he's leaving his wife. One thing led to another, and before you know it we had our clothes off and were doing it right in the recording studio. I must admit, it was my secret sex fantasy come true.

Counselor: And since then?

Luz: We've been able to get together only a few times since then, because he's been on vacation in California with his family for the last couple of weeks. He wasn't around much for my pregnancy scare.

Counselor: Does he know about it?

Luz: Yeah, I thought he got me pregnant. Boy, was he relieved when he found out I wasn't. That was the final thing to get me in here. I can't screw around any more taking all these chances. I don't want to ruin my whole future and wind up being pregnant with some married man's child.

Paraphrasing, Reflection of Feelings, and Summarizing

Paraphrasing, reflection of feelings, and summarizing all work similarly for birth control clients as they do for other types of clients. Paraphrasing liberally throughout clients' stories helps counselors get a clear understanding of the events discussed before moving on to other issues and the feelings associated with the story. Effective paraphrasing leads to reflecting clients' feelings toward themselves, their partners, and the situation. Getting to the feelings associated with using a method consistently and correctly is essential if counselors are to help clients make truly informed choices about contraceptive methods.

   Remember that paraphrasing and reflecting feelings should occur throughout the responding part of the interview. After counselors have established trust with clients and given them ample opportunity to discuss their stories by using general attending skills and minimal encouragers, they should use paraphrasing and reflection of feelings regularly to make sure they understand the part of the story just discussed before moving on. Don't forget the three parts of effective paraphrases: (1) a shortened restatement of the client's statement in the counselor's words, (2) the use of key words from the client's story, and (3) the use of a "check it out" strategy by counselors (Engen & Albert, 1995).

Once clients' thoughts and feelings about their sexual lifestyles have been expressed, summarization helps clarify what they are thinking and feeling. Summarization provides another opportunity for them to hear the story again and decide whether anything needs to be added, deleted, or clarified. It also shows clients how well counselors are following their stories.

Example: Paraphrase (One Example of One Thing Discussed by Luz)

Counselor: Luz, let me be sure I understand what you are saying about Raul. You've known him a long time, but the first time you "hooked up" was last year after you broke up with Tommy. Is that right?

Luz: Yes, that's right.

Example: Reflection of Feelings (One Example)

Counselor: Luz, you seem pretty worried that your luck might be running out as far as not getting pregnant because you are not using birth control consistently.

Luz: (Nods her head affirmatively without speaking)

Example Summarization of the Entire Story

Counselor: Luz, before we move on to talk about anything else, let me make sure I understand where you are coming from. It seems that there are three main guys you've had sex with over the past couple of years. There's your ex-boyfriend, Tommy, with whom you haven't had sex in a year. Since your break-up, you've been having sex a few times a week with another old friend Raul and Randi, your boss, with whom you've had sex only a few times in the past two months. You like to get high when you have sex, and you use birth control less than half the time you have intercourse. You came in because your pregnancy scare was a final wake-up call to do something. Does this sound accurate?

Luz: Yeah, but when I hear it from someone else it sounds much worse.

Counselor: Much worse?

Luz: Yeah, I come across like some kind of dope-fiend sex addict or something.

Counselor: Is that how you feel?

Luz: No, I mean I like to get high once in a while and I like sex—I'm not denying this. In the past four years, though, I've really been with only three guys. Two of them—Tommy and Raul—I knew very well and was faithful to. This thing with Randi kind of swept me off my feet but I think I've landed. I mean, I've got big plans. I am going to make something of myself. I've worked too hard to let anything get in the way.

Counselor: Okay, Luz, I understand.

Influencing Skills

As mentioned earlier, the overall goal of counseling clients about birth control is to help them pick methods that they will use consistently and correctly every time they have sexual intercourse (Planned Parenthood, 2002). All of the influencing skills described in Chapter 5 come into play in trying to achieve this goal for clients.

Feedback and self-disclosure are both subtle influencing skills. They are used to help clients gain new insights into their own behavior and their counselor's experiences. Clients such as Luz, who seem concerned about how they are perceived by others, benefit from hearing objective feedback about their behavior. Such information, when presented in a supportive way, can be a source of strength in overcoming their problems or making positive lifestyle changes (Ivey & Ivey, 2003). Counselor self-disclosure about similar problems helps clients see their problems differently. Their struggles are no longer viewed as obstacles that cannot be overcome. Instead, clients see that even their counselors (who in clients' eyes are role models for mental health) had similar problems and overcame them. This leveling of the playing field between clients and counselors is empowering (Engen & Albert, 1995).

Feedback

Feedback consists of objective information about how the client is behaving. It differs from paraphrasing and summarizing in that the information counselors "feed back" to clients isn't about their stories, but rather about how they act and come off to others when telling their stories. Feedback can be positive or negative in nature. "Feeding back" can be a very powerful technique when clients hear things about themselves and the way they appear to others that they might never have considered or are new to them. In the last section of dialogue between Luz and her counselor, hearing the counselor's summary of her story was, in a sense, a form of feedback. Luz's reaction to it showed the counselor that she cared about how she came off to others. Clients who don't really care about such things will be less influenced by feedback than those who share Luz's concerns.

Example

Counselor: Luz, it's interesting because the words you use to describe my summary of your sexual lifestyle are "Yeah, I come across like some kind of dope-fiend sex addict or something." I don't believe you are either, but you do mix sex, drugs, and lack of birth control a lot, and those three things add up to a pretty high risk of unintended pregnancy.

Luz: I know. That is why I am here. I need to make some changes.

Self-disclosure

Recall from Chapter 5 that self-disclosure is the intentional sharing of counselors' personal information about themselves with their clients. It is not the same as the unintentional self-disclosure that goes on nonverbally between counselors and clients as they size each other up as a normal part of the counseling process. That kind of self-disclosure goes on despite the best efforts of counselors to remain neutral.

Counselors should keep the four guidelines for effective self-disclosure (see Counseling Hints 5.2) in mind when applying it to influencing birth control clients: Be intentional; keep it simple; stay parallel; and do not lie. Counselors need to remember that inappropriate self-disclosure shifts the focus of the story away from the client and toward the counselor.

Example: Appropriate Self-disclosure

Counselor: Luz, I know what you are feeling. I was in high school in the late sixties and in college during the seventies. Everyone was experimenting with drugs and sex, and it was pretty easy to get caught up in all of it. I went through more than one pregnancy scare myself after taking too many chances after getting high.

Luz: (In astonishment) I'd never have thought that. You kind of remind me of my grandmother.

Counselor: (Laughing) I'll take that as a compliment.

Luz: Sorry, I didn't mean to insult you.

Counselor: No insult taken, it's okay.

Changing the Focal Point

As discussed in Chapter 5, changing the focal point of the story is an excellent way to influence clients. Remember—focusing the narrative is a subtle skill designed to help clients open their minds to different ways of viewing their issue. Any (or all) of the seven major focal points discussed in Chapter 5 can be used to help clients see their problem from a variety of perspectives: (1) the individual focus, (2) the main theme or problem focus, (3) the family focus, (4) the other individual focus, (5) the mutuality focus, (6) the interviewer/counselor focus, and (7) the cultural or environmental context focus (Ivey & Ivey, 2003). Counselors decide which focal point(s) to explore based on information derived from their clients' stories. In Luz's case, it would be interesting for her to explore how the record industry or college campus culture/environments factor into her combining drugs, sex, and lack of birth control. It might also be interesting to ask her how she thinks her sex partners view these issues.

Example

Counselor: Luz, let's shift gears for a moment. I want you to think about your pattern of combining drug use with sex and nonuse of birth control. Tell me a little about sex, drugs, and rock and roll on campus nowadays.

Luz: Wow, I'm not really sure. I mean, I don't really party there much any more. I used to be so much more involved on campus than I am now. When I was a freshman and sophomore, I was really involved in the Latina Students Organization and a Latina sorority. I used to go to all of their functions and hang out at the student center with the girls. I've been way too busy to get involved with that for the past two years. I've been superbusy doing internships, working, and going to school full-time. I am really not that close to the sorority anymore. I mean, I still live on campus, but I am rarely there from Friday to Monday and I've been spending lots of nights sleeping in Raul's room.

Counselor: What is that like?

Luz: He shares a suite with three other guys. They are real low key because they sell pot and don't want to draw attention to their room. They all have girlfriends and don't throw loud parties or anything like that. I will usually smoke some herb with Raul and just hang out there. It is very mellow.

Counselor: Tell me about the music business.

Luz: Now that is another story. It is very wild. There are all kinds of drugs all over the place. There is this big cross-over with the business of making music and the business of distributing music. Our place is both a production studio and the headquarters for the record label, so we do everything from mix CDs to produce music videos to host gala release parties. There is always something happening 24 hours a day, seven days a week. The people who come in and out do all kinds of drugs to stay awake or mellow out. The drugs are not out in the open or on the table or anything like that, but everyone has access to a lot of different things at a moment's notice.

Counselor: How does that affect you?

Luz: It blew me away last semester. I got kind of into it but Randi sat me down after a month and told me I was starting to let him down. I wasn't doing my job. He let me know that although he couldn't control all of the outside people, he did have rules for his own staff: No drugs, nothing illegal on work time in his studio.

Counselor: What about his personal use of cocaine with you?

Luz: That was different. There was nobody around, just he and I, and it was kind of a spontaneous thing.

Counselor: Uh huh.

Confrontation

Ivey and Ivey (2003) view confrontation as "supportive challenge"—a skill used to help clarify clients' stories by pointing out any discrepancies, incongruities, or mixed messages that come up. As discussed in Chapter 5, many intentional and unintentional reasons explain why clients present discrepancies, incongruities, and mixed messages in their stories. Often, confronting these mismatches will illuminate the reasons for their use. In other cases, the reasons why clients use them are less important than their actual confrontation of those issues. Confrontation helps clients become more congruent by pointing out discrepancies, seeking clarification, and forcing them to rethink their behavior (Ivey & Ivey, 2003). If counselors use confrontation effectively, clients learn that incongruities, discrepancies, or mixed messages will not go unnoticed by counselors and they begin to become more genuine and less discrepant in their thoughts, feelings, and actions (Ivey et al., 1997a, 1997b; Engen & Albert, 1995). Ideally, this growth in learning how to deal with birth control issues will carry over into learning how to deal with other issues in their lives. A good way to employ confrontation is to use Ivey and Ivey's (2003) one hand, other hand technique.

Example

Counselor: (Continuing with Luz's story) Luz, on the one hand, you say that you don't party much when you are on campus. On the other hand, you spend a few nights a week smoking pot with a guy who deals drugs from his dorm suite. What does that mean?

Luz: Well, I guess because it is only the two of us, and sometimes maybe one of his roommates and his girl, it doesn't seem like a party to me.

Example

Counselor: Luz, on the one hand, you say that your drug use and partying on campus don't have a lot to do with your nonuse of birth control. On the other hand, you say that you are a lot less likely to use birth control when you are high.

Luz: Yeah, I guess I did say that. It almost seems that I get high and have unprotected sex more than I thought I did.

Example

Counselor: Luz, on the one hand, you say that Randi has these no-drug standards for his workplace. On the other hand, he produces some coke and the two of you get high and have sex at the studio?

Luz: I don't know what to say. I never really thought about it that way. I guess he had his own private stash at work.

As a result of these confrontations, Luz begins to see some of the discrepancies and incongruities in her life. The next step involves tying some of these threads together.

Eliciting and Reflecting Meaning

Eliciting and reflecting the meaning of a client's story is a skill that is used to get clients to uncover the meaning of their problems for themselves. Counselors ask clients to reflect on their thoughts, feelings, and behaviors and to interpret what all of it means to them. This technique is very similar to interpretation of meaning, in which counselors add their own interpretations of clients' stories. Eliciting and reflecting meaning are supposed to go beyond the mere restatement of the explicit facts of the stories and delve into their implicit meaning.

Example

Counselor: Luz, what do you think your current lack of use of birth control is all about?

Luz: I think I have never really assumed any responsibility for my behavior. I've always relied on the men in my life to do something to prevent me from getting pregnant. You know, using condoms and pulling out are the two things I've always used, and both of them rely on the guy.

Counselor: How do you feel about that?

Luz: I'm kind of embarrassed. Here I am, a senior in college, ready to make my mark on the world, and I haven't taken responsibility for my own body yet.

Counselor: That's okay. That is why you came in. You're ready to start taking charge.

Interpretation and Reframing

Interpretation of meaning and reframing are separate skills that are used together to influence clients. As noted earlier, interpretation of meaning is very similar to eliciting and reflecting feelings but is counselor directed. Reframing entails retelling the story with different meanings. It presents new meanings for clients to consider and helps them consider alternative ways of viewing and managing their problems. When interpreting and reframing clients' stories, counselors draw from their personal life experiences, their clinical experience, and the theoretical frameworks that guide their counseling. Different counselors will interpret and reframe clients' stories in different ways.

Example: Interpretation and Reframing

Counselor: Luz, I hear what you are saying about how you have never really taken responsibility for your birth control needs.

From what you have told me, I would agree with your assessment. I think the issue goes beyond this, however, and is compounded by your drug use. It is not uncommon for people to lose their inhibitions and self-control when under the influence of drugs. In fact, that is a major reason why people take psychoactive drugs, from alcohol to LSD—to lose control. You seem much less likely to use birth control when you use drugs, so I'd like you to consider the idea of combining these two issues. I want you to start viewing your drug use as part of your birth control needs, and not as a separate issue. How does that sound?

Luz: It makes sense, especially since I do like to combine the two. I rarely get high just to get high. I'd say about 90% of the time I've used drugs over the past year, it has been related to sex.

Counselor: Exactly. Maybe you can start thinking about methods that you can use that won't conflict with this aspect of your lifestyle. It also brings up a couple of other issues, like HIV and STD risk and how your illegal drug use can lead to other problems, such as getting arrested. I wouldn't be doing you any good if we didn't discuss these things in addition to birth control methods.

Luz: I understand.

Directives and Logical Consequences

Information giving, directives, and instruction giving form the heart of health counseling and distinguish it from more generic counseling. The main focus of health counseling is teaching clients how to manage, cure, or cope with their health problems.

A great deal of information related to birth control is readily available. The key to effective birth control counseling is delimiting that information. The type and quantity of information given to clients should focus on the goal of birth control counseling: helping clients pick methods that they will use consistently and correctly every time they have sexual intercourse.

Birth counselors can delimit the sheer volume of information without any loss of service to their clients by tailoring their information giving to clients' lifestyles. For instance, Luz clearly needs a birth control method that is very effective and continuous. She doesn't want to take any more chances and doesn't want a pregnancy to interrupt her future plans. It also seems that relying on situational methods, such as barrier methods, is not a good idea because of her mixing of drugs and sex. She also needs to think about her risk of acquiring an STD because she is not monogamous and both of her partners use drugs. Although Luz has not said anything about her partners (or herself) using injection drugs, she needs to assess these risks. The counselor needs to discuss the role of barrier methods with Luz (perhaps as an add-on STD prevention strategy). Discussing birth control methods such as sterilization, IUDs, and natural family planning would not be a good use of the counselor's time. Luz's counselor could give her a brochure that discusses these other methods if Luz is interested.

Directives for Choosing a Birth Control Method

As mentioned several times in this chapter, the overall goal of counseling clients about birth control is to help them pick methods that they will use consistently and correctly every time they have sexual intercourse. To meet this goal, counselors must discuss the following directives:

1. Help clients find methods that are safe for them based on their personal health risks.
2. Help clients find methods that meet their criteria for acceptable levels of effectiveness and risk.
3. Help clients find methods that are a good fit with their sexual lifestyles.
4. Help clients find methods they can afford to use.
5. Help clients find methods that are culturally acceptable to them.

Directive 1: Help Clients Find Safe Methods Based on Their Health Risks

1. Discuss the results of the medical examination and sexual medical history.

2. Discuss any contraindications based on these factors.

Logical Consequences of Finding Safe and Effective Methods

1. Discussing medical contraindications with clients will help them understand which methods would be unavailable because of their health risks.
2. Giving clients information about the theoretical and actual use effectiveness of a variety of methods and then discussing these data with them will help clients decide which methods are acceptable.
3. Having clients determine their acceptable level of pregnancy risk ensures a better fit between method and client.

Specific Instructions for Finding Safe and Effective Methods

1. Go over the medical chart.
2. Go over any lifestyle behaviors, such as smoking, that did not appear on the chart.

Example

Counselor: Luz, I need to verify a few things from your medical history before we talk about methods.

Luz: Okay.

Counselor: Luz, there doesn't seem to be anything unusual in your medical history. You report that you have none of the cardiovascular risk factors, such as blood clots, or other issues that would interfere with you using oral contraceptives. You also don't have diabetes or any chronic disease. Your weight is normal, and you don't smoke. Is that right?

Luz: Yes, I used to smoke when I was a teenager, but I stopped five years ago.

Counselor: Good.

Directive 2: Help Clients Find Methods That Meet Their Criteria for Acceptable Effectiveness and Risk

1. Discuss the nature of risk.
2. Show clients the risks associated with various methods.

3. Have clients indicate their acceptable level of risk.

Logical Consequence of Clients Finding Methods That Meet Their Criteria for Acceptable Effectiveness and Risk

1. Clients will be much more likely to use methods that meet their parameters for safety and effectiveness.
2. Clients will accept failure based on their acceptance of a certain level of risk.

Specific Instructions for Finding Methods That Meet Their Criteria for Acceptable Effectiveness and Risk

1. Define theoretical and actual use effectiveness.
2. Describe the nature of risk.
3. Go over the methods chart (see Table 7.1) that indicates levels of effectiveness.
4. Ask the client what an acceptable level of risk is.
5. Have the client decide what his or her acceptable level of risk is.

Example

Counselor: Luz, did the doctor who examined you talk about theoretical and actual use effectiveness?

Luz: No, what is that?

Counselor: The theoretical effectiveness of a birth control method is the estimate of how it should work if a person uses it consistently and correctly. It is really a measure of the best-case scenario for how effective it could be when studied in the laboratory. Theoretical effectiveness estimates the lowest expected percentage of women who will get pregnant while using the method. For instance, a method might be said to have a 99% theoretical use effectiveness, meaning that there is a 1% theoretical risk of getting pregnant while using it. Do you understand?

Luz: Yes.

Counselor: Good. The actual use effectiveness of a birth control method is a more accurate measure of how it actually works when real people use it under normal circumstances. It estimates the number of women who actually use the method for one year and get pregnant while on it. Here is a chart that shows the difference. (Shows Luz Table 7.1.)

Luz: Wow, there is a big difference in some of the methods. Look at condoms. They jump almost 20%. Why the difference?

Counselor: Good observation. Methods like condoms rely on people to use them consistently and correctly every time they have sex. There is a lot of room for human error in storing them properly, remembering to use them each time, and putting them on properly. Other methods, like sterilization, have very little difference in the two types of effectiveness.

Luz: I can see that. I guess once you're sterilized, there is nothing more to do.

Counselor: Remember, a method like the male condom can actually be more than 90% effective if you use it properly every time you have intercourse.

Luz: I understand, but I think I want something that is closer to 99% effective, like the pill.

Counselor: So what you are saying is that your desired level of effectiveness is around 99% actual use effectiveness?

Luz: Yes.

Directives 3, 4, and 5: Help Clients Find Methods That Fit Their Sexual Lifestyles, Are Affordable, and Are Culturally Acceptable

1. Help the client match methods to his or her sexual lifestyle.
2. Help the client match methods to his or her financial needs.
3. Help the client match methods to his or her cultural needs.

Logical Consequences of Clients Finding Methods That Fit Their Sexual Lifestyles, Are Affordable, and Are Culturally Acceptable

Clients are much more likely to use methods consistently and correctly every time they have intercourse if they find methods that fit their lifestyles,

are affordable, and are culturally acceptable to them.

Specific Instructions for Helping Clients Find Methods That Fit Their Sexual Lifestyles, Are Affordable, and Are Culturally Acceptable

1. Assess how the client's choice of method matches the demands of his or her sexual lifestyle.
2. Assess how the method fits with the client's comfort level.
3. Assess how the method matches the client's STD risk.
4. Assess the client's ability to pay for the method.
5. Assess how the method matches the client's religious/cultural beliefs.

Example

Counselor: Luz, it seems that you like the effectiveness offered by oral contraceptives. They are good choices for women who have sex frequently and don't want to use methods that need to be reapplied each time they have sex, like spermicides or condoms. Take a look at this table [shows her **Table 7.3**] and fill it out for me. It will help us assess your comfort level with different kinds of fertility control methods.

Luz completes the table and hands it to the counselor.

Counselor: From what you have indicated on this table and told me about your sexual activity, the pill seems consistent with your lifestyle. What do you think?

Luz: I agree. I like the pill because sometimes I like to make love two or three times in one night. I wouldn't want to have to get out of bed and get new condoms or have to use that messy spermicide every time.

Counselor: The only thing I really worry about, though, is that the pill doesn't give you any protection against STDs. Right now

Is This the Right Method for Me?

It Is Important to Choose a Method of Birth Control That Works Well to Prevent Pregnancy. It Is also Important to Choose a Method You Will Like! Ask Yourself These Questions so You Can Judge Carefully.

What type of birth control are you thinking about? _____

Have you ever used it before? _____ yes _____ no

If yes, how long did you use it? _____

		Circle Your Answer	
Are you afraid of using this method?	yes	no	don't know
Would you rather not use this method?	yes	no	don't know
Will you have trouble remembering to use this method?	yes	no	don't know
Have you ever become pregnant while using this method?	yes	no	don't know
Will you have trouble using this method carefully?	yes	no	don't know
Do you have unanswered questions about this method?	yes	no	don't know
Does this method make menstrual periods longer or more painful?	yes	no	don't know
Does this method cost more than you can afford?	yes	no	don't know
Does this method ever cause serious health problems?	yes	no	don't know
Do you object to this method because of religious beliefs?	yes	no	don't know
Have you already had problems using this method?	yes	no	don't know
Is your partner opposed to this method?	yes	no	don't know
Are you using this method without your partner's knowledge?	yes	no	don't know
Will using this method embarrass you?	yes	no	don't know
Will using this method embarrass your partner?	yes	no	don't know
Will you enjoy intercourse less because of this method?	yes	no	don't know
Will this method interrupt lovemaking?	yes	no	don't know
Has a nurse or doctor ever told you *not* to use this method?	yes	no	don't know

Do you have any "don't know" answers? Ask your instructor or physician to help you with more information.

Do you have any "yes" answers? "Yes" answers mean you may not like this method. If you have several "yes" answers, chances go up that you might not like this method; you may need to think about another method.

Source: Adapted from Hatcher R, Guest F, Stewart G, et al. (1998). *Contraceptive Technology,* 17th ed., New York: Ardent.

you are having sex with two guys who use drugs and are into both the drug and music cultures. Using condoms with them would definitely reduce your risks for getting infected with an STD. What do you think about this?

Luz: I really don't worry about that too much. I know both of these guys.

Counselor: Do you really? Each of these guys comes from a high-risk area and is involved in illegal drug use. How do you know what they are doing when they are not with you?

Luz: I guess you are right.

Counselor: Have the three of you been tested for HIV or other STDs?

Luz: No.

Counselor: I think you should consider not only getting on birth control pills, but also using condoms with these guys until all of you have HIV tests and they agree to limit their sexual activity to only you. This might not be possible with Randi, who you say is married.

Luz: I know. I need to sit and talk to him and maybe stop having sex with him until he leaves his wife and settles down with me.

Counselor: What about Raul?

Luz: I'm going to tell him that we need to get an HIV test before we have any more sex.

Counselor: How about using both condoms and the pill in the meantime?

Luz: It makes sense. I'll do it.

Counselor: One last thing. How does using the pill conflict with any cultural religious beliefs you have?

Luz: It really doesn't. I am kind of my own person and don't pay attention to those kind of things.

Counselor: Okay. I want to refer you to a colleague of mine to talk about your drug use. I think she might be able to help you understand this a little bit better than I could. How do you feel about that?

Luz: Okay, but I'm not guaranteeing I will never use drugs again.

Counselor: I understand. Here is her name and phone number. I will call her and tell her to expect your call. Can you call her after we are finished?

Luz: Yes.

Counselor: Good, make an appointment with the clinic secretary to see me in two weeks. I want to see how you are doing with your condoms and pills. You can also set up an appointment with her for HIV and STD tests. I'll see you in two weeks.

Luz: Goodbye.

Summary

This chapter began with a discussion of the terminology associated with birth control counseling, including the subtle differences between the terms "birth control," "family planning," "contraception," and "fertility control." Of these terms, fertility control is probably the least controversial. A discussion of theoretical and actual use effectiveness followed.

Next, the categories and mechanisms of action of fertility control methods were discussed. Blonna and Levitan's (2005) categorization method was used to explain how the various methods worked. The chapter then moved into a discussion of how to counsel clients about birth control. The primary goal of such counseling is to help clients find a method that they will use consistently and correctly every time they have sexual intercourse. The application of the microskills model was demonstrated with regard to counseling clients about fertility control.

Study Questions

1. What are the differences between *birth control, contraception,* and *family planning?*
2. What are the five mechanisms of action for fertility control methods?
3. What is an acceptable level of risk of pregnancy for a fertility control method? Why is it considered acceptable?
4. What are the risks associated with pregnancy and childbirth for the various fertility control methods?
5. What category of fertility control methods offers the best protection against STDs? What are the differences in STD protection found among the methods in this category?
6. How do hormonal contraception measures work?
7. What risks are associated with use of the pill?
8. How do a person's (or a couple's) fertility control needs change over the course of a lifetime?
9. What key questions should you ask yourself when evaluating any fertility control method?
10. What makes communicating about sex different from communicating about other subjects?

11. How does language level influence sexual communication?
12. What is the primary goal of birth control counseling?
13. How can a counselor use sexual self-disclosure effectively when counseling clients about birth control?
14. How can changing the focal point help clients appraise their birth control needs?
15. What are the key directives for each of the goals of birth control counseling?

References

Blonna R, Levitan J (2005). *Healthy Sexuality*. Belmont, CA: Thomson/Wadsworth.

Consumer Reports (1995). How reliable are condoms? *Consumer Reports* May:320–325.

Davis C, Blank J, Lin HY, Bonillas C (1996). Characteristics of vibrator use among women. *Journal of Sex Research*, 33:4, 313–321.

Engen H, Albert M (1995). *Microcounseling* (four-part videotape series). Iowa City, IA: University of Iowa.

Hatcher RA, Trussel J, Stewart F, et al. (1998). *Contraceptive Technology*, 17th ed. New York: Arden Media.

Ivey AE, Gluckstern NB, Ivey MB (1997a). *Basic Influencing Skills*, 3rd ed. North Amherst, MA: Microtraining Associates.

Ivey AE, Gluckstern NB, Ivey MB (1997b). *Basic Influencing Skills*, 3rd ed. (videotape). North Amherst, MA: Microtraining Associates.

Ivey AE, Ivey MB (2003). *Intentional Interviewing and Counseling: Facilitating Client Development in a Multicultural Society*, 5th ed. Belmont, CA: Thomson/Wadsworth.

Machaud SL, Warner RM (1997). Gender differences in self-reported troubles talk. *Sex Roles: A Journal of Research* 37:527–541.

Mandel B (1981). Communication: a four part process. *Hotliner* 4:6.

McDonough P (1995). The safest sex. *Psychology Today* Sept/Oct:47–49.

McGinty K, Knox D, Zusman ME (2003). Nonverbal and verbal communication in "involved" and "casual" relationships among college students. *College Student Journal* 37:68–72.

Nelson A, Hatcher R, Zieman M, et al. (2000). *Managing Contraception*. Tiger, GA: Bridging the Gap Foundation.

Noller P, Fitzpatrick MA (1991). Marital communication. In Booth A. *Contemporary Families: Looking Forward, Looking Backward*. Minneapolis: Council on Family Relations.

Norris K (1996). Celibate passion. *Utne Reader* Sept:51–53.

Ortho-McNeil Pharmaceutical (2003). *Ortho Evra*. http://birthcontrol.orthoevra/faqs/faqs.html.

Planned Parenthood Federation of America (2002). Abortion. www.plannedparenthood.org/abortion.

Tannen D (1990). *You Just Don't Know: Women and Men in Conversation*. New York: William Morrow.

United States Department of Health and Human Services (USDHHS), Office of Disease Prevention and Health Promotion (ODPHP) (2003). *Healthy People 2010: A Systematic Approach to Health Improvement*. www.healthypeople.gov/Document/html/uih/uih_bw/uih_2.htm#obj.

Learning Objectives

By the end of the chapter students will:

1. Understand the nature and extent of the asthma problem in the United States

2. Describe the goals of asthma counseling

3. Compare and contrast asthma with other chronic diseases

4. Describe the risk factors for asthma

5. Discuss the nature of "triggers" for asthma attacks

6. Describe the actions of long-term and acute asthma medications

7. Discuss some common emotional responses to having asthma

8. Explain why counselors, in their introductions, should use words such as "manage" and "control" instead of "cure" and "treat" when helping clients set reasonable therapeutic goals

9. Describe how counselors with asthma can use self-disclosure effectively

10. Discuss how changing the focal point can help clients view their asthma differently

11. List and describe the key directives and logical consequences for each of the asthma management counseling goals

Health Counseling for Secondary Prevention

Chapters 8, 9, and 10 focus on health counseling for secondary prevention of asthma, hypertension, and STDs, respectively. As discussed in Chapter 1, health counseling, like health promotion and health education, can target any of the three levels of prevention: primary, secondary, and tertiary. Health counseling for secondary prevention focuses on two issues: ensuring adherence to treatment regimens and preventing reinfection or the reoccurrence of health problems.

A major feature of secondary prevention at the community level is finding asymptomatic disease in susceptible populations. At the individual level, health counseling involves working with these asymptomatic clients on a one-on-one basis. A first step in secondary prevention counseling often involves convincing clients that they even have a problem. Many clients with conditions such as hypertension remain unaware of their problems until they are detected through screening activities. Before counselors can help them control their conditions, they must first convince clients of the severity of their illnesses, even though they do not present noticeable symptoms.

The intention of health counseling for secondary prevention is to prevent the progression of health problems. Counselors must ensure that clients adhere to treatment regimens prescribed by their physicians. Health counselors must also teach clients ways to reduce future reinfection (as in the case of STDs) or reoccurrence of episodes of their current illness (as in preventing future asthma attacks or episodes of high blood pressure) (Mausner & Kramer, 1985).

Overview of Asthma

Epidemiology

Asthma accounts for more than 14 million lost work days for adults and 14 million missed school days for children annually (ALA, 2003a). It is the leading chronic cause of school absenteeism among children ages 5–15 in the United States (Mannino, Homa, Akinbami, et al., 2002). The most current asthma prevalence data show that more than 20 million Americans had asthma in 2001 (more than 73 people per 1000) and that 31 million Americans (more than 113 per 1000) were diagnosed with asthma at some point in their lives. The highest prevalence rates for asthma, both for lifetime diagnosis and current disease, are found among children ages 5–17 and among blacks. Current prevalence among children ages 5–17 in 2001 was 98.1 per 1000, as compared to 73.4 per 1000 for the overall population. Rates for boys ages 0–17 are approximately 30% higher than those for girls (99 per 1000 versus 74.4 per 1000) (ALA, 2003a; NCHS, 2003). In adults, however, asthma rates for women are consistently higher than those for men. Possible reasons for this difference include differences in hormones, obesity, or other factors (CDC, 2001).

Asthma prevalence rates for blacks have consistently been higher than those for whites. The latest data indicate that prevalence among blacks is 22% higher than prevalence among whites (ALA, 2003a). While the disparity may appear to be racial, in fact it may be more related to urban living (Aligne, Auinger, Byrd, & Weitzman, 2000). Increased rates of asthma are closely associated with poverty, poor air quality, greater exposure to indoor allergens (in particular, cockroaches and their droppings), insufficient patient education, and inadequate medical care (AAFA, 2003).

Diagnosis

Asthma is a chronic respiratory disease that affects the large airways. Its pathology is rooted in the inflammatory response. The immune system, for reasons still unknown, becomes hypersensitive to stimuli that normally would not produce such a reaction. When the lungs of people with asthma are exposed to such stimuli, the musculature of the bronchi constrict, and the mucous membrane lining produces copious amounts of secretions. These two reactions lead to a reduction in the size of the airway, and hence to a reduction in the volume of air that can be inhaled and exhaled (see **Figure 8.1**). If the constriction is severe enough and occurs for a prolonged period of time, death from hypoxia can result.

The diagnosis of asthma is made based on medical history, physical examination, family history (a family history of allergies increases the likelihood of asthma), and pulmonary (lung) function testing. Once the diagnosis of asthma is made, further evaluation is needed to identify the asthma triggers. **Triggers** are the stimuli that initi-

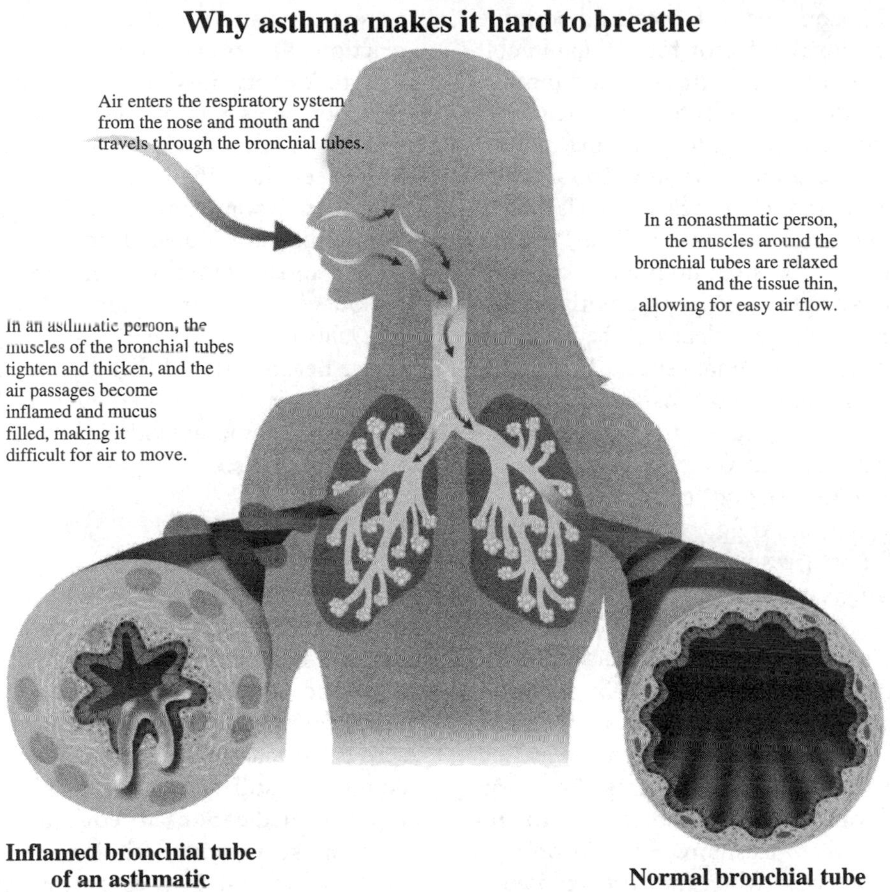

Why asthma makes it hard to breathe

Air enters the respiratory system from the nose and mouth and travels through the bronchial tubes.

In a nonasthmatic person, the muscles around the bronchial tubes are relaxed and the tissue thin, allowing for easy air flow.

In an asthmatic person, the muscles of the bronchial tubes tighten and thicken, and the air passages become inflamed and mucus filled, making it difficult for air to move.

Inflamed bronchial tube of an asthmatic

Normal bronchial tube

Figure 8.1 During an asthma attack airways become inflamed and mucus filled. (*Source:* Image provided by the American Academy of Allergy, Asthma and Innunology. www.aaaai.org. All rights reserved.)

ate an asthma episode or attack. They can be either allergens or irritants.

Allergens are particles of protein matter such as pollen or molds, dust mite or cockroach droppings, and dog or cat dander, urine, or saliva, to name the more common ones. Microscopic organisms called dust mites thrive on small particles of plant and animal material that make up house dust. Their droppings are the most common indoor allergen that can trigger asthma symptoms. Indoor molds send out small spores that can trigger allergy symptoms. These molds thrive in high-humidity areas of the home, such as in bathrooms and damp basements. Unlike allergens such as an-

imal dander, indoor molds are easily eliminated once they are discovered. **Animal dander** is a protein found in the saliva, dead skin flakes, and urine of fur-bearing animals. These tiny airborne protein particles can cause an immune response after landing on the moist lining of the eyes or nose or being inhaled into the lungs. In many people with asthma, the same substances that cause allergy symptoms can also trigger an asthma episode. These allergens may be things that are inhaled, such as pollen or dust, or things that are eaten, such as shellfish.

Irritants are substances that "irritate" the lungs such as cigarette smoke (first- or second-hand), cold air, ozone, paint fumes, and perfume. Smoking is a major risk factor for asthma in children, and a common trigger of asthma symptoms for people of all ages. All forms of cigarette smoke are capable of triggering asthma attacks. People with asthma should not only stop smoking to minimize their risk of attacks, but also avoid the smoke from others' cigarettes. This "second-hand" smoke, or "passive smoking," can also trigger asthma symptoms in people with the disease. Studies have shown a clear link between second-hand smoke and asthma, especially in young people. Passive smoking worsens asthma in children and teens and may cause as many as 26,000 new cases of asthma each year (AAFA, 2003).

In some people, strong emotions, such as laughing or crying, can trigger an asthma episode, as can a viral upper respiratory infection. Exposure to cold air, drugs such as aspirin, food and food additives or preservatives such as sulfites, and exercise (exercise-induced asthma) are also triggers for some people (AAFA, 2003).

Triggers vary from person to person, so knowing an individual's triggers is key to counseling, treatment, and control. People with asthma react in a variety of ways to triggers. Some react to only a few triggers, others to many. Some people get asthma symptoms only when they are exposed to more than one factor or trigger at the same time. Others experience more severe episodes in response to multiple factors or triggers. In addition, asthma episodes do not always occur immediately after a person is exposed to a trigger. Depending on the type of trigger and a person's level of sensitivity to it, asthma episodes may be delayed. It is important for clients to be aware of the things in their environment that tend to spur asthma attacks or make chronic asthma symptoms worse. Because people with asthma react differently to triggers and combinations of triggers, an important step in asthma management is the assessment of triggers (ALA, 2003a).

Identification of triggers includes skin sensitivity testing for allergens, in which small amounts of potential allergens are placed on the skin and then "pricked" or injected just under the skin. If the person is sensitive to the allergen, a hive-like local reaction will occur. Sometimes blood testing is used to identify possible allergens, but this method may not be as reliable (National Jewish Medical and Research Center, 2003). Once the triggers have been identified, a treatment plan that includes environmental control, trigger avoidance, and medication is developed.

The most common symptoms of an asthma episode (attack) are frequent coughing, wheezing, shortness of breath, and tightness in the chest. Because it is difficult to breathe during an asthma episode, the person may be anxious as well. An asthma episode is brought on by exposure to triggers.

Treatment

Asthma cannot be cured. For this reason, the goal of asthma therapy is controlling the condition through a combination of medication and trigger avoidance (environmental control). Only licensed healthcare providers, such as physicians, can prescribe asthma medications. However, nonmedical counselors still need to understand the different types of medications to educate clients and help them make informed choices about their therapeutic regimens. Two categories of asthma medications exist: **long- term controllers** and **quick relief rescuers.**

Long-Term Controllers

Long-term controller medications are used daily to minimize the risk of attacks by reducing inflammation and irritation of the airways (AAFA, 2003). These drugs, which are also called "maintenance medicines," help prevent symptoms from occurring in the first place. When taken regularly, they reduce the constriction (narrowing of airways in the lungs) and/or the inflammation (underlying swelling and irritation in the airways of the lungs). Many people need to treat both the constriction and the inflammation for optimal asthma control. Three types of long-term controllers exist: corticosteroids, antileukotrienes, and mast cell stabilizers.

Corticosteroids are a type of steroid used to reduce inflammation and irritation of the airways. They can be inhaled or taken in a pill form and are the most commonly prescribed long-term controllers. These drugs are the most effective anti-inflammatory agents available and are considered an essential treatment for moderate to severe asthma. Corticosteroids shouldn't be confused with anabolic steroids, which increase muscle mass (AAFA, 2003).

Antileukotrienes are oral medications that work by blocking leukotrienes, powerful chemicals that are involved in the constriction and swelling of airways associated with asthma (AAFA, 2003).

Mast cell stabilizers are nonsteroidal long-term controllers that work by stabilizing the membranes of mast cells. Mast cells produce histamine, a chemical released during the allergic reactions that result in the inflammation of airways. By stabilizing the mast cells, these drugs may prevent some of the allergic and inflammatory components of asthma.

Mast cell stabilizers are commonly prescribed as long-term therapy in children or people with very mild asthma. They are also sometimes prescribed for administration prior to exercise or allergy exposure. These agents have very mild side effects (AAFA, 2003).

Quick Relief Rescuers

Quick relief rescuers are used to treat asthma attacks. Also referred to as bronchodilators, they work by quickly relaxing and dilating constricted airways. Quick relief rescuers do not reduce the underlying inflammation associated with asthma, so they do not prevent future asthma attacks.

The most common and effective quick relief rescuers are the **beta-agonists**. These agents stimulate beta-receptors, thereby relaxing smooth muscle and opening the bronchioles. Beta-agonists are available in short- and long-acting forms. Most are inhaled directly into the lungs through inhalers, also known as puffers.

Short-term, inhaled beta-agonists are fast acting and provide relief for four to six hours. Also known as rescue inhalers, they should be taken only when sudden asthma symptoms occur. They work quickly to open the airways by relaxing airway muscles. They do not provide long-term asthma control or help prevent future attacks.

Long-term beta-agonists are available in inhaler or pill form. They help keep the airways open by relaxing the muscles surrounding the airways for 12 hours or longer. This effect can also help prevent airway constriction from occurring in the first place. Inhaled long-acting bronchodilators should not be used to relieve sudden asthma symptoms.

Hypo-sensitization

Hypo-sensitization, also known as "allergy shots," may also be helpful in treating asthma attacks that are triggered by allergies. This treatment involves the systematic desensitization of the body to allergens through direct exposure to controlled levels of the substances to which clients are allergic. Not all experts agree about the usefulness of allergy shots (AAFA, 2003).

Control and Prevention

An asthma attack is defined as an emergency department visit, a hospital admission, an unscheduled office visit, or a need for oral, intravenous, or intramuscular corticosteroids. Much of the control of asthma depends on the patient's disease self-management. Controlling asthma is defined as experiencing 24 hours without an attack, a nighttime awakening due to asthma, or the use of more than two puffs of a rescue inhaler (AAFA, 2003). Achieving such control requires adherence to an individualized asthma management plan that is based on overt symptoms and peak flow lung function readings. Peak flow lung function readings are taken with a meter (see **Figure 8.2**).

A peak flow meter is a portable, inexpensive, hand-held device that measures the volume of expired air. Peak flow readings are taken by clients daily to monitor their lung function. Normal peak flows vary depending on age, height, sex,

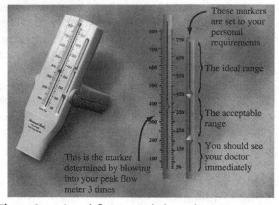

Figure 8.2 A peak flow meter helps asthmatics monitor their lung functioning. (*Source:* www.medimagery.com/asthma/flow.jpg.)

Peak Flow		Symptoms	Advice
Green Zone	> 80% of usual best	No change	Continue usual treatment
Yellow Zone	60%–80% of usual best	Increased or at onset of upper respiratory tract infection	Resume or double dose of preventer
Orange Zone	40%–60% of usual best	Nocturnal waking, frequent need for bronchodilators (3–4 hourly), or no response to increased treatment	Start/resume oral corticosteroid and contact your doctor as soon as possible
Red Zone	<40% of usual best	No relief with bronchodilators	Call an ambulance and continue use of reliever

Figure 8.3 Charting one's peak flow helps reduce the risk of life-threatening attacks. (*Source:* ALA (2003b).)

and race (ALA, 2003b). While standardized "normal" readings are available, it is the individual's personal best readings that are used in developing treatment plans. The peak flow readings are broken into three ranges: green, yellow, and red (see **Figure 8.3**).

The green zone readings are usually 80% to 100% of the usual or "normal" peak flow rate

for the person. A reading in this zone means that the individual's asthma is under reasonably good control.

Readings in the yellow zone, typically 50% to 80% of the usual or "normal" peak flow rate, signal a need for caution. This reduction in peak

Environmental Air Quality

Health Implications of Poor Air Quality

Two indicators of air quality are ozone (outdoor) and indoor environmental tobacco smoke (ETS). While dramatic improvements in air quality in the United States have occurred over the past three decades, millions of tons of toxic pollutants are still released into the air each year from automobiles, industry, and other sources. Nearly half of all Americans live in areas that failed to attain established health-based standards for ozone.

More than half of all nonsmoking Americans are exposed to ETS. Home and workplace environments are both major sources of exposure. Approximately 15 million children are estimated to be exposed to secondhand smoke in their homes. Both exposure to ozone and ETS

can trigger asthma attacks. Poor air quality also contributes to other respiratory illnesses, cardiovascular disease, and cancer. Exposure to ETS increases the risk of heart disease and respiratory infections in children and is responsible for an estimated 3000 cancer-related deaths of adult nonsmokers. The overall death rate from asthma increased 57% between 1980 and 1993; for children, it increased 67% over the same period (USDHHS, 2003).

Objectives for the Nation

- Reduce the proportion of persons exposed to air that does not meet the U.S. Environmental Protection Agency's health-based standards for ozone
- Reduce the proportion of nonsmokers exposed to environmental tobacco smoke

flow may indicate airway narrowing and may require extra treatment.

A reading in the red zone is typically less than 50% of the normal personal best and usually indicates severe narrowing of the airways. Readings in the red zone require immediate use of rescue medications to open the airways and follow-up with a physician (ALA, 2003b).

The peak flow readings and/or symptoms in the three color zones serve as the basis for the asthma action plans that are developed by clients and their physicians. Asthma action plans are individualized for clients based on their personal best peak flow readings and symptoms.

As a lifelong chronic disease, asthma impacts every dimension of health. People with asthma often report how the disease has shaped their lives and influenced them in ways that extend beyond their physical well-being.

Case Study 8.1
Carlos

Carlos is 52 and identifies as Cuban American. He has had asthma all of his life. He is a professor of health studies, has been married for 32 years, and has two sons, ages 17 and 20. Carlos believes that having asthma has shaped his entire life, from his earliest recollections. We will use this belief as a starting point for his discussion of how asthma has affected every facet of his life.

Counselor: Carlos, you mentioned that your earliest recollections of childhood were as a person with asthma. Can you explain this?

Carlos: Sure. I just never remember *not* having asthma. I guess my two most vivid recollections were getting allergy tests and being unable to play with the other kids.

Counselor: Tell me about this.

Carlos: I remember wearing long sleeves one summer to hide my allergy tests. It was in the late 1950s, and my mother used to take me on the bus (two buses, actually) across town

to go to the allergist for testing. I remember hating the place; it smelled of disinfectant and he had these trays and trays of long, thin hypodermic syringes filled with all of his patients' allergens. I just remember seeing these hundreds of needles all neatly lined up in stainless steel shallow trays.

Counselor: Tell me more.

Carlos: I used to dread going in and having the doctor pull out my tray and inject 30 or 40 of these needles into the sensitive inside part of my forearm. He would inject little bubbles of each prepared allergen to see if my body would react to them, indicating that I was allergic to them. I would cry because I was so afraid of this. The doctor had big, hairy forearms and lots of nose hair. That is all I remember about him. Oh yeah, he had very rough hands and he used to yank my arm to hold it still. All week I would dread going to school because I was embarrassed about the rows of neat little bubbles that would itch and drive me crazy. All the kids would make fun of me and pick on me, calling me "scab boy" and other horrible names. I hated it, and it went on for months. I hated going to school because of this. I was very self-conscious.

Counselor: You mentioned being unable to play with the other kids. Tell me about that.

Carlos: There were lots of things. The most vivid picture I recall is a winter scene. It was the middle of the winter, and it had snowed at least a foot the night before. We had a day off school and all the kids, my brother included, were in the backyard behind the house. We had a big yard that adjoined a small business with a parking area for trucks. It was about the size of a football field. I was standing on a kitchen chair watching all of the other kids running around, screaming and yelling, throwing snowballs, making snow forts, being kids. My mother would not allow me to go out because I might get an asthma attack. I stood on that kitchen chair for hours, tears streaming down my face, hating "being an asthmatic." I also hated my mother.

Counselor: Hated your mother?

Carlos: Yeah, there she was, smoking her cigarettes, windows closed, probably contributing more to my asthma than all the cold air and snow in the world, keeping me inside like some kind of a freak.

Counselor: Is that what you felt like, some kind of a freak?

Carlos: Yeah, for years I always felt different, like some freak who couldn't do the simplest things without getting sick. I couldn't play sports, couldn't run around too much, couldn't camp out in the backyard without getting sick. I hated my childhood. I was a weak, pathetic, sickly, pasty-faced little "asthmatic." I was also an easy target for bullies who used to terrorize me on my way to school.

Counselor: Wow, you seem such a healthy, vibrant man now. What changed?

Carlos: When I was in eighth grade we moved to a different part of town, a suburb really. I used it as an opportunity to change. I was very interested in health and determined—driven really—to get better, and prepare to leave my family and life as soon as I was able.

Counselor: Driven?

Carlos: Yeah, I knew at 10 or 11 that the only way I would get better was to do it myself and that eventually I'd have to leave my parents and home because they were not going to change their lifestyle for me. They still smoked, had a dog, refused to go to new doctors or do anything else for my asthma. They claimed that they just couldn't afford to "keep going to doctors and spending money on drugs for me." It was a wake-up call.

Counselor: What did you do?

Carlos: My eighth-grade year was devoted to reading about health and asthma, changing my diet, starting to exercise, getting healthier. The couple of new friends I had nicknamed me "wheat germ" because of my passion for health. I went from being a sickly, overweight weakling in eighth grade to being the second strongest kid (we used to take the President's Council on Physical Fitness test every year) in the freshman class. I lost 25 pounds and could run a mile without having an asthma attack.

Counselor: How did that make you feel?

Carlos: For the first time in my life, I had some positive self-esteem. I was still very shy and insecure. I also still had attacks almost every day, but they didn't freak me out as much and they weren't as severe. My medication worked better with my improved level of health. This reinforced my interest in health even more. I still carried around a lot of anger directed toward my parents, but I was on my way and never intended to look back.

Counselor: (We jump to Carlos's college years.) Tell me about your college years.

Carlos: I was driven. My parents had put nothing aside for me for college. I didn't really expect anything anyway, so I went to junior college and lived at home for one year. At 19, I got married and for the first time in my life I could control my environment. I was looking for a way out, and falling in love and getting married really was an attractive option. My wife was great and worked with me to keep our place clean and keep allergens to a minimum. I worked, went to class, came home, and studied, exercised, planned for our future.

Counselor: Sounds like you missed out on a lot of the typical college experience.

Carlos: I guess so, but I don't regret it. I couldn't smoke pot and party and live like many of my friends, because my body couldn't take it. I remember hanging out one night and smoking some pot, drinking, and crashing on the floor of my friend's fraternity house. I woke up in the middle of the night with an incredible asthma attack, and it convinced me that I just couldn't do those things. The next 20 years was really a reflection of this realization. I carved out a life based on healthy practices and tried my best to keep getting healthier while minimizing as many triggers as I could. I also got more interested in health and chose it as a career, working for a state health department for 15 years before coming to the university.

Counselor: Sounds like your asthma, to use your words, made you "driven."

Carlos: Yeah, I was driven to succeed. I wanted to control my asthma but also be financially well off. I never wanted to feel that I couldn't afford to be healthy or take care of my kids' health needs. I didn't ever want to feel helpless again. My asthma forced me to grow up, be strong, and take care of myself.

Goals of Asthma Counseling

As mentioned earlier, asthma is an incurable, chronic disease. As such, treatment of people with asthma focuses on reducing or eliminating the occurrence of asthma attacks and optimizing lung function using the least amount of medication. Asthma control requires reducing exposure to triggers and increasing adherence to asthma action plans that combine the monitoring of lung function with medication administration. Managing asthma effectively requires a long-term commitment to behavioral changes that affect every major dimension of health and lifestyle. Asthma control is influenced by the physical, social, emotional, intellectual, occupational, environmental, and even spiritual dimensions of clients' health. There are four goals for asthma counseling: (1) reducing the frequency and severity of clients' future attacks, (2) helping clients adhere to medications prescribed by their healthcare providers, (3) reducing clients' need to rely on medication to control their asthma, and (4) developing lifestyle-modification plans that help clients control triggers and build resistance to attacks. In addition to these primary goals, counselors must assess clients' goals regarding their infections.

Counseling Clients with Asthma Using Microskills

Counseling clients with asthma begins with an overall understanding of what the disease means to clients and ends with specific directives and instructions to help them control triggers and manage their action plans. Because asthma management depends so heavily on proper medication use, unless counselors are also licensed healthcare professionals (e.g., physician, nurse, respiratory therapist) or Certified Asthma Educators (CA-E), they should work in concert with these medical providers to ensure optimal patient care and the avoidance of liability.

Case Study 8.2
Peter: Coming to Terms with His Asthma

Peter is 21, a senior in college, married, and white. Peter was a student of Dr. Blonna's several years ago. He described his asthma story over the course of a semester in class and in private meetings with Dr. Blonna. We will provide a brief overview of his case initially and use him to illustrate the three sets of microskills.

At 21, Peter made a decision to try to finally gain control over his asthma. He was about 35 pounds overweight, had very low endurance, and suffered from asthma attacks on a regular basis. Recently married, Peter was determined, with the help of his wife, to finally take control of his health and his asthma.

Peter had asthma his entire life. Prior to getting married and moving into a new apartment with his wife, he lived at home with his parents for 21 years. Neither of his parents were college graduates. Both worked in manufacturing jobs—his dad at one of the last automakers left in New Jersey, his mom for a large pharmaceutical company. Both of Peter's parents smoked. His mom smoked cigarettes. His father smoked cigars. Peter's mother smoked throughout her entire pregnancy. They lived in an older house and had a dog (a golden retriever) and a bird as pets. Peter's maternal grandfather died from emphysema.

Born one month premature, Peter had pneumonia as a newborn. He suffered a collapsed left lung and had to remain in the hospital for several weeks before being released to go home. His earliest recollections of childhood are of having asthma.

Peter refers to himself as an "asthmatic." His overall recollection of his childhood (and life in general) is of "missing out" on all the things he couldn't do, ranging from playing in the snow to going out for youth sports.

Peter harbored a great deal of anger and resentment toward his parents and life in general. He blamed his parents for not doing enough to help him deal with his asthma. Although he had made a personal commitment to get better and felt responsible for his health, he still looked back frequently at how matters were handled by his parents up until this point.

Introductory Skills

A good introduction is essential to gaining clients' trust. Clients are often reluctant to discuss their problems and must be won over early in the interview.

Identify Yourself and Explain Your Role

Living with asthma can be a very emotional experience. Many people with asthma have experienced life-threatening attacks and serious physical symptoms that have affected their emotional health. Counseling people with asthma requires that counselors explore these emotional issues in addition to the purely physical aspects of the disease. This approach needs to be explained to clients up front, so that they will have no misconceptions about what will be brought up and why

it needs to be discussed. Try writing a script for this part of the introduction, and practice it until it becomes second nature to you. When introducing yourself, it is very important to make a concerted effort to establish a skin-to-skin human connection with the client. A firm handshake is a good way to do so. Extend your hand, make eye contact, and smile as you give the client a firm (but not crushing) handshake.

Example

Counselor: (Extending hand, smiling) Hi, I'm [name]. I'm one of the counselors at the clinic. My job is to make sure you understand why you are here, and what you need to know to manage your asthma and live a full and productive life.

You have asthma, and I understand that this can be a very emotion-laden condition. To understand what having asthma means to you, I must talk to you about some very personal issues related to your background and family life. I am not here to judge you or your family in terms of how you handled your asthma in the past or the things that have contributed to your attacks. My job is to help you make the best decisions for yourself regarding how to manage your asthma from this point forward. Together, we will work out a plan for making sure that you gain control of your asthma so that you have fewer attacks and need to rely less on medication to control it if possible. I want you to understand that everything we say is confidential and that your name and anything we talk about cannot be shared with anyone else.

Clarify the Client's Name

A simple way to verify the client's name is to use an open-ended statement following your introduction. Do this while you are still standing and immediately following your handshake and self-identification.

Example

Counselor: (Before sitting and explaining his role) And your name is . . . ?

Explain the Client's Role

After exchanging names and describing your role, start to explain the client's role. A simple explanation should include the three key elements discussed in Chapter 3: (1) active participation, (2) self-responsibility, and (3) honesty.

Example

Counselor: Peter, your role in this process is to be as open and honest as possible when talking to me. The only way I can help you is if you tell me exactly what is going on with you and everyone involved in your illness. You'll have to take an active role in this process and take responsibility for getting better. Together, we can work out a therapeutic plan that includes adhering to the medication your healthcare provider prescribed as well as coming up with ways to minimize exposure to your personal asthma triggers.

Set Goals for the Session(s)

As an asthma counselor, you have four primary goals for your clients: (1) reducing the frequency and severity of future attacks, (2) helping clients adhere to medications prescribed by their healthcare providers, (3) reducing their need to rely on medication to control their asthma, and (4) developing lifestyle-modification plans that help control triggers and build resistance to attacks. In addition to these primary goals, counselors must assess clients' goals regarding their infections.

Example

Counselor: Peter, there are four things I *must* discuss with you today regarding your asthma. First, we need to figure out how to help you reduce the frequency and severity of future attacks. Second, we need to discuss how to help you adhere to the medication(s) prescribed by your healthcare provider. Third, we must decide how you can reduce your need to rely on medication to control your asthma. Fourth, we need to develop a lifestyle-modification plan to control your triggers and build resistance to attacks. What goals do you have for our sessions?

Give the client time to think this through before moving into the next part of the session.

Transition to the Client's Story

A good way to make the transition from the introduction to getting clients to tell their stories is to use open-ended statements regarding what happened. Here are a few examples:

"Peter, why don't you tell me what led to you being here today."
"Peter, tell me a little bit about what you know about asthma."
"Peter, tell me a little bit about your asthma for the past month."

The idea in using such open-ended statements is to get clients talking about their asthma as well as their overall lifestyles. You can start with either topic, but recognize that understanding both of these components of the overall story is essential to meeting your four asthma counseling goals.

Attending Skills

Listening to clients tell their asthma stories will give you insights into the nature of their history and lifestyles in general as well as how these factors relate to their current asthma condition. It is essential that you set a nonjudgmental tone from the start while attending.

Nonverbal Skills

Be aware of both your own and your clients' body language. Be particularly aware of tension in individual body parts or major areas or aversion of eye contact. Clenching and unclenching the hands, tension across the chest and shoulders, and facial tension (e.g., tight jaw muscles, furrowed brow) are sure signs of discomfort. More obvious is averting eye contact. While it is normal to look away and periodically break eye contact when you are talking, averting eye contact when the other person is talking may indicate that something is wrong.

Verbal Following

A key aspect of verbally following asthma clients' stories is paying particular attention to the issue of control of the condition. Clients will often give you clues regarding how they feel about being able to control and manage their asthma by shifting to the third person while talking about their disease. For instance, they might talk about how hard it is for "people" to manage a disease like asthma. They will also use labels that identify people with the disease, such as stating how unfair it is that "asthmatics" get this disease while others are spared.

Examples

Peter: Yeah, you know how hard it is for people to live with asthma. They always have to watch out for things like being around cats that other people don't even think about.

Peter: Most people don't know what asthmatics go through trying to live in a world full of triggers.

Such subtle nuances in language are often intentional and serve as a way for clients to test counselors' sensitivity about their condition. They are sometimes used as "bait," thrown out to see if counselors "bite" by responding in sympathetic or other ways.

Additionally, the use of the third person or labeling as clients tell their stories gives counselors a sense of whether clients feel in control of their asthma. Clients who are in control tend to talk about "my asthma," taking responsibility for it and seeing it as a condition that they have. Clients who identify as "asthmatics" use stereotypes to describe what they are experiencing and tend to take less personal responsibility for their health. This distinction is important for counselors to notice because it will affect the directives discussed later in the session(s). Such personal descriptions and use of the third person can serve as take-off points for verbal following. In other words, follow these threads in the story to see how they unfold.

Examples

Counselor: Peter, I notice that you refer to yourself as an "asthmatic." What does that mean to you?

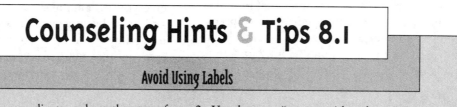

Counseling Hints & Tips 8.1

Avoid Using Labels

A good way to empower clients and set the stage for gaining control over their asthma is to avoid labeling the person with the disease. This practice applies to other conditions besides asthma.

1. Avoid the term "asthmatics."
   - Calling someone an "asthmatic" creates a stereotypical picture of someone by lumping all people with the condition together.
   - Calling someone an "asthmatic" equates the person with the disease.
   - Using terms such as "asthmatic" reduces individual responsibility for managing the condition.

2. Use the term "person with asthma."
   - Calling someone a "person with asthma" creates a picture of an individual with many attributes, one of which is having asthma.
   - Calling someone a "person with asthma" does not make the person one with the disease (he or she is a person first).
   - Calling someone a "person with asthma" increases personal responsibility for managing the problem (just as with a person with a family, a person with a career, or a person with a mortgage, for example).

Counselor: Peter, I notice that you tend to refer to yourself as an "asthmatic." Tell me more about this.

Counselor: Peter, tell me what it is like for people to live with asthma.

Counselor: Peter, what is it like for people who have asthma to manage the condition?

Peter: It is very difficult. It feels like you can never let your guard down. If you're an asthmatic, you go over someone's house to visit and you have to worry if they have a cat or if their house is moldy. You go away for a weekend and you have to worry if the hotel has feather pillows or if the housekeeper dusted under the bed. Little, stupid things like this affect asthmatics every day.

Counselor: It seems that these things in the environment are very unpredictable.

Peter: Exactly. People with asthma are always worrying over the things they can't control, over the unpredictable.

By following up on Peter's use of the word "asthmatics" and the phrase "people with asthma," the counselor gets Peter to provide an overview of some things in his environment that act as personal asthma triggers. The counselor also encourages Peter to share some of his feelings regarding his perceived lack of control of this condition. Because Peter sensed the counselor's nonjudgmental tone, he felt comfortable going into more detail regarding his story.

Vocal Tone

Try to match the pace and tone of clients' stories. Asthma patients experience a range of emotions regarding their infections, and they express these emotions in the way they tell their stories. Peter's tone is tinged with emotion as he discusses being an "asthmatic." His pace is disjointed and his vocal tone is uneven. He bounces between bursts of rapid speech followed by measured pauses (apparently to recollect his thoughts). His voice is very animated as he makes a point or tries to illustrate something.

He raises his voice often to make points and vent his emotions.

Another client might respond to being infected with asthma entirely differently, and his or her story might be told with less emotion and a more even pace and volume. Other clients might speak more softly and adopt a more submissive tone, implying embarrassment, guilt, or shame. Don't respond to their stories with your own tone and pace. Instead, let their emotions and style dictate yours. Try to capture the "vocals" of the client so as to encourage them to continue.

Another interesting thing about talking to clients with asthma is the way the disease can manifest itself in their breathing. Wheezing, shortness of breath, and faintness in speech are commonly associated with asthma. People with asthma become so accustomed to breathing that they become acute observers of others' breathing patterns. Case Study 8.3 illustrates this phenomenon.

Case Study 8.3
Donald: Youth Football Player

Donald is an 11-year-old African American middle school student and youth football player.

A few years ago, Dr. Blonna was coaching a youth football team for 10- and 11-year-olds. He would run laps with the players and take them through a series of warm-up exercises and stretches. It was the first week of the preseason and a new boy, Donald, showed up. Dr. Blonna noticed Donald lagging behind the group. When he ran up next to Donald, he noticed his hunched posture and labored breathing as he ran. This is how the scenario played out.

Dr. Blonna: Hey, Donald, how are you doing?
Donald: (As he averts eye contact and tries to straighten up and catch his breath) Okay, coach, I'm just out of shape.
Dr. Blonna: Not a problem. Walk with me a while.

The two slowed to a gentle walk outside of the running area as the rest of the teams and players kept running around the field.

Donald: Okay, coach, I could use a rest.

Dr. Blonna: Tell me, Donald, how do you like football so far?

Donald: (Averts eye contact, stops his shoulders slightly) It's okay, I guess.

Dr. Blonna: It's a lot of running, huh?

Donald: (Whimsically) Yeah, more than I thought it would be.

Dr. Blonna: So, Donald, how long have you had asthma?

Donald: (Looking up, startled) How did you know?

Dr. Blonna: I can always tell by the breathing. You see, I have asthma and I still get that way sometimes. I have my inhaler right here in my pocket. (Pulls out inhaler to show Donald.)

Donald: Wow, how long have you had asthma?

Dr. Blonna: Ever since I can remember. I had it my whole life.

Donald: I hate having it. It is so embarrassing. I don't want anybody to know I use an inhaler.

Dr. Blonna: Yeah, I can understand that. I wish I didn't have to use mine either, but I do so I try to make the best of it. What do you take for it, Donald?

Donald: I'm on two different inhalers, but I left the one I use for attacks at home.

Dr. Blonna: Is that your mom over there? The lady waving to us?

Donald: Yeah, she just dropped me off.

Dr. Blonna: Let's go ask her if she can get your inhaler for you. In the meantime, you can help me out with some other stuff until she comes back. We don't have to mention this to the other guys if you don't want.

Donald: Okay, coach. Let's go talk to my mom.

After practice, Donald, his mother, and Dr. Blonna had a long talk about Donald's asthma, how football would impact it, and the need for Donald to have his inhaler with him at practice. They worked out a reasonable plan for working around Donald's asthma while still allowing him to participate in youth football. Having asthma himself, Dr. Blonna was quick to recognize it in Donald and talk to him about it.

Responding Skills

Nonverbal and Verbal Minimal Encouragers

As illustrated by Donald, when you are uncomfortable with certain issues, your body language and eye contact will often give you away. In Donald's case, it was really a combination of the physical posturing associated with labored breathing as well as the body language associated with being embarrassed and feeling awkward. Just as Donald did on the practice field, clients in counseling send out nonverbal messages about how they feel about their stories. Pay attention to the same attributes in your clients that you do with yourself. Aversion of eye contact, tension, and closed body posture all might indicate unspoken problems that you may need to address at the appropriate time. They could also represent discrepancies between *what* is being said and *how* it is being said.

Conversely, a relaxed, open, approachable body language indicates acceptance and an openness to communicate. Try to encourage clients to continue talking by maintaining a relaxed posture and periodically scanning your own body for signs of any tension that might be transmitted to clients

As mentioned in Chapter 3, simple "uh huhs," key words, and mirroring are important tools for encouraging clients to continue their stories. They are especially helpful with sensitive subjects because they demonstrate acceptance and assist in keeping clients talking.

Open Invitation to Talk

Using questions to clarify asthma-related information is very important because of the way the disease is so interwoven into all of the dimensions of health and lifestyle. No two people experience asthma in the same way, and understanding the meaning of the disease for individual clients takes careful questioning to gather and clarify information.

Open-Ended Statements and Questions

One helpful way to clarify information with asthma patients is to use open-ended statements liberally in an effort to create a more relaxed, conversational tone. It is better to get the answers to a series of individual questions by asking clients one or two open-ended statements than by asking them a slew of yes/no questions.

When counseling clients with asthma, such as Peter, it is important to understand exactly what triggers their asthma attacks. Knowledge of these triggers plays a big part in developing specific directives and instructions about how clients can abolish, avoid, or alter them. The way you uncover this information about triggers can vary drastically depending on the types of questions you employ. For instance, the following short list (there are many more) includes closed questions that could be used with Peter:

"Peter, does animal dander trigger your asthma attacks?"
"Peter, does cat dander trigger your asthma attacks?"
"Peter, does dog dander trigger your asthma attacks?"
"Peter, does exercise trigger your asthma attacks?"
"Peter, does dust trigger your asthma attacks?"
"Peter, do certain foods trigger your asthma attacks?"
"Peter, does stress trigger your asthma attacks?"
"Peter, do extremes in temperature trigger your asthma attacks?"

You can get the answers to these questions by asking each one directly, or you can ask one or two indirect, open-ended questions and listen to the client respond. If clients miss one or two questions, you can follow up your open-ended question with specific closed questions.

Example: Open-Ended Statements
"Peter, tell me about the kinds of things that trigger your asthma attacks."
"Peter, can you tell me about some of the things that trigger your asthma?"

Peter: Well, it's kind of changed since I was a young kid, and especially since I moved out of my parents' house. As a kid, almost anything out of the ordinary could trigger an attack. I couldn't really play with my dog too much because his dander would sometimes trigger an attack. This was especially true if I was in the same room with my parents and they were smoking. It is different now.
Counselor: How is it different?
Peter: I have begun to exercise a little in the past few months, and my lungs seem to feel better because of it. I don't automatically get an attack anymore if I just run around a little. I also think it is due to moving out of my parents' house. My wife doesn't smoke. We have no pets, and we have only a couple of area rugs in the bedroom and living room. I haven't had an attack from just hanging around the house since I moved out.
Counselor: What else?
Peter: I have to be careful when doing things like shoveling snow in the real cold air in the winter, cutting the grass in the summer, and raking leaves in the fall. All of these are triggers for me.
Counselor: Well, at least you are now living in an apartment and you don't have to worry about those things.
Peter: Yeah, I never thought about that.

Using open-ended questions to get the same needed "trigger" information is a less intrusive way to gather the data than asking a laundry list of questions. It also allows counselors focus more on clients, to listen and observe how they come across. Rather than having to concentrate on which closed question to ask next, using open-ended statements allows counselors to focus completely on clients' stories. Counselors can always go back and use closed questions to clarify any information that is missing or unclear.

Example

Counselor: Peter, you mentioned that when you were in the same room with your parents and the dog, and your parents were smoking, you usually had asthma attacks. Did they stop smoking when you had an attack?

Peter: No, they just told me to go into my bedroom or the family room and use my inhaler.

Counselor: Peter, you mentioned that shoveling snow, mowing the lawn, and raking leaves used to trigger your attacks. Were you the one responsible for doing these chores around your house?

Peter: Yes, my parents expected me to do these things and thought I was using my asthma as a excuse to get out of my chores.

Paraphrasing, Reflection of Feelings, and Summarizing

Paraphrasing and reflection of feelings work similarly for asthma patients as they do for other clients. The major difference is the wide range of emotions associated with asthma, ranging from poor self-image to anger to feelings of helplessness.

Asthma patients (such as Peter) often direct their anger and other strong emotions at parents or others whose behavior affects their ability to control the disease. Persons with asthma often blame their parents for passing this disease on to them. Feelings of anger and hostility are common toward those who are blamed for being the source of their affliction.

Paraphrasing judiciously throughout the client's story will help you clarify how the person views the disease and its relationship to parents and caretakers. Once clients' thoughts and feelings about suffering from asthma are expressed, summarization can help clarify what the client is thinking and feeling. The summary provides an opportunity for the client to hear the story again and decide if anything needs to be added, deleted, or clarified. It also shows the client how well you are following and your assessment of the situation.

Example: Paraphrase

Counselor: Peter, let me make sure I understand what you are saying. You have had asthma all of your life and it pretty much stayed the same until you moved out of your parents' house. Is that right?

Peter: Yeah, that's right.

Example: Reflection of Feelings

Counselor: Peter, you seem very angry at your parents because they continued to smoke and did little to help you reduce your triggers to the disease.

Peter: Yeah, I am very angry with them. I suffered all of those years, and I don't think I'll ever forgive them.

Example: Summary

Counselor: Peter, let me make sure I understand where we are up until this point. Your asthma is triggered by a host of things, ranging from tobacco smoke to raking leaves in the fall. You have had this disease all your life but have noticed an improvement in your condition since you moved out of your parents' house. You are feeling pretty positive and seem to be ready to take control of your asthma, but you still get angry when you think about how your parents didn't seem to care about you. Is this accurate?

Peter: Yeah, I guess so. I also have very mixed feelings about my parents. I think they loved me, and they did take me to doctors to try to help me, but it just seems that they were never willing to make any big sacrifices to help me get better.

Influencing Skills

As mentioned earlier, there are four primary goals for counseling people with asthma: (1) reducing the frequency and severity of future attacks, (2) helping clients adhere to medications prescribed by their healthcare providers, (3) reducing their need to rely on medication to control their asthma, and (4) developing lifestyle-modification plans that help control triggers and build resistance to attacks. In addition to these primary goals, counselors must assess clients' goals regarding their disease. Many of the influencing skills can be used to achieve these goals.

Self-disclosure

As you saw in Case Study 8.3 with Donald, self-disclosure is an excellent technique for demonstrating empathy with clients and helping them build confidence in their perceived ability to change. Self-disclosing to clients that you, the counselor, know what they are going through because you have asthma is one way to do so. When counselors describe how they have successfully managed to achieve their professional and personal goals while learning how to control their asthma, clients can begin to view their own asthma differently. Rather than seeing it as a condition that prohibits them from living a full life, they can see it as something that is within their ability to manage.

Example

Counselor: Peter, I kind of know what you are going through. I have asthma and remember what it was like when I was first learning how to manage it. I often felt that life was unfair and blamed my parents for "doing this to me." Over time, though, I learned how to manage it, and I no longer feel asthma controls my life. I definitely think it has shaped who I am to a certain extent, but I no longer feel it controls my destiny.

Peter: I didn't know you had asthma. I would never have guessed that. I hope I can learn how to manage it as well as you do.

Counselor: Give it time, Peter. You will learn how to manage it.

Confrontation

Confrontation will come into play extensively in asthma counseling, just as it does in all health counseling. Clients will present inconsistencies in their stories for a variety of reasons, ranging from embarrassment over having the illness to simply being unable to accurately recount events from their past. As with all other health problems, counselors can use these inconsistencies to challenge clients in gentle, supportive ways.

Example

Counselor: Peter, on the one hand you say you think your parents loved you because they took you to a doctor to treat your asthma but on the other hand you question their love because they didn't seem willing to make the big sacrifices necessary to help you. What do you mean?

Peter: I guess I have mixed feelings about them. I am thankful that they did something but resent them for not doing enough for me.

Counselor: Okay, I understand. It is common for people to have mixed feelings about issues. You can learn how to manage your asthma despite these mixed feelings towards your parents.

Changing the Focal Point

Changing the focal point is an excellent way to help clients see their problems through the eyes of other people who are intimately involved in their problems. Sometimes clients find this exercise helpful, particularly in changing their personal constructs related to the illness. They may not be able to change anything in the story, but they might find some relief in their emotional response to it if they can see it through the eyes of other people. Peter's reaction to his parents perfectly illustrates this possibility.

Example

Counselor: Peter, I understand your anger and resentment of your parents regarding your asthma, and I don't want to deny you those feelings. What I'd like to do today is to get you to try to see your asthma through their eyes. Close your eyes and step back 20 years, to a time when most of the information we have about asthma and smoking was less well accepted and poorly understood. I also want you to try to imagine what it is like to be addicted to a drug like nicotine, the powerful drug your parents are addicted to. [Counselor pauses for a few seconds and then continues.] Good. Now try to put yourself in your parents' shoes and visualize how they might respond to finding out that their child has asthma and that their smoking plays a part in it by triggering attacks.

Peter: Okay, I can do that.

Counselor: How do you think they viewed it?

Peter: I think they'd be skeptical and want to deny the connection.

Counselor: What are they denying?

Peter: I think they want to deny that they had anything to do with it. I think admitting this connection would have been too painful for them. I think it would have meant that they would have to stop smoking. My mom was a two-pack-a-day smoker and my dad was pretty addicted to cigars.

Counselor: What else do you see?

Peter: I see fear. Neither one of them is too bright, so I think they were afraid of this disease and what it meant for me and for them. I think by denying it, they wouldn't have to face their fears.

Counselor: Good. How can you use this different viewpoint to help yourself deal with your feelings toward them?

Peter: I guess I can use it to get a better sense of their weaknesses and to see that maybe they didn't hate me so much as they were just weak and not able to deal with my asthma. It still doesn't mean that I am going to let them off the hook all of a sudden or start feeling just wonderful about them. I suffered through too many attacks for that to happen.

Counselor: Okay, Peter, but every once in a while when you feel this anger and resentment toward them, try to step back and put yourself in their shoes just to get a sense of who they are and what they were and still are feeling about your asthma.

Directives and Logical Consequences

As mentioned earlier, there are four primary goals for counseling people with asthma: (1) reducing the frequency and severity of future attacks, (2) helping clients adhere to medications prescribed by their healthcare providers, (3) reducing their need to rely on medication to control their asthma, and (4) developing lifestyle-modification plans that help control triggers and build resistance to attacks. Consequently, the key directives for influencing clients with asthma revolve around these four goals.

Directive 1: Assessment of Lung Function Using a Peak Flow Meter

Assessing lung function with a peak flow meter is an essential first step in the development of an asthma action plan and any systematic attempt to manage clients' asthma.

1. Clients will know how to use a peak flow meter.
2. Clients will understand the role played by peak flow assessment in an asthma action plan.
3. Clients will assess their lung function using a peak flow meter.

Logical Consequences of Assessing Lung Function Using a Peak Flow Meter

1. Measurements with a peak flow meter can help clients and their doctors monitor asthma. These measurements are an important source of information in helping doctors prescribe appropriate medications for their clients.
2. Monitoring peak flow rates can help clients recognize changes or trends in their asthma.
3. Peak flow readings may signal the need to change medications.
4. Documentation of peak flow patterns provides a visual aid to help patients understand the air flow changes brought about by their asthma.

Specific Instructions for Assessing Lung Function Using a Peak Flow Meter

1. Before each use, make sure the sliding marker or arrow on the peak flow meter (see Figure 8.2) is at the bottom of the numbered scale (zero or the lowest number on the scale).

2. Stand up straight. Remove gum or any food from the mouth.
3. Take as deep a breath as possible and then hold it.
4. Put the mouthpiece of the peak flow meter into the mouth and close lips tightly around the mouthpiece. Be sure to keep the tongue away from the mouthpiece.
5. In one breath, blow out as hard and as quickly as possible. Blow a "fast hard blast" rather than "slowly blowing" until all of the air in the lungs is emptied.
6. Write down the number where the sliding marker stopped. It indicates the peak flow.
7. Repeat the entire routine three times.
8. Record the highest of the three ratings. Do not calculate an average.
9. Measure the peak flow rate close to the same time each day. Clients can measure the peak flow rate before or after using medication. Some people measure it both before and after taking medication. Try to do it the same way each time.
10. Keep a chart of peak flow rates and discuss the readings with the doctor (ALA, 2003b).

Example

Counselor: Peter, the first thing we need to do is make sure you understand how to use a peak flow meter and why it is an important part of your asthma action plan. Keeping track of your air flow can help you and your doctors monitor your asthma. The readings are a very important source of information that can help your doctor prescribe the best medication for you. Keeping track of your air flow can give you a visual picture of your asthma and help you feel more in control of it. What do you think?

Peter: Okay, I can see that.

Counselor: Good. Let's start by going over a few things about your peak flow meter. I'll write these steps down as we go along. Before each use, make sure the sliding marker or arrow on your peak flow meter is at the bottom of the numbered scale. This point is repre-

sented by zero, or the lowest number on the scale. Do you see that?

Peter: Yes, mine says zero.

Counselor: Good. Now you need to stand up straight and remove gum or food from your mouth.

Peter: (Stands up straight) I have no gum or food.

Counselor: Okay, now take as deep a breath as possible and then hold it [demonstrates this to Peter]. After you take that breath, you put the mouthpiece of the peak flow meter into your mouth and close your lips tightly around the mouthpiece. Be sure to keep your tongue away from the mouthpiece [demonstrates this to Peter]. In one breath, blow out as hard and as quickly as you can. Try to blow a "fast hard blast" rather than "slowly blowing" until all of the air in the lungs is emptied [demonstrates this to Peter]. Okay, you try it this far. Tell me what you are going to do. (Patient quiz)

Peter: I am going to empty my lungs of air, and then take as deep a breath as possible and hold it. Then I am going to put the mouthpiece of the meter in my mouth, make a good seal, and blow out in a hard blast.

Counselor: Good. Now let's see you do it.

Peter: Okay [successfully demonstrates the technique]. Now what?

Counselor: When you have expelled your blast of air, look at the meter and write down the number where the sliding marker stopped. It indicates your peak flow [shows Peter his reading]. Then you need to repeat this entire routine three times and write down the highest of your three ratings. Do not calculate an average of the three.

Peter: Okay, I do this three times, keep track of the number where my marker stops, and write down the highest of the three recordings [Peter demonstrates this successfully].

Counselor: Good. The only thing left is to make sure you do this close to the same time each day. You also can measure your peak flow rate before or after using your medication. It doesn't matter which you choose, as long as you do it the same way each time. Keep a chart of your peak flow rates and bring them each time you see me or your doctor. It's a good idea to go over them periodically with your doctor in case he or she needs to change your medications. What questions do you have?

Peter: None.

Counselor: Before we move on, why don't you go over the entire procedure one more time and demonstrate it again for me. I know this is hard to remember. (Repetition, patient quiz)

Peter: Okay [goes over the entire sequence and demonstrates it successfully].

Directive 2: Taking Prescribed Drugs as Directed

It is important to remember that nonmedical counselors do not prescribe asthma medications for clients. Their sole role in this directive is to help clients achieve maximum compliance with the medication regimens prescribed by their physicians. Counselors must be sure to make this role clear to both clients and their physicians before discussing medication-taking instructions.

Counselors need to know how different types of asthma medications work and are administered so they can help clients adhere to their therapeutic regimens. They should work in concert with licensed healthcare providers to help clients adhere to their asthma action plans.

1. *Know the two primary categories of asthma drugs.* Many drugs to control asthma are available. Most are either long-term controllers or quick relief rescuers.
2. *Take drugs as prescribed.* It's important that clients take their drugs as prescribed.
3. *Be aware of side effects.* If clients experience side effects, they should tell their doctors so that the drugs can be changed or the dose adjusted.
4. *Be aware of the need for multiple drugs.* Many people need to take two or more drugs to control their asthma.

Logical Consequences of Taking Prescribed Drugs as Directed

1. Taking long-term controller medication regularly will help prevent asthma attacks by treating constriction and inflammation of the airways in the lungs.
2. Taking quick relief rescuer medications as prescribed will stop immediate symptoms of an asthma attack.
3. If clients do not take their medication properly, their symptoms may worsen.

Specific Instructions for Taking Prescribed Drugs as Directed

1. Discuss how quick relief rescuers and long-term controllers work.
2. Describe how long-term controllers often do not provide immediate relief, but rather help lessen the frequency and severity of episodes over time and must be taken regularly, even in the absence of symptoms.
3. Discuss the importance of keeping quick relief rescuers handy at all times.
4. Name the medication. Clients need to know the names of their medication(s).
5. Discuss the medication's efficacy. Clients need to believe that their medications are the best available for their particular problems, especially if the treatment is difficult to take or produces side effects.
6. Explain the dosage and schedule. To take medications correctly, clients need to know how many puffs/pills to take each day, how doses should be spaced, and how long to take them.
7. Note any potential side effects. Clients need to know what side effects to expect or they will discontinue taking their medications when these side effects occur.
8. Determine any contraindications. Clients need to know what to avoid while taking their medications or they might experience unanticipated side effects or reduction in efficacy.
9. Describe the expected symptom response. Clients need to know how long each type of

medication takes to work and how the effects of the different types of drugs are evaluated.

10. Consider the possibility of missed doses. Clients need to know what to do if they miss a dose.

Example

Counselor: Peter, the next thing we need to do is make sure you understand how to take your medications correctly. I see that your doctor has put you on two medications, [*Drug A*], a pill, and [*Drug B*], an inhaler. Is that correct?

Peter: Yes, that is correct.

Counselor: Okay, do you know the difference between the two drugs?

Peter: Yes, the doctor told me that [*Drug A*] is designed to be taken every day and will help relax my airways and reduce the risks of having an asthma attack in the first place. [*Drug B*] is my emergency inhaler, to be used when I am having an attack. It will open up my airways.

Counselor: You seem to have a good understanding of the different types of medications you have been prescribed and their use. I need to go over a few more details and be sure you know how to use them correctly. I can't prescribe medication for you, but I can help you learn how to use it consistently and correctly.

Peter: Okay.

Counselor: [*Drug A*] is a long-term controller medication called a leukotriene receptor antagonist. *It is not a steroid.* It works by blocking leukotrienes, substances associated with the inflammatory process of asthma. It will not provide immediate relief, like your inhaler. Rather, it is designed to help lessen the frequency and severity of your attacks over time. It must be taken daily, even in the absence of symptoms. You should not stop

taking or change the dose of your inhaler because you are taking [*Drug A*]. It should not be used to stop an attack that has already begun. You should always have your inhaler handy for that.

Peter: Okay.

Counselor: Your doctor has determined that [*Drug A*] is the best available long-term controller medication for you. You need to take one [*x*]-milligram tablet every day. This is the perfect dose for you. Do not take more than one pill, even when you are having an attack. Use your inhaler to control attacks [writes these instructions down on a patient education sheet for Peter]. Do you understand?

Peter: Yes, I do.

Counselor: Why don't you just repeat it back to me one time. (Patient quiz)

Peter: Okay [repeats how to take medication].

Counselor: Peter, in clinical studies, the side effects experienced by people taking medications such as yours were found to be mild and they varied by age. They included headache, ear infection, sore throat, and upper respiratory infection. In most cases, these side effects generally did not stop patients from taking the drug. If you experience any of these problems, continue taking your medication but see your doctor immediately.

Peter: Okay.

Counselor: There are really no contraindications for this medicine. You can eat whatever you want and go about your normal routine. The only two contraindications would be if you if you were pregnant or nursing. I don't expect you'll be experiencing either condition in the near future [lame attempt at counselor humor].

Peter: Not if I can help it. Ha, ha.

Counselor: Peter, you probably won't notice any dramatic effects once you begin taking [*Drug A*]. Within a couple of weeks, however, you should see a reduction in the frequency and severity of your attacks. If you miss a dose, just pick up with taking the medication the next day. Do not take two doses at one time.

Drug A denotes a long-term controller medication.
Drug B denotes a quick-relief rescuer.

Peter: Okay.

Counselor: Before we move on to [Drug B], why don't you just repeat to me how you will take [Drug A] and what to avoid, or what to do if you miss a dose or experience side effects. (Patient quiz)

Peter: All right [explains entire regimen correctly].

Counselor: Good. Now let's talk a little bit about [Drug B], which is a quick relief rescue inhaler—a form of albuterol. It is designed for use when you are experiencing an asthma attack. It is a form of albuterol and the effects are designed to last for six hours or longer. Do not use this inhaler more frequently than it was prescribed by the doctor. If you find that you need to use it more than every six hours, you should speak to your doctor about perhaps switching your long-term controller or doing something else to help you control your asthma. Do you understand?

Peter: Yes.

Counselor: I see from your inhaler [Peter had handed it to the counselor] that you are instructed to take two puffs every six hours as needed. How has that been working out?

Peter: Pretty good. The doctor had originally given me a spacer to use with the inhaler, but I like it better without using the spacer.

Counselor: That is okay. Tell me how you take your puffs. (Patient quiz)

Peter: It is real similar to using the peak flow meter. I completely empty my lungs, put the inhaler in my mouth, and simultaneously push down the plunger and inhale deeply. I then hold the medicine in my lungs deeply for at least 10 seconds.

Counselor: The only thing I'd add is to store it at room temperature and shake it vigorously before each use. How long do you wait between puffs?

Peter: I wait about a minute and then repeat the procedure.

Counselor: Good. Once again, make sure you shake the inhaler between puffs.

Peter: Okay.

Counselor: Common side effects of using [Drug B], and other forms of albuterol, include palpitations, chest pain, rapid heart rate, and tremors or nervousness. The only contraindications for using albuterol are being pregnant or nursing. Peter, most quick relief rescue inhalers last for about 200 puffs. This information is listed on your canister [shows this to Peter]. If you divide 200 by 8 puffs per day, you'll see that the canister will last about 25 days. Keep track of when your canister will run out so you can be sure to have another one available (RxList, 2004).

Directive 3: Following an Asthma Action Plan

An asthma action plan combines peak flow readings with medication taking. As discussed earlier, it uses a "zone system" (see Figure 8.3) to help clients assess their lung function and medicate accordingly. If clients adhere to this plan, they can prevent inflammation and constriction of their lungs, thereby reducing the risk of suffering from an attack (AAFA, 2003).

1. Review (the plan should originally be presented by a physician) the asthma action plan concept with clients.
2. Make sure clients understand how peak flow readings are related to medication needs.
3. Make sure clients discuss their action plans with their physicians on a regular basis.

Logical Consequences of Following an Asthma Action Plan

1. Following the directives as indicated based on peak flow readings under each zone as well as regular symptoms should provide immediate relief.
2. Monitoring peak flow allows for a visual assessment of how medications are working and indicates to clients whether medications should be increased or decreased.
3. If clients do not follow their action plans, they have a greater chance of symptoms worsening or of suffering severe asthma attacks.

Specific Instructions for Following
an Asthma Action Plan

1. Describe what each color in the zone represents.
2. Describe the symptoms associated with each zone.
3. Explain what to do regarding medication taking for each zone.
4. Emphasize the importance of seeking medical care when in the yellow and red zones (ALA, 2003b).

Example

Counselor: Peter, your doctor should have talked to you about developing an asthma action plan based on your daily peak flow readings and medication use. Did he or she do this?

Peter: Yes, he did.

Counselor: Tell me what the doctor told you.

Peter: He said that I needed to chart my peak flow readings and monitor them. When my peak flow is in a certain color zone, it represents a different need for medication.

Counselor: What do the zones represent?

Peter: Here is the chart the doctor gave me [shows the counselor the Figure 8.3 asthma action plan]. When my peak flow readings are in the green zone, everything is okay and I should just keep doing what I am doing. When they hit the yellow zone, I need to continue taking my medication and double up on my inhaler dose as I need it. If I move into the orange zone, I need to start taking the steroid pills my doctor gave me. I should also contact him immediately. If I ever fall into the red zone, I should get to a hospital quickly and call my doctor.

Counselor: Excellent.

Directive 4: Assess Asthma Triggers

It is important for clients to be aware of the things in their environment that tend to trigger asthma attacks and make chronic asthma symptoms worse. Because people with asthma react differently to triggers and combinations of triggers, an important step in asthma management is the assessment of triggers.

1. Teach clients how to use a log to identify their asthma triggers.
2. Teach clients how to monitor their asthma triggers.
3. Teach clients how to use the information from their logs to control triggers.

Logical Consequences of Assessing
Asthma Triggers

1. If clients can monitor their asthma triggers by using logs, they can feel more in control over their disease.
2. If clients can monitor their asthma triggers by using logs, they can learn how to manage triggers and reduce the number of asthma attacks they have.

Specific Instructions for Assessing
Asthma Triggers

1. Keep a daily asthma trigger log (see **Figure 8.4**).
   - Every day, log in any trigger that initiated asthma symptoms (from labored breathing to a full-blown attack).
   - If there are no triggers for any particular day, note this by writing "no triggers today."
   - When triggers initiate asthma symptoms, take a peak flow reading and record it in the log.
   - Indicate the severity of the symptoms on a scale of 1 to 10 (with 10 being the worst).
   - Indicate which medication and what dose you took to alleviate symptoms.
   - Indicate whether the medication worked.
2. Review this log weekly to identify personal triggers.
3. Review this log with your doctor every few months to help modify your asthma action plan.

Example

Counselor: Peter, here is an example of an asthma triggers daily log [shows Peter the log]. I'd like you to start keeping it today.

Peter: What is it used for?

Day	Trigger	Peak Flow Reading	Severity of Symptoms 1—10	Medication	Response to Medication
12/21	Cat	400	Difficulty breathing (8)	2 puffs albuterol	Stopped attack
12/23	Cigar smoke	390	Difficulty breathing (7)	2 puffs albuterol	Stopped attack
12/24	Cold air	460	Shortness of breath (9)	Stopped exercise	Stopped attack
12/25	Overeating	390	Very hard to breathe (7)	4 puffs albuterol	Stopped attack

Figure 8.4 Monitoring triggers is an excellent way to begin to reduce exposure to them.

Counselor: It will help you identify and monitor your personal asthma triggers. By understanding your triggers, you can begin to eliminate some of them that are within your control.

Peter: Okay.

Counselor: Peter, you won't be able to eliminate all of your triggers, because some things, such as air pollution and seasonal allergies, are beyond your control. Even so, those types of triggers can be modified, if not eliminated completely.

Peter: What do I need to do?

Counselor: Keep the daily log every day. If you look at the sample, you'll see that each day you need to fill in any trigger that initiated your asthma symptoms. These symptoms could range from mild labored breathing to a full-blown attack. If you have no triggers on any particular day, note that by writing "no triggers today."

Peter: That sounds easy enough.

Counselor: Good. When your triggers initiate any asthma symptoms, take a peak flow reading and record it in the log. Be sure to indicate the severity of the symptoms on a scale of 1 to 10. Ten is the worst. Then I want you to indicate which medication you took and what the dose was. Lastly, please indicate whether the medication worked. Peter, I expect you to keep this log faithfully and bring it back next week when we meet again.

Peter: I'll definitely do it.

Counselor: Good. Besides showing it to me, you need to bring the log to discuss with your doctor, especially if it seems that your medications are not working in controlling your asthma.

Directive 5: Controlling Asthma Triggers

Many different categories of asthma triggers exist, some of which are easier to control than others. Some, such as exercise behavior, are personal and can be controlled through individual action. Others, such as family pets, are related to family lifestyle and may not be so easy to change. Often (as we saw in Carlos's and Peter's case studies), problems associated with controlling triggers can lead to emotional distress and interpersonal stress. Sometimes it is necessary to involve the entire family in asthma counseling so they can understand the dynamics associated with a family member's disease.

1. Use an asthma triggers log to identify triggers.
2. Organize triggers into definable categories.
3. Identify triggers that can be eliminated or minimized.
4. Identify triggers that can't be eliminated or minimized but must be modified.
5. Develop strategies for controlling triggers.
6. Implement strategies for controlling triggers.

Logical Consequences of Controlling Asthma Triggers

1. Reducing or removing as many asthma and allergy triggers as possible from homes will reduce the frequency and severity of asthma symptoms and attacks.
2. Reducing or removing as many asthma and allergy triggers as possible from work sites and other environmental areas will reduce the frequency and severity of asthma symptoms and attacks.
3. Failing to reduce or remove triggers will result in increased frequency and severity of attacks and the inability to successfully implement an asthma action plan.

Specific Instructions for Controlling Asthma Triggers: Allergen-Related Triggers

1. Consider meeting with an allergist to get tested for allergens and begin a program of desensitization.
2. During your allergy season, you should do the following:
   - Keep your windows closed.
   - Minimize time spent outdoors during the midday and afternoon, if possible, because pollen and some mold spore counts are highest then.
3. Install an air cleaner in your forced-air central heating/cooling system.
4. If you do not have forced-air central heating and cooling, use a stand-alone air cleaner to remove allergens from the air (AAFA, 2003).

Specific Instructions for Controlling Asthma Triggers: Illness-Related Triggers

1. Be aware that sinus symptoms, such as runny nose, coughing up mucus, fever, or sore throat, can trigger asthma attacks.
2. Take prompt action to treat even the mildest cold symptoms with over-the-counter cold remedies, vaporizers, and other medications before they worsen.
3. Avoid visitors with colds or the flu for similar reasons.

4. Practice good hand-washing technique to reduce the risk of disease transmission.

Specific Instructions for Controlling Asthma Triggers: Dust-Related Triggers

1. Reduce humidity to less than 50% by using a dehumidifier or an air conditioner.
2. Remove as much wall-to-wall carpeting as possible, especially in the bedroom.
3. Remove venetian blinds, especially in the bedroom.
4. Encase mattresses, box springs, and pillows in airtight, zippered, plastic, or special allergen-proof fabric covers.

Counseling Hints & Tips 8.2

Proper Hand-Washing Technique

Many people are not familiar with proper hand-washing technique as a way to reduce risks associated with communicable diseases. This technique avoids touching the sink with the hands. It is preferable to have water controls and soap dispensers that use knee or foot controls. If not available, use clean paper towels to touch faucet controls. Hand washing may be followed by drying with paper towels, but contact with the outside of the towel dispenser must be avoided.

1. Turn on the faucet with a clean paper towel.
2. Operate the soap control with a foot control or use a clean paper towel.
3. Wash between the fingers for 30 seconds.
4. Rinse hands thoroughly under flowing water, but do not make contact with the faucet or sink.
5. If contact is made, hand washing must be restarted.
6. Allow water to run toward the elbows; do not allow water from the arm to run down to the hands.
7. Dry hands with clean paper towels and *then* turn off water with paper towels.

5. Wash sheets and blankets weekly in hot water (130°F) and dry them in a hot dryer.
6. Replace comforters and pillows made of natural materials (such as down, feathers, or cotton) with items made from synthetic fibers, or encase the natural materials in allergen-proof covers.
7. Control clutter by picking things up and putting them away.
8. Keep clothing in drawers.
9. Vacuum the bedroom once a week, using a vacuum with a HEPA filter or a double bag.
10. Wear a dust mask, and remember to change the filter regularly (Nguyen, Chen, Gill, & Gill, 2001).

Specific Instructions for Controlling Asthma Triggers: Mold-Related Triggers

1. Ventilate and clean basements, bathrooms, and kitchens regularly.
2. Use air conditioners to control excess moisture during warm-weather months.
3. Clean the area with a solution containing one part bleach to 20 parts water and a small amount of detergent.
4. Remove carpeting or wallpaper that shows visible signs of mold or mildew. Repair and seal leaking roofs or pipes promptly.
5. Remove carpeting from concrete or damp floors.
6. Avoid storing clothes, bedding, papers, or other items in damp areas.
7. Use a dehumidifier in a damp basement. Empty and clean the unit regularly to prevent mildew from forming inside the dehumidifier.
8. Seal openings where water is seeping into the basement.
9. Install exhaust fans in the kitchen and bathrooms.
10. Keep houseplants out of bedrooms (Nguyen et al., 2001).

Specific Instructions for Controlling Asthma Triggers: Pet-Related Triggers

1. Avoid pets that cause allergies.
2. Keep the pet out of the rooms where you spend much of your time, such as the bedroom and the family room.
3. Try giving your dog or cat a weekly bath. Although not all experts are convinced of its effectiveness, some studies have shown benefits to this practice.
4. Let only nonallergic family members groom the pet.
5. Remove your rugs or vacuum them weekly with a special vacuum; animal allergens cannot be removed from the lower levels of the rug with a conventional vacuum cleaner. Use a vacuum with a HEPA filter or a double bag. Be sure to change the filter often.
6. Clean regularly. Even after a pet has been removed from your house, it can take weeks, months, or even a year or more for the animal allergens to be eliminated from fabrics (Nguyen et al., 2001).

Specific Instructions for Controlling Asthma Triggers: Air-Related Triggers

1. Ban smoking in your home, and do your best to avoid enclosed places that are smoky.
2. Avoid other airborne irritants, such as perfumes, fumes from paint and cleaning products, and any other strong fumes or odors.
3. To remove other airborne particles from your home that may trigger your asthma symptoms, use air conditioners, HEPA filters (replace them regularly), and electrostatic air purifiers.
4. If possible, do not use a wood-burning stove, kerosene heater, or fireplace.
5. Avoid using aerosol sprays that allow irritating particles to enter the lungs. Use non-aerosol pump containers.
6. Limit outdoor activities in smog-infested areas.
7. Minimize exposure to high-traffic areas where auto exhaust can trigger an attack. Use air conditioning or roll up windows to avoid exhaust fumes.
8. Avoid extreme cold-air weather conditions or cover the nose and mouth with a scarf or other clothing article (Nguyen et al., 2001).

Specific Instructions for Controlling Asthma Triggers: Exercise-Related Triggers

1. Always use pre-exercise inhaled medications before beginning vigorous exercise.
2. Warm up before exercising. To warm up, walk at a slow pace for 5 to 10 minutes and then stretch your muscles.
3. Cool down when you are finished. The cool-down period allows your body (including your lungs) to adjust to temperature changes, thereby decreasing the risk that your asthma symptoms will flare up.
4. Keep your quick relief inhaler with you while exercising.
5. Set exercise goals you can reach. Reaching a goal will give you a sense of accomplishment. Once you've reached your goal, reward yourself.
6. Exercise at a moderate pace until you become fit.

diverse perspectives 8.1

Poverty, Cockroaches, and Asthma

The role of cockroach allergen as an asthma trigger was first discovered by Bernton et al. (1972). Over the past 30 years, other studies have confirmed a positive association for allergy and asthma with cockroach proteins. Skin tests have been used to show positive reactions to cockroaches in asthma sufferers for more than three decades (Kang, 1976; Kang, Vellody, Homburger, & Yunginger, 1979; Hulett & Dockhorn, 1979; Call, Smith, Morris, et al., 1992). Pollart et al. (1989) found that the level of cockroach antibodies in the blood of people with asthma was significantly higher than that in the serum of a control group of individuals without asthma.

A more recent study published in the *New England Journal of Medicine* found that the combination of cockroach allergy and exposure to cockroach debris made asthma attacks worse in inner-city children (Rosenstreich, Eggleston, Kattan, et al., 1997). The children in this study were mostly poor and lived in older, multiple-family, inner-city dwellings. Children who were both allergic to cockroach allergen and exposed to high levels of this allergen had three times as many hospitalizations, twice as many hospital visits, and more missed schooldays than other students without similar allergies. According to Rosenstreich et al. (1997), cockroach exposure might be an even more significant trigger of severe asthma attacks than exposure to dust mites and cat dander.

In the United States, the rising incidence of asthma is especially notable in inner cities, where exposure to cockroaches is almost universal. The combination of substandard housing and multiple urban dwellings promote high cockroach populations in these areas (Koehler, Patterson, & Brewer, 1987). Sarpong et al. (1996a) found statistically significant associations between cockroach allergen sensitization and lower socioeconomic status, cockroach exposure at home, and African American ethnicity. Clearly, exposure to cockroach allergens is a risk factor for the higher prevalence of asthma in poor urban areas (Call et al., 1992).

Sarpong et al. (1996b) recommend that avoidance of cockroach allergens be included in management of any person with asthma. While weekly vacuum cleaning combined with examination of cockroach parts and residue can reduce the level of cockroach allergens, these researchers found that reducing exposure to cockroach allergens could be achieved only through extermination of what they termed the "resident cockroach populations."

Currently available pesticides can reduce cockroach populations by 85% to 100% and maintain these reductions for at least three months (Wright & Dupree, 1988; Kaakeh, Scharf, & Bennett, 1997a, 1997b). Cockroaches, however, are very resilient and are capable of adapting behaviorally, physiologically, and genetically. As a consequence, their control requires constant monitoring. Such extermination and monitoring poses a daunting challenge for residents of the United States' inner cities.

7. If it is cold outdoors, exercise indoors or wear a mask or scarf over your nose and mouth.
8. If you have known allergies, avoid exercising outdoors when pollen counts or air pollution levels are high.
9. Restrict exercise when you have a viral infection.
10. If you have an asthma attack while exercising, stop and repeat the pre-exercise inhaled medication.
11. If your symptoms go away, restart the exercise.

Specific Instructions for Controlling Asthma Triggers: Cockroach-Induced Triggers
1. Seal potential points of entry for cockroaches, such as wall cracks; gaps in windows, floors, and doors; and around drains.
2. Fix and seal all leaky faucets and pipes.
3. Keep food in tightly closed containers.
4. Sweep or vacuum the floor after meals.
5. Wash dishes in hot, soapy water immediately after meals.
6. Clean kitchen surfaces and cupboards regularly.
7. Clean under the stove, refrigerator, and toaster to get rid of loose crumbs.
8. Hire a trained exterminator to treat the interior of your home while you and your family and pets are out.
9. Take out the garbage and recyclables frequently, and use lidded garbage containers in the kitchen (Nguyen et al., 2001).

Example (Using Reducing Exercise Triggers)
Counselor: Peter, you mentioned that you would like to start exercising. Let's look at how we can work to control exercise-related triggers.

Peter: I'd like that. I really want to build my lungs up.

Counselor: The first thing you need to do is to set exercise goals that you can reach. Reaching a goal will give you a sense of accomplishment. Don't try to advance too quickly. Give yourself a few months to get into shape.

When starting out, exercise at a moderate pace until you become fit.

Peter: I've got some good exercise guidelines from my doctor.

Counselor: Good. Just remember to always use your inhaler before beginning to exercise. This consideration is especially important for aerobic exercise, because it places a greater demand on your lungs. Make sure you warm up before exercising. To warm up, walk at a slow pace for 5 to 10 minutes and then stretch your muscles.

Peter: Okay.

Counselor: Keep your quick relief inhaler with you while exercising, just in case you need it, and always cool down when you are finished exercising. The cool-down period allows your body and your lungs time to adjust to temperature changes. It will help decrease the risk that your asthma symptoms will flare up. If it is cold outdoors, exercise indoors or wear a mask or scarf over your nose and mouth. If you are allergic to pollen, avoid exercising outdoors when pollen counts or air pollution levels are high. Any questions?

Peter: No, I understand.

Counselor: If you have an asthma attack while exercising, stop and use your inhaler. If your symptoms go away, you can resume exercising. If they don't, stop exercising for the day. I know this is a lot to remember, so why don't you repeat the instructions back to me.

Peter: I should set reasonable goals and take a few months to get into shape. I need to be sure to use my inhaler before I work out, and I should stop and use it if I develop any symptoms during my workout. If the symptoms don't go away, I should stop exercising for the day. I should also warm up and cool down before and after exercising and be careful about exercising in the cold weather or when my allergies are kicking up.

Counselor: Sounds good. Good luck.

Peter: Thanks.

Summary

Asthma has become a major public health threat, whose prevalence has increased dramatically over the past 30 years. This incurable, chronic disease affects every facet of patients' life and health. Although asthma is not typically thought of as a fatal disease, asthmatic attacks, if uncontrolled, can lead to death.

Asthma is a major force in shaping the lives of people who have it. The disease forces them to look at their world differently and make many adaptations and adjustments to their lifestyle in an effort to live in a world full of triggers.

The microskills model can be applied to counseling people with asthma. In this chapter, the authors work through the application of introductory, attending, responding, and listening skills to show how to counsel someone with this disease.

Study Questions

1. Describe the epidemiologic trends for asthma over the past 20 years.
2. Why is asthma such a serious personal and public health problem?
3. What is the main goal of asthma counseling?
4. How is asthma similar to and different from other chronic diseases?
5. List and describe the risk factors for acquiring asthma.
6. List and describe three common environmental triggers for asthma attacks.
7. List and describe three triggers for asthma attacks other than those listed in Study Question 6.
8. Describe how to control the triggers in Study Questions 6 and 7.
9. How do long-term asthma medications work in reducing the occurrence of attacks?
10. How do short-term medications work in stopping attacks once they begin?
11. Why should counselors use words such as "manage" and "control" instead of "cure" and "treat" when working with clients with asthma?
12. How can counselor self-disclosure influence patients with asthma in a positive way?
13. How can counselors use focusing the narrative to help clients view their asthma in a more positive light?
14. List and describe the key directives and logical consequences for each of the asthma management counseling goals.

References

Aligne CA, Auinger P, Byrd RS, & Weitzman M (2000). Risk factors for pediatric asthma contributions of poverty, race, and urban residence. *American Journal of Respiratory Critical Care Medicine*, 162:873–877.

American Lung Association (ALA) (2003a). *Trends in Asthma Morbidity and Mortality*. www.lungusa.org/data/asthma/ASTHMAdt.pdf.

American Lung Association (ALA) (2003b). *Peak Flow Meters*. www.lungusa.org/asthma/astpeakflow.html.

Asthma and Allergy Foundation of America (AAFA) (2003). *What Is Asthma?* www.aafa.org/templ/display.cfm?id=2&sub=25.

Bernton HS, McMahon TF, Brown H (1972). Cockroach asthma. *British Journal of Diseases of the Chest* 66:61–66.

Call RS, Smith E, Morris MD, et al. (1992). Risk factors for asthma in inner-city children. *Journal of Pediatrics* 121:826–866.

Centers for Disease Control and Prevention (CDC) (2001). Self-reported asthma prevalence among adults in the United States, 2000. *Mortality and Morbidity Weekly Report* 50:682–686. www.cdc.gov/mmwr/preview/mmwrhtml/mm5032a3.htm.

Hulett AC, Dockhorn RJ (1979). House dust mite *(D. farinae)* and cockroach allergy in a Midwestern population. *Annals of Allergy* 42:160–165.

Kaakeh WM, Scharf E, Bennett GW (1997a). Efficacy of conventional insecticide and juvenoid mixtures on an insecticide-resistant field population of German cockroach *(Dictyoptera: Blattellidae)*. *Journal of Agricultural Entomology* 14:339–348.

Kaakeh WM, Scharf E, Bennett GW (1997b). Evaluation of trapping and vacuuming compared with low-impact insecticide tactics for managing German cockroaches in residences. *Journal of Economic Entomology* 90:976–982.

Kang B (1976). Study on cockroach antigen as probable causative agent in bronchial asthma. *Journal of Allergy and Clinical Immunology* 58:357–365.

Kang B, Vellody D, Homburger H, Yunginger JW (1979). Cockroach cause of allergic asthma: its specificity and immunological profile. *Journal of Allergy and Clinical Immunology* 63:80–86.

Koehler PG, Patterson RS, Brewer JR (1987). German cockroach infestation in low income apartments. *Journal of Economic Entomology* 80:446–448.

Mannino DM, Homa DM, Akinbami LJ, et al. (2002). Surveillance for Asthma—United States, 1980–1999. *Morbidity and Mortality Weekly Report Surveillance Summary* 51:1–13.

Mausner JS, Kramer S (1985). *Epidemiology: An Introductory Text*. Philadelphia: W. B. Saunders.

National Center for Health Statistics (NCHS) (2003). *Asthma Prevalence, Health Care Use and Mortality, 2000–2001*. www.cdc.gov/nchs.

National Jewish Medical and Research Center (2003). *Medfacts: Allergy Testing*. www.nationaljewish.org/medfacts/testing.html.

Nguyen P, Chen S, Gill C, Gill M (2001). Counseling patients on management of asthma. *Insights* Nov:9–18.

Pollart SM, Chapman MD, Fiocco GP, et al. (1989). Epidemiology of acute asthma: IgE antibodies to common inhalant allergens as a risk factor for emergency room visits. *Journal of Allergy and Clinical Immunology* 83:875–882.

Rosenstreich DL, Eggleston P, Kattan M, et al. (1997). The role of cockroach allergy and exposure to cockroach allergen in causing morbidity among inner-city children with asthma. *New England Journal of Medicine* 336:1356–1363.

RxList (2004). *Rx List: The Internet Drug Index*. www.rxlist.com/cgi/generic/albut1_pi.htm.

Sarpong SB, Hamilton RG, Eggleston PA, Adkinson NF (1996a). Socioeconomic status and race as risk factors for cockroach allergen exposure and sensitization in children with asthma. *Journal of Allergy and Clinical Immunology* 97:1393–1401.

Sarpong SB, Wood RA, Eggleston PA (1996b). Short-term effects of extermination and cleaning on cockroach allergen Bla g 2 in settled dust. *Annals of Allergy, Asthma, and Immunology* 76:257–260.

United States Department of Health and Human Services (USDHHS), Office of Disease Prevention and Health Promotion (ODPHP) (2003). *Healthy People 2010: A Systematic Approach to Health Improvement*. www.healthypeople.gov/Document/html/uih/uih_bw/uih_2.htm#obj.

Wright CG, Dupree NE (1988). Single family dwellings: evaluation of insecticides for controlling German cockroaches. *Insecticide and Acaricide Tests* 15:355.

Learning Objectives

By the end of the chapter students will:

1. Understand the nature and extent of the hypertension problem in the United States

2. Describe the goals of hypertension counseling

3. Compare and contrast hypertension with other chronic diseases

4. Describe the risk factors for hypertension

5. Describe the actions of a variety of hypertension medications

6. Discuss some common emotional responses to having high blood pressure

7. Describe how counselors with hypertension can use self-disclosure effectively

8. Discuss how changing the focal point can help clients view their hypertension differently

9. List and describe the key directives and logical consequences for each of the hypertension counseling goals

Overview of Blood Pressure and Hypertension

To understand high blood pressure, one must first understand something about how the cardiovascular system operates. Blood pressure is determined by the actions of the blood, the heart, and the blood vessels working in concert. The heart, blood, and blood vessels create a closed system, with the three parts working to-gether to pump blood, under pressure, throughout the body. This pressure is influenced by the overall level of health of the heart and blood vessels as well as the volume of blood in the system. The volume of blood that the heart is able to pump into the arteries is determined, in part, by how much blood fills the heart prior to each beat, how strongly the heart contracts during each beat, and how flexible (or stiff) the blood vessels are. The less flexible and more blocked the blood vessels, the greater the pressure needed to move blood through the system. The more pliable and open the blood vessels, the less pressure is needed to pump blood through them.

The stiffness of the blood vessels is influenced by **atherosclerosis** and other changes associated with lifestyle and aging. Blood pressure and pulse pressure increase as a normal part of aging, because the large arteries become stiff due to changes in proteins such as **collagen** and **elastin** that affect their composition and that of the surrounding tissue.

The kidneys also exert a tremendous influence on blood pressure because of their role in regulating blood volume. During normal operations, the arteries within kidneys sense the volume of blood in the body. When the volume is low, the kidneys secrete **renin,** an enzyme, which triggers production of **angiotensin,** a hormone. Angiotensin triggers the release of **aldosterone,** another hormone that helps regulate the sodium and water balance by retaining sodium and water and excreting potassium. This process increases water retention and hence blood volume.

Blood pressure is a measure of the force that blood exerts on the inner walls of the arteries at two points in the cardiac cycle: when the heart beats and when it is at rest and filling with blood. As just mentioned, blood pressure is dependent upon and is determined by the volume of blood within the heart and arteries, the condition of the blood vessels, and the mechanics of the heart as it pumps blood through the system. Blood pressure is measured in millimeters of mercury (mm Hg) using a **sphygmomanometer,** or blood pressure cuff (see **Figure 9.1**). When the heart pumps blood into the arteries during each heartbeat, the pressure within the arteries increases rapidly. The greatest pressure—the peak level exerted on the artery walls—is called the **systolic blood pressure (SBP).** This pressure is recorded as the top (i.e., larger) of the two numbers included in a blood pressure reading. When the heart muscle relaxes and fills with blood to get ready for the next heartbeat, arterial pressure decreases because the blood is draining out of the large arteries into the

body's organs. The lowest level to which blood pressure decreases between heartbeats is called the **diastolic blood pressure (DBP).** It is the lower reading, or bottom number, in a blood pressure reading. The systolic minus the diastolic is considered the **pulse.**

Diagnosis

Normal blood pressure is considered to be a systolic blood pressure of less than 120 mm Hg and a diastolic blood pressure of less than 80 mm Hg. Systolic blood pressure of 120–139 mm Hg or diastolic readings of 80–89 mm Hg are considered **pre-hypertension.** Patients with pre-hypertension (those in the 130–139/80–89 mm Hg blood pres-

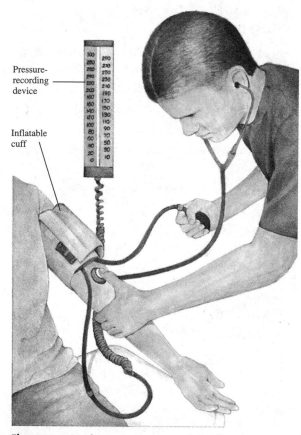

Pressure-recording device

Inflatable cuff

Figure 9.1 A sphygmomanometer (blood pressure cuff) is used to determine blood pressure.

sure range) have twice the risk of developing hypertension as those with lower values (NIH, 2003b). Systolic readings above 140 mm Hg or diastolic readings above 90 mm Hg constitute **hypertension** (NIH, 2003b). (See **Table 9.1.**) Hypertension is diagnosed when two or more blood pressure readings are elevated. One isolated elevated blood pressure reading is not sufficient for diagnosing hypertension, as many things can elevate blood pressure in normal individuals, ranging from exercise to strong emotions such as surprise, fear, or anger. Consequently, sustained elevation in blood pressure represents the criterion for diagnosis.

Hypertension is often referred to as "the silent killer" because it does its damage quietly, without obvious symptoms. The only way people find out that they have hypertension is by having their blood pressure checked. This fact explains why millions of Americans are currently walking around with undiagnosed hypertension and why it is so important for people at risk to have their blood pressure checked at least once a year (NIH, 2003a).

There are two types of hypertension: essential and secondary. **Essential hypertension,** also known as idiopathic or systemic hypertension of unknown cause, accounts for more than 95% of all cases (Dosh, 2001). It is caused by a complex interaction of controllable (e.g., obesity, smoking, sedentary lifestyle) and uncontrollable (e.g., genetic predisposition) risk factors. (See **Table 9.2.**)

The remaining cases of high blood pressure are referred to as **secondary hypertension** and have a clearly identifiable cause. The elevation of blood pressure associated with secondary hypertension is the result of having another illness or condition or of using certain medications or products (Onusco, 2003). Treating the illness or condition, or ceasing use of the medication or product, usually resolves this type of hypertension. For example, people with kidney disease often have high blood pressure. When their kidney disease is controlled, their blood pressure returns to normal levels. Likewise, pregnancy often causes elevated blood pressure. In most cases, the cessation of pregnancy results in the mother's blood pressure returning to normal levels. Products such as oral

---

——————[**Table 9.1**]——————

Hypertension Diagnoses

High Blood Pressure (Hypertension) Is Diagnosed when Multiple Blood Pressure Readings Exceed 140/90 mm Hg.

Blood Pressure Levels for Adults*

Category	Systolic† (mm Hg)‡		Diastolic† (mm Hg)‡	Result
Normal	Less than 120	*and*	Less than 80	Good for you!
Pre-hypertension	120–139	*or*	80–89	Your blood pressure could be a problem. Make changes in what you eat and drink, be physically active, and lose extra weight. If you also have diabetes, see your doctor.
Hypertension	140 or higher	*or*	90 or higher	You have high blood pressure. Ask your doctor or nurse how to control it.

*For adults ages 18 and older who are not on medicine for high blood pressure and do not have a short-term serious illness. (*Source: The Seventh Report of the Joint National Committee on Prevention, Detection, Evaluation, and Treatment of High Blood Pressure*, NIH Publication no. 03–5230, National High Blood Pressure Education Program, May 2003).
†If systolic and diastolic pressures fall into different categories, overall status is the higher category.
‡Millimeters of mercury.

Table 9.2	
Hypertension Risk Factors	
Some High Blood Pressure Risks Are Beyond Your Control. Most, However, Can Be Minimized Through Lifestyle Modifications	
Risk Factors You Can Control	**Risk Factors Beyond Your Control**
High blood pressure	Age (55 or older for men;
Abnormal cholesterol	65 or older for women)
Tobacco use	Family history of early heart
Diabetes	disease (having a father or
Overweight	brother diagnosed with
Physical inactivity	heart disease before age
	55 or having a mother or
	sister diagnosed before
	age 65)

crease with age. For men, the risk begins to rise significantly at the age of 45. For women, the risk escalates at age 55. Individuals who have normal blood pressure at age 55 have a 90% lifetime risk for developing hypertension. The prevalence of hypertension increases with age and is more than 70% among people 65 years and older (Dosh, 2001). As the U.S. population ages, the prevalence of hypertension will increase even further unless broad and effective preventive measures are implemented. In persons older than 50 years, systolic blood pressure greater than 140 mm Hg is a much more important cardiovascular disease (CVD) risk factor than diastolic blood pressure. The risk of CVD beginning at 115/75 mm Hg doubles with each increment of 20/10 mm Hg (AHA, 2003).

Gender

In young adulthood and early middle age, more men develop high blood pressure than women do. Men continue to be more likely to have hypertension than women until women reach menopause. For men and women ages 55 to 64, rates are roughly equal. At ages 65 and older, however, hypertension rates for women surpass those for men (AHA, 2003; see **Table 9.3**). Women ultimately

contraceptives can increase the risk of hypertension as well (NIH, 2003b).

Epidemiology

Hypertension is the most common primary diagnosis in the United States, affecting approximately 50 million adults and accounting for more than 35 million physician office visits annually as the primary diagnosis (NIH, 2003a). Among principal diagnoses given by family physicians for outpatient visits, only acute respiratory tract infection (7%) is more common than hypertension (6%). The annual direct medical costs of caring for patients with hypertension exceed $10 billion (Dosh, 2001). Hypertension affects approximately 24% of the U.S. population. From 1991 to 2001, the number of deaths rose 53.0% (AHA, 2003).

Uncontrollable Hypertension Risk Factors

Age

Although it is usually associated with older adults, hypertension can occur at any age. For most Americans, it is likely that their blood pressure will in-

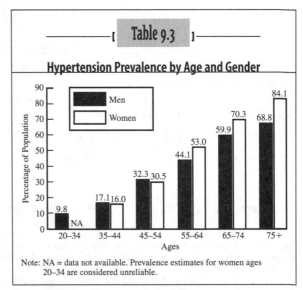

Table 9.3

Hypertension Prevalence by Age and Gender

Note: NA = data not available. Prevalence estimates for women ages 20–34 are considered unreliable.

Source: *Health, United States, 2003*, CDC/NCHS.

have the same risk of cardiovascular disease as men, but generally develop it 10 years later. Despite the gender-related difference, coronary heart disease is the leading cause of death for both men and women (Mayo Clinic, 2003).

Race

The American Heart Association estimates that approximately 37% of all African American men and women have hypertension. About 24% of non-Hispanic white men and 21% of non-Hispanic white women have high blood pressure. Among Hispanic men and women, 24% and 22%, respectively, have hypertension. Americans of Asian and Pacific Island descent have the lowest incidence of hypertension, with 10% of the men and 8% of the women being affected (AHA, 2003; see **Table 9.4**).

African Americans are twice as likely to develop high blood pressure as whites. They are also more likely to develop serious complications from the disease or to die of a stroke or heart attack related to high blood pressure. Hypertension risks vary dramatically within the African Ameri-

can community. The highest rates of hypertension among African Americans are found in people who are middle-aged or older, less educated, overweight or obese, physically inactive, and have diabetes. The lowest rates are found among younger, but also overweight or obese, African Americans (AHA, 2003). In 2001, the death rates per 100,000 people from high blood pressure were 13.7 for white males, 47.8 for black males, 13.4 for white females, and 38.9 for black females (AHA, 2003).

Family History

People with a father or brother who had a heart attack or stroke before turning 55, or a mother or sister who had a heart attack or stroke before the age of 65, are at greater risk of developing hypertension than individuals without such family histories. Heredity does not necessarily mean someone will follow his or her family's path, however. By modifying other risk factors, a person can reduce his or her chance of developing hypertension regardless of family history (NIH, 2003b).

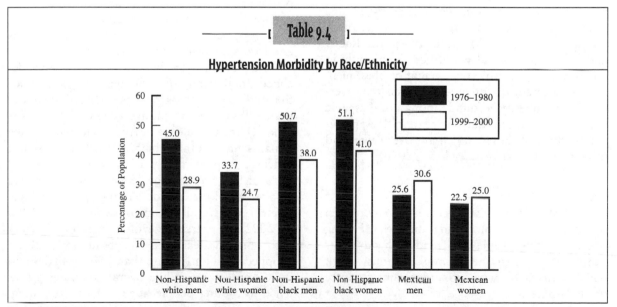

Table 9.4

Hypertension Morbidity by Race/Ethnicity

Source: CDC/NCHS. Data based on a single measure of blood pressure. Health, United States, 2003.

Controllable Hypertension Risk Factors

Obesity

The more body mass a person has, the more blood the individual needs to supply oxygen and nutrients to the tissues. The volume of blood circulating through the blood vessels increases and creates extra force on the arterial walls. People who are overweight and obese are more likely to have high blood pressure than those whose weight is under control. The prevalence of overweight and obese Americans has increased steadily in recent decades. The prevalence of Americans who are overweight, defined as having a **body mass index (BMI)** of 25 or higher, increased from approximately 56% of the population in 1988–1994 to 65% of the population in 1999–2000. The prevalence of obese Americans (BMI of 30 or higher) also increased during this time period, from approximately 23% of the population to 31%. In one year, between 2000 and 2001, the prevalence of obesity increased almost 6%. The percentage of extremely obese Americans (BMI of 40 or higher) increased from approximately 3% of the population to almost 5% (AHA, 2003).

These increases in all periods analyzed were noted for both men and women, across all age groups, and for non-Hispanic whites, non-Hispanic blacks, and Mexican Americans. Racial and ethnic groups did not differ significantly in the prevalence of either overweight or obese men. Among women, the greatest prevalence of overweight and obesity is found among non-Hispanic black women more than 40 years old. Approximately 80% of these women are overweight and more than 40% are obese (AHA, 2003).

Sedentary Lifestyle

Lack of physical activity increases the risk of high blood pressure by increasing the risk of being obese. Inactive people also tend to have higher heart rates. Their heart muscles must work harder with each contraction, increasing the force on the arteries.

Data from national risk factor surveys reveal that approximately 55% of Americans aged 18 and older are not physically active enough to meet the minimal standards recommended by the U.S. Surgeon General (AHA, 2003). About 38% of all Americans aged 18 or older report never engaging in physical activity. Approximately 62% engage in at least some physical activity, and about 23% engage in light to moderate physical activity at least five times per week. Men, young people, non-Hispanic whites, and Asian/Pacific Islander non-Hispanic adults are more likely to engage in at least some physical activity as compared to women, older people, and non-Hispanic blacks and Hispanics (AHA, 2003). Other variables related to an increased level of physical activity include having a college education, earning a higher income, living in the West, and being married (AHA, 2003). Physical inactivity is more prevalent among women than men, among blacks and Hispanics than whites, among older adults than younger adults, and among those with lower incomes than higher earners (AHA, 2003).

Tobacco Use

The chemicals in tobacco can damage the lining of the artery walls, causing the arteries to accumulate fatty deposits that contain cholesterol plaques. Nicotine also constricts blood vessels and forces the heart to work harder.

Smoking rates in the United States have declined dramatically over the past 30 years. Since the mid-1960s, smoking has declined by more than 40% among people age 18 and older. Unfortunately, the prevalence of Americans who smoke remains unacceptably high, according to health officials. Approximately 25% of U.S. men and 21% of U.S. women age 18 years and older still smoke. Smoking trends among young people point to an overall decline, however. From 1980 to 2002, the percentage of high school seniors who smoked decreased by about 13%. Rates dropped by slightly more than 2% for males and 24% for females. While overall smoking prevalence for young people appears to be declining, about 39% of male students in grades 9–12 and 30% of female students in high school still smoke (AHA, 2003).

Stress

Chronic and acute stress can elevate blood pressure and keep it high as long as the source of stress is not handled successfully. During the alarm stress response, blood pressure rises in response to perceived threats in an attempt to mobilize energy to fight or flee. If the individual successfully copes with the source of threat (the stressor), blood pressure will return to normal. Exposure to chronic, long-term stressors results in a continual activation of the stress response, which can damage the body's regulatory systems by keeping blood pressure high for long periods of time (Blonna, 2005).

Sodium and Potassium

People who are sodium sensitive retain sodium too easily, leading to fluid retention and increased blood pressure. Most Americans consume far more salt (sodium) than their bodies need. High sodium consumption increases blood pressure in some people, leading to hypertension. The National Institutes of Health (2003a) recommends that people restrict their consumption to about 2.4 g of sodium or 6 g of sodium chloride (common table salt) daily.

Potassium is a mineral that helps balance the amount of sodium in the cells. If people don't consume or retain enough potassium, they can accumulate too much sodium. Following the Dietary Approaches to Stop Hypertension (DASH) diet can help reduce blood pressure by increasing intake of foods that are high in potassium, calcium, magnesium, protein, and fiber while lowering consumption of saturated fat, total fat, and cholesterol. The DASH diet includes whole grains, poultry, fish, and nuts, but low amounts of fats, red meats, sweets, and sugared beverages (NIH, 2003a).

Alcohol

No one knows exactly how or why alcohol increases blood pressure. Some evidence, however, suggests that heavy drinking can damage the heart muscle and increase blood pressure. It can also harm the liver and brain. Alcoholic drinks contain high amounts of calories, which matters if you are trying to lose weight (NIH, 2003a).

Hypertension as a Risk Factor

Hypertension is both a form of cardiovascular disease and a risk factor for other forms of CVD such as heart attack and stroke. Hypertension is also a risk factor for other illnesses such as kidney failure. Stroke is the third leading cause of death in the United States, affecting 700,000 people each year and killing more than 160,000 of them (AHA, 2003); hypertension is the leading cause of stroke. The small arteries in the brain, when put under constant elevated pressure, may rupture or form a clot along the inside wall. Both of these processes interrupt the flow of blood to brain cells, resulting in cell death. Because brain cells do not regenerate, stroke survivors are left with permanent, irreparable neurological damage. Half of all people who have a first heart attack and two-thirds who have a first stroke have blood pressures higher than 160/95 mm Hg (AHA, 2003). People with systolic blood pressure of 160 mm Hg or higher and/or diastolic blood pressure of 95 mm Hg or higher have a relative risk for stroke about four times greater than the risk for individuals with normal blood pressure (AHA, 2003).

One of the many controllable risk factors for heart attack is hypertension. Similar to the process that occurs in the brain, when the coronary arteries are put under constant elevated pressure, the rate of plaque formation inside the arteries accelerates, and the risk of clot formation greatly increases. As the blockage enlarges, or when a clot forms, the blood flow to the heart muscle is interrupted. This lack of blood flow leads to death of heart cells—that is, a heart attack. The size of the area affected and the location of the damage will determine whether the person survives the heart attack or dies from it.

Uncontrolled hypertension can also affect the kidneys. Hypertension is a leading cause of kidney failure, resulting in more than 15,000 new cases each year (NIH, 2003b). Elevated pressure in the blood vessels damages these organs and renders the kidneys unable to filter the blood, leading to kidney failure. Patients with kidney failure must either have a transplant or receive dialysis for the rest of their lives (NIH, 2003b).

Prevention and Control

The relationship between hypertension and risk of CVD events such as heart attack and stroke is continuous, consistent, and independent of other risk factors such as obesity and smoking. The higher a person's blood pressure, the greater his or her risk of heart attack, heart failure, stroke, and kidney disease (NIH, 2003a). For those people with hypertension who are 40–70 years of age, each increment of 20 mm Hg in systolic blood pressure or 10 mm Hg in diastolic blood pressure doubles the risk of CVD across the entire blood pressure range from 115/75 to 185/115 mm Hg (NIH, 2003b).

Conversely, reducing high blood pressure reduces one's risk for cardiovascular disease complications. Antihypertension therapy has been as-sociated with reductions in stroke incidence averaging 35%–40%; myocardial infarction, 20%–25%; and heart failure, more than 50% (NIH, 2003b). It is estimated that in patients with stage 1 hypertension (SBP 140–159 mm Hg and/or DBP 90–99 mm Hg) and additional cardiovascular risk factors, achieving a sustained 12 mm Hg reduction in systolic blood pressure over 10 years will prevent 1 death for every 11 patients treated (NIH, 2003b).

Although current blood pressure control rates (SBP < 140 mm Hg and DBP < 90 mm Hg) have improved over the past three decades, they remain far below the Healthy People 2010 goal of 50% (see **Table 9.5**). While 70% of Americans are aware of their hypertension, only 59% are receiving treatment for it and just 34% have their disease under control. While high blood pressure cannot be cured, it can be controlled. Achieving adequate control means that blood pressure can be lowered and kept at a normal level if treatment is followed. The goal of treatment is to reduce further illness or death due to kidney or cardiovascular disease (NIH, 2003b). This goal is best attained by identifying people at risk for hypertension at the pre-hypertension stage and helping them make lifestyle modifications in controllable risk factors (see **Table 9.6**).

[Table 9.5]

Hypertension Awareness

Trends in Awareness, Treatment, and Control of High Blood Pressure in Adults Ages 18–74*

	National Health and Nutrition Examination Survey (%)			
	II (1976–1980)	III (Phase 1 1988–1991)	III (Phase 2 1991–1994)	1999–2000
Awareness	51	73	68	70
Treatment	31	55	54	59
Control†	10	29	27	34

*High blood pressure is systolic blood pressure (SBP) ≥ 140 mm Hg or diastolic blood pressure (DBP) ≥ 90 mm Hg or taking antihypertensive medication.
†SBP < 140 mm Hg and DBP < 90 mm Hg.
Sources: Unpublished data for 1999–2000 computed by M. Wolz, National Heart, Lung, and Blood Institute.

Table 9.6

Lifestyle Modifications to Manage Hypertension*†

Modification	Recommendation	Approximate SBP Reduction (Range)
Weight reduction	Maintain normal body weight (body mass index 18.5–24.9 kg/m²).	5–20 mm Hg/10 kg weight loss
Adopt DASH eating plan	Consume a diet rich in fruits, vegetables, and low-fat dairy products with a reduced content of saturated and total fat.	8–14 mm Hg
Dietary sodium reduction	Reduce dietary sodium intake to no more than 100 mmol per day (2.4 g sodium or 6 g sodium chloride).	2–8 mm Hg
Physical activity	Engage in regular aerobic physical activity such as brisk walking (at least 30 minutes per day, most days of the week).	4–9 mm Hg
Moderation of alcohol consumption	Limit consumption to no more than two drinks (1 oz or 30 mL ethanol; e.g., 24 oz beer, 10 oz wine, or 3 oz 80-proof whiskey) per day in most men and to no more than one drink per day in women and lighter-weight persons.	2–4 mm Hg

DASH: Dietary Approaches to Stop Hypertension.
*For overall cardiovascular risk reduction, stop smoking.
†The effects of implementing these modifications are dose and time dependent, and could be greater for some individuals.

These changes include reducing to or maintaining normal weight, reducing sodium intake to no more than 2400 mg per day, consuming a diet rich in potassium (more than 3500 mg/day) and calcium in the form of low-fat dairy products (adopting the DASH eating plan), engaging in at least 30 minutes of aerobic exercise on most days of the week, and limiting alcohol intake to no more than two drinks per day for men and one drink per day for women.

For many people, these changes suffice to bring blood pressure back to more normal levels. However, these changes must be permanent. If they are not, blood pressure will simply increase again. These activities do not cure the problem, but rather help to control it. If lifestyle changes alone cannot reduce high blood pressure, then medications are added.

Antihypertensive medications work by targeting the specific mechanisms within the body that regulate blood pressure. These mechanisms control blood volume, arterial stiffness, and the heart's contraction. These mechanisms and the categories of drugs that act on them are described in **Table 9.7**.

The various categories of hypertension medications have contraindications and side effects that make them more or less appropriate for specific patients. Physicians begin by selecting what they consider to be an appropriate drug to prescribe as initial therapy. This decision will be influenced by the patient's age, his or her race, and the presence of coexisting diseases or conditions, such as kidney disease, that may contraindicate a certain drug or, conversely, indicate one drug over another. The doctor considers many other factors

Table 9.7

Blood Pressure Drugs

Drug Category	How They Work
Diuretics	These are sometimes called "water pills" because they work in the kidney and flush excess water and sodium from the body through urine.
Beta blockers	These reduce nerve impulses to the heart and blood vessels. This makes the heart beat less often and with less force. Blood pressure drops, and the heart works less hard.
Angiotensin-converting enzyme inhibitors	These prevent the formation of a hormone called angiotensin II, which normally causes blood vessels to narrow. The blood vessels relax, and pressure goes down.
Angiotensin antagonists	These shield blood vessels from angiotensin II. As a result, the blood vessels open wider, and pressure goes down.
Calcium-channel blockers	These keep calcium from entering the muscle cells of the heart and blood vessels. Blood vessels relax, and pressure goes down.
Alpha blockers	These reduce nerve impulses to blood vessels, allowing blood to pass more easily.
Alpha-beta blockers	These work the same way as alpha blockers but also slow the heartbeat, as beta blockers do.
Nervous system inhibitors	These relax blood vessels by controlling nerve impulses.
Vasodilators	These directly open blood vessels by relaxing the muscle in the vessel walls.

as well. If the first-choice drug is ineffective or only partially effective, or if it causes intolerable side effects, another drug can be tried. Sometimes, if the first drug is only partially effective but the client tolerates it well, the dose can be increased, or a second drug can be added.

Hypertension medications have many side effects, ranging from minor ones such as fatigue, coughing, or skin rash, to severe ones such as sexual dysfunction, depression, or electrolyte abnormalities. Many different medications can be substituted that may achieve the same results but not carry the same side effects. The major goal of hypertension medication is to lower blood pressure effectively while causing the fewest side effects.

It is not unusual for physicians to prescribe several different medications before finding one that works well for a patient. Often, medications from different categories are used in combination, especially in stage 2 hypertension, where excessive blood pressure and **compelling indications** such as diabetes merit more drastic efforts.

Controlling hypertension through medication requires frequent, open communication among clients and medical professionals to ensure that patients adhere to their treatment regimens. Counselors, working in concert with physicians, can play a vital role in this process, helping empower clients and teaching them how to communicate with their physicians.

Goals of Hypertension Counseling

The National Institutes of Health (2003b) has set six goals for hypertension prevention and control:

1. Follow a healthy eating plan.
2. Be physically active.
3. Reduce the amount of sodium in your diet.
4. Drink alcohol only in moderation.
5. Maintain a healthy weight.
6. Take prescribed drugs as directed.

Following these goals will help clients keep their blood pressure within normal limits and reduce

The following hints can help ensure that you understand your medications and feel good about taking them properly:

1. Take responsibility for your own health by talking freely with your doctor about your medications. Remember—you are the one who is taking the medicines.
2. Carry a record of all your medications at all times and bring it to each visit.
3. Know what you take and why you take it.
4. Tell you doctor about any nonprescription (over-the-counter) drugs or dietary supplements (herbs, vitamins) you are taking.
5. Take notes if it helps you.
6. Ask about the cost of prescriptions. Perhaps a generic drug could be prescribed instead.
7. If you are taking drugs at several different times during the day, ask whether it is possible to take any of your medications as a single daily dose. Ask what will happen if you miss a dose and how you should make it up.
8. Ask about any possible side effects and what to do if they occur.
9. Ask if any special instructions apply to a particular medicine (e.g., taking it at a particular time of day, or with or without food or drink) or if you should avoid any activities while on the drug.
10. If you don't understand something, ask for an explanation—don't be shy!

Don't pressure your doctor to prescribe a drug just because you saw it advertised on TV or in a magazine. Discuss alternatives to drugs, if appropriate. Certain conditions can be lessened or even reversed by alterations in diet, exercise, or other behaviors. Don't be embarrassed about asking questions. You are the main person responsible for monitoring your health and taking medicines safely, so the more knowledge you have, the more effectively you can make decisions about your health care.

Source: De la Valle (2003).

---

their risks of hypertension-associated kidney and cardiovascular disease.

Counseling Clients with Hypertension Using Microskills

Hypertension control requires adherence to lifestyle changes and medication compliance. Achieving these goals is especially difficult because hypertension is usually asymptomatic—it does not cause obvious symptoms. The main way clients know that their blood pressure is elevated is through daily monitoring.

Counselors must be sure that clients understand the asymptomatic nature of this disease and can correctly monitor their blood pressure. Additionally, counselors must teach clients how to identify health behaviors that contribute to their high blood pressure, develop action plans to change those behaviors, and create lifestyles to maintain those changes. Perhaps the key issue in successful hypertension control is getting the patient to understand that hypertension control is a lifelong commitment because treatment does not cure it. If treatment is stopped, patients must recognize that their blood pressure will rise again, along with their risk of complications.

Case Study 9.1
Ida

Ida, 44, is heterosexual and identifies as a Puerto Rican American. Ida is a recently separated mother of three boys, aged 21, 19, and 14. Her oldest son is a junior in college, her middle child is a freshman in college, and her youngest son is a freshman in high school. Ida and her husband separated because of tensions in the marriage that had been brewing for at least a decade. Her husband continues to split the cost of maintaining the house and funding the boys' college expenses while he and Ida proceed with their divorce.

Ida works as a manager for a major insurance company. She earns a good salary, so she will be able to maintain the house once the divorce is final. Her job is very pressure-packed and filled with deadlines and demands.

Ida is about 50 pounds overweight, is sedentary, eats a diet high in fat, and has a very stressful life. She is a nonsmoker. Her blood pressure, which has been "borderline" for several years, has been consistently high over the past few weeks. Her doctor recently put her on medication to lower her blood pressure and referred her for counseling to one of the staff members of his practice. The counselor also runs a group for patients with hypertension.

Introductory Skills

A good introduction is essential to gaining clients' trust. As discussed earlier in the text, clients are often reluctant to discuss their problems and must be won over early in the interview. When counseling hypertension patients, counselors must maintain the highest level of credibility and trust because they are working with clients who have an asymptomatic condition that requires long-term lifestyle modifications to manage.

Identify Yourself and Explain Your Role

The key issue in working with hypertension patients is realizing that for most of them, hypertension is a very difficult disease to conceptualize. The notion of blood pressure and its effects can be quite challenging to grasp. Couple this with the asymptomatic nature of hypertension, and the fact that it is both a disease and a risk factor, and

you have a very confusing condition. For these reasons, it is easy for clients to become skeptical about their condition and therapeutic plan.

Counseling people with hypertension requires that counselors explore these issues and use empathy to connect with clients' skepticism. Try writing a script for this part of the introduction and practice it until it becomes second nature to you. When introducing yourself, it is very important to make a concerted effort to establish a skin-to-skin human connection with the client. A firm handshake (ungloved) is a good way to do so. Extend your hand, make eye contact, and smile as you give the client a firm (but not crushing) handshake.

Example

Counselor: (Extending hand, smiling) Hi, I'm [name]. I'm one of the counselors at the clinic. My job is to make sure you understand why you are here, and what you need to know to manage your hypertension and live a full and productive life.

You have hypertension, also known as high blood pressure, which can be a very confusing condition to understand. You feel normal, you don't see any signs and symptoms on your body, and yet you are being told that you have a life-threatening condition and will need to change your lifestyle to manage it.

To understand what having high blood pressure means to you, I will have to talk to you about a variety of issues related to your background and family life and ask you lots of questions. I am not here to judge you or your family in terms of your lifestyle or the things that have contributed to your high blood pressure. My job is to help you make the best decisions for yourself regarding how to control your blood pressure from this point forward. Together, we will work out a plan for making sure that you gain control of your high blood pressure so that you can lower your risks for problems such as kidney failure, heart attack, and stroke—three of the major diseases related to high blood pressure. I want you to understand that everything we say is confidential and that your name and anything we talk about cannot be shared with anyone else.

Clarify the Client's Name

A simple way to verify the client's name is to use an open-ended statement following your introduction. Do so while you are still standing and immediately following your handshake and self-identification.

Example

Counselor: (Before sitting and explaining his role) And your name is . . . ?

Explain the Client's Role

After exchanging names and describing your role, start to explain the client's role. A simple explanation should include the three key elements of the client role discussed in Chapter 3: (1) active participation, (2) self-responsibility, and (3) honesty.

Example

Counselor: Ida, your role in this process is to be as open and honest as possible when talking to me. The only way I can help you is if you tell me exactly what is going on with you and everyone involved in your illness. You'll have to take an active role in this process and take responsibility for getting better. Together, we can work out the therapeutic plan that will work best for you in getting better in the future.

Set Goals for the Session(s)

As a hypertension counselor you must emphasize the six goals for hypertension prevention and control: (1) maintain a healthy weight, (2) be physically active, (3) follow a healthy eating plan, (4) reduce the amount of sodium in the diet, (5) drink alcohol only in moderation, and (6) take prescribed drugs as directed (NIH, 2003b). In addition to these primary goals, counselors must assess clients' goals regarding their disease. The best way to do so is to describe your goals and assess clients' needs.

Example

Counselor: Ida, there are six things I *must* discuss with you today regarding your hypertension. First, how to maintain a healthy weight. Second, how to be more physically active. Third, how to develop and follow a healthy eating plan. Fourth, how to reduce the amount of sodium in your diet. Fifth, how to drink alcohol only in moderation. Sixth, how to take your prescribed drugs as directed. What goals do you have for our sessions?

Give the client time to think this through before moving into the next part of the session.

Ida: I don't have any other goals.

Transition to the Client's Story

A good way to make the transition from the introduction to getting clients to tell their stories is to use open-ended statements regarding what happened. Here are a few examples:

"Ida, why don't you tell me what led to you being here today."
"Ida, tell me a little bit about what you know about high blood pressure."
"Ida, tell me a little bit about your high blood pressure for the past few months."

The idea in using these open-ended statements is to get clients talking about their hypertension as well as their overall lifestyles. You can start with either topic, but understanding both components of the overall story is essential to meeting the hypertension counseling goals.

Attending Skills

Listening to clients tell their hypertension stories will give you insights into the nature of their histories and lifestyles in general as well as how these factors relate to their current high blood pressure problems. It is essential that you set a nonjudgmental tone from the start while attending.

Nonverbal Skills

Be aware of both your own and your clients' body language. Be particularly attuned to any tension in individual body parts or major areas or the aversion of eye contact. Clenching and unclenching the hands, tension across the chest and shoulders, and facial tension (e.g., tight jaw muscles, furrowed brow) are sure signs of discomfort. More obvious is averting eye contact. While it is normal to look away and periodically break eye contact when you are talking, averting eye contact when the other person is talking may indicate that something is wrong.

Verbal Following

A key aspect of verbally following hypertension clients' stories is paying particular attention to any hint of skepticism and disbelief about having the condition. This consideration is specifically related to the asymptomatic nature of the problem and its control. Clients will often give verbal and nonverbal clues regarding how they feel about having a problem they can neither see nor feel. They will talk about how "people" have a hard time understanding and controlling something they neither see nor feel while rolling their eyes or shaking their heads.

Example

Counselor: Ida, tell me a little bit about what it is like having high blood pressure.

Ida: (Rolling her eyes) I don't know, maybe somebody made a mistake. I don't feel any different.

Counselor: Different?

Ida: Yeah, you know. It's not like I have any more aches and pains or lumps or anything like that. I don't feel any different than I did last year when the doctor told me I was "borderline."

Ida: (Shaking her head) It's a lot to expect, you know, for people to pay all that money for those pills and make all these changes in their lives.

The counselor should file this information away until later in the interview, when it is appro-priate to confront Ida with this discrepancy between how she expects to feel and how she actually feels.

Vocal Tone

Try to match the pace and tone of clients' stories. People with high blood pressure experience a range of emotions regarding their disease and express these emotions in the way they tell their stories. Ida's tone belies her skepticism about having hypertension. It also contains anger at having this condition.

Example

Counselor: Tell me more.

Ida: I'm just so aggravated at having this condition on top of everything else.

Counselor: Everything else?

Ida: Yeah, the separation, the college expenses, the pressure at work. I'm just so angry I could burst. It's just so hard to believe.

Other clients might respond to having hypertension entirely differently, and their stories might be told with much less emotion. More fearful clients might speak more softly and adopt a more submissive tone, underscoring their fears. Don't respond to their stories with your own tone and pace, but rather let their emotions and style dictate yours. Try to capture the "vocals" of the client to encourage them to continue.

Responding Skills

Nonverbal and Verbal Minimal Encouragers

Clients in counseling send out nonverbal messages about how they feel about their stories. Pay attention to the same attributes in your clients that you notice with yourself. Aversion of eye contact, tension, and closed body posture all might indicate unspoken problems that you may need to address at the appropriate time. They could also represent discrepancies between *what* is being said and *how* it is being said.

Conversely, a relaxed, open, approachable body language indicates acceptance and an openness to communicate. Try to encourage clients to continue talking by maintaining a relaxed posture and periodically scanning your own body for signs of any tension that might be transmitted to clients.

Simple "uh huhs," key words, and mirroring are very important tools that can be used to encourage clients to continue their stories. They are especially helpful with sensitive subjects, because they demonstrate acceptance and assist in keeping clients talking.

Open Invitation to Talk

Using questions to clarify hypertension-related information is very important because of the way the disease is so interwoven into all of the dimensions of health and lifestyle. No two people experience it the same way, and understanding the meaning of the disease for individual clients takes careful questioning to gather and clarify information.

Open-Ended Statements and Questions

One helpful way to clarify information with high blood pressure patients is to use open-ended statements liberally to create a more relaxed, conversational tone. It is better to get the answers to a series of individual questions by asking one or two open-ended statements than by asking clients a slew of yes/no questions.

When counseling clients with hypertension, such as Ida, it is important to understand exactly what their lifestyles are like. Knowledge of their lifestyles plays a major part in developing specific directives and instructions about how clients can manage their high blood pressure. Using open-ended statements to find out about clients' lifestyles is preferable to using a list of closed questions.

For instance, the following closed lifestyle-related questions could be used with Ida:

"Ida, do you exercise?"
"Ida, do you run, walk, swim, or do other types of exercise?"
"Ida, do you do anything to control your work stress?"

"Ida, have you ever practiced meditation on a regular basis?"
"Ida, have you ever done any diaphragmatic breathing?"
"Ida, do you watch what you eat?"
"Ida, do you count the calories in your meals?"

You can get the answers to these and many more lifestyle-related questions by asking each directly, or you can ask a few indirect, open-ended questions and listen to clients describe their lifestyles. If clients miss one or two questions, you can follow up your open-ended question with specific closed questions.

Example Open-Ended Statements

Counselor: Ida, tell me a little about your exercise behavior over the past few months.

Counselor: Ida, tell me a little about your stress management activities over the past few months.

Counselor: Ida, tell me a little about your diet over the past year.

Ida: I've really let my health slip over the past couple of years. I mean, it's not like I have ever been a health nut or anything. I've never really liked exercise or really watched what I've eaten. This past year things between Pedro [her husband] and myself have been really bad, and I've just kind of let everything slip.

Counselor: Slip?

Ida: Yeah, I have been using food as a way to deal with the stress of our separation. I have been spending a lot of time just feeling sorry for myself or worrying about the future. When I do that, I eat. Even before that, however, I always found it hard to eat healthy and keep my weight down. I grew up in Puerto Rico, and my family always felt that food and enjoying life were more important than exercise and watching what you ate. I remember my mother saying how a man liked a woman "with a little meat on her bones." I guess I've had a little extra "meat on my bones" my whole life. When I came to the United States to go to college, I lived with my aunt Rosa and she was just like my mother. Every day we'd feast on the foods of my country. Every day it was some kind of pork or chicken with beans and rice cooked the old-country way with lard, not canola oil.

Counselor: Sounds like you've spent some time thinking about eating healthy. You mention canola oil as compared with lard.

Ida: Oh yeah, I went through a few years trying to cut back on fat and start eating a little healthier, but Pedro always fought me. He was always the one to call my mother and tell her that I was becoming too much like these skinny American women. The irony is that he began having an affair with a tall, athletic blond Anglo woman from his office. Go figure.

Paraphrasing, Reflection of Feelings, and Summarizing

Paraphrasing and reflection of feelings work similarly for hypertension patients as they do for other counseling clients. As we've seen with asthma and other conditions, patients often direct their anger and other strong emotions at parents or others whose behavior affects their ability to control the disease. Ida, for example, has strong feelings of anger toward Pedro regarding her weight. Such feelings of anger and hostility toward those who are blamed for being the source of health problems are common.

Paraphrasing judiciously throughout the client's story will help you clarify how the person views his or her disease and its relationship to parents and caretakers. Once clients' thoughts and feelings are expressed, summarization helps clarify what clients are thinking and feeling. It is an opportunity for them to hear their stories again and decide whether anything needs to be added, deleted, or clarified. It also shows them how well you are following and your assessment of the situation.

Example: Paraphrase

Counselor: Ida, it seems that your struggle with maintaining a healthier lifestyle has a lot to do with the way you were brought up and your current problems with Pedro. Is that accurate?

Ida: I guess so. I still take responsibility for my behavior, though.

Example: Reflection of Feelings

Counselor: Ida, you seem very angry at Pedro because of his betrayal and relationship with someone who seems to be the opposite of what he told you attracted him for all of these years. Is that true?

Ida: Yeah, I am very angry with both of them. I not only feel betrayed, but I also feel like a fool for not seeing this coming.

Example: Summary

Counselor: Ida, let's step back for a moment before we continue, just so I'm sure I completely understand what you are telling me. It seems that your problems with maintaining a healthy weight have a lot to do with the messages you have received all of your life from your family, your culture, and your husband regarding what an attractive woman should look like. Also, attempts to improve your diet and change your lifestyle have been met with resistance by your family. On top of this, your husband winds up leaving you for a woman who is kind of your polar opposite, and you are feeling very angry and betrayed. Is that pretty much on target?

Ida: I'd say that sums it up. Nice life, huh?

Influencing Skills

As mentioned previously, the goals for hypertension prevention and control (NIH, 2003b) are sixfold: (1) maintain a healthy weight, (2) be physically active, (3) follow a healthy eating plan, (4) reduce the amount of sodium in the diet, (5) drink alcohol only in moderation, and (6) take prescribed drugs as directed. In addition to these primary goals, clients such as Ida often bring other issues to counseling that should be addressed. In her case, Ida needs to work through the issues related to her self-concept, body image, relationship, and betrayal to gain more control of her life and make the lifestyle changes necessary to reduce her blood pressure and keep it in control. Ida's counselor would apply the various influencing skills to help Ida meet these goals.

Self-disclosure

Self-disclosure is an excellent technique for building confidence in clients regarding their perceived ability to change. Self-disclosing to clients about your own struggles (in this case, they could be related to either lifestyle or relationship issues) shows clients that you empathize with them and know what they are going through because you have been there yourself. Counselors serve as powerful role models when they show clients that they have successfully managed similar issues.

Example

Counselor: Ida, I kind of know what you are going through. I had hypertension associated mostly with being obese and sedentary. I have struggled with my weight my entire life. It took a couple of years for me to overcome the habits of my past and learn how to manage my weight. For a while, it seemed that every time I took one step forward in my weight-loss program, I took two steps backward. In time, however, I got control of my eating and exercise and stopped feeling out of control.

Ida: I'm surprised to hear that you have had problems with your weight. You look so trim.

Counselor: Someday I'll show you a picture of what I looked like 20 years ago. If I could learn how to manage my weight, I know you can do it.

Confrontation

Confrontation will come into play in hypertension counseling, just as it does in all health counseling. Clients will present inconsistencies in their stories for a variety of reasons. As you can see with her story, Ida's struggles with her weight extend over her entire lifetime and are interwoven with mixed feelings for her husband, mother, and culture. Inconsistencies in clients' stories are inevitable with lifestyle-based health problems that have evolved over time. Counselors must be gentle and nonjudgmental when confronting clients about these discrepancies. Confrontation should be used as a supportive challenge to help clients such as Ida see the discrepancies in their lives and behaviors and grow from them—not as a way to make them feel as if they are being punished for their behavior. Using Ivey and Ivey's (2003) "one hand, other hand" confrontation technique is a good way to achieve this goal.

Example

Counselor: Ida, on the one hand, it seems that Pedro told you that he liked you with "a little meat on your bones." On the other hand, you seemed to want to lose weight and get in shape. Can you explain this?

Ida: Sure, this has been part of my problem for several years. I knew that the way I had been raised and taught to look and behave was not good for my health. I really wanted to lose weight and get healthy years ago, but my husband and mother fought me every step of the way. I guess this is why I am so angry. I didn't listen to myself and do what I know I should have done, and I wound up both getting high blood pressure and losing my husband.

Changing the Focal Point

Changing the focal point is an excellent way to help clients see their problems through the eyes of other people who are intimately involved in their problems. It is also an effective technique for helping counselors understand the dynamics of clients' stories. Counselors can use this information to direct their influencing more accurately.

Changing the focal point often helps clients modify their personal constructs related to the illnesses. These personal constructs may be related to their own self-esteem, their feelings and expectations of others, or a variety of other issues that factor into their ability to gain control over their health problems.

Example: Changing the Focus to Other Family Members

Counselor: Ida, I'm sure your prior attempts to change your eating and exercise behavior have affected your boys over the years. Tell me how your sons have reacted to your attempts at controlling your weight and making the lifestyle changes we have talked about.

Ida: It's funny that you mention this. All three of my boys are very Americanized. They really are not that interested in our Puerto Rican heritage, especially when it comes to food. For the most part, they are really not into things like beans and rice and fried plantains [a form of banana]. Over the past few years, they have really nagged me about my weight and have tried to get me to go running with them as they have exercised to stay in shape for sports. They all play soccer and baseball. Pedro is the one who has fought it. He has insisted on me cooking a certain way and has always ridiculed me for trying to get in shape. If it were up to the boys, we would have switched to a low-fat diet as a family years ago. In fact, I really cooked two meals for dinner each night: one meal for Pedro and me and a lower-calorie version for the boys.

Counselor: It seems that the idea of modifying your diet isn't totally new. You've looked into this issue in the past.

Ida: Yeah, I guess I have.

By changing the focus to the boys, the counselor has gained valuable information about Ida's willingness to make some of the changes necessary to gain control of her weight. This information will help Ida's counselor work with her in structuring her directives for gaining control of her hypertension. Together, they should be able to work out a diet relatively easily because of her past experience and obvious willingness to change.

Directives and Logical Consequences

The directives and instructions of hypertension counseling emanate from the goals for hypertension prevention and control (NIH, 2003b): (1) follow a healthy eating plan, (2) be physically active, (3) reduce the amount of sodium in the diet, (4) drink alcohol only in moderation, (5) maintain a healthy weight, and (6) take prescribed drugs as directed.

Directive 1: Follow a Healthy Eating Plan

1. *Initial assessment.* Instruct clients to keep a daily eating log to assess current eating patterns.

2. *Construction of a healthy eating plan.* Teach clients about the DASH (Dietary Approaches to Stop Hypertension) eating plan, which emphasizes eating foods low in saturated fat, total fat, and cholesterol, and high

consumption of fruits, vegetables, and low-fat dairy foods.

3. *Ongoing assessment.* Instruct clients to continue writing down everything that they eat and drink and to note areas that are healthy as well as those that need improvement.

Logical Consequences of Following a Healthy Eating Plan

1. Clients will understand the components of their current diets.
2. Clients will understand the strengths and weaknesses of their current diets.
3. Clients will set reasonable healthy eating goals based on the DASH plan.

4. Clients will tailor their diets to meet their needs while adhering to the basic tenets of the DASH plan.
5. Clients will learn how to follow a healthy eating plan.

Specific Instructions for Following a Healthy Eating Plan

1. Start keeping a diary of current eating habits. This diary should include what is eaten, how much, when, and in what context. The context includes things like snacking on high-fat foods to cope with stress or eating while watching television (see **Figure 9.2**).

Food or Drink						
How Much	**What Kind**	**Time**	**Where**	**Alone or with Whom**	**Activity**	**Mood**
3	Chocolate chip cookies	3:25 P.M.	Office	Alone	Working on report	Bored
1	Cheeseburger	6:15 P.M.	Burger King	Claire, Jackie	Talking	Happy
1	Regular french fries					
1	Vanilla shake					
1 cup	Haagen-Daz ice cream	10:00 P.M.	Kitchen	Alone	Watching TV	Tired

Figure 9.2 Sample food diary.

2. Instruct clients to bring their diaries to future sessions. Explain that you will go over the diary at the next visit to help them assess their current eating patterns.
3. Describe the DASH plan to clients.
4. Set reasonable eating goals based on the DASH plan.
5. Tailor the DASH plan to each client's specific needs.

Example

Counselor: Ida, the first thing you need to do to learn how to follow a healthy eating plan is to take an honest look at your current eating style. I'd like you to keep a diet diary for the next few weeks. Here is an example of one [hands Ida a sample blank and completed diary; see Figure 9.2]. You can see that you should fill in everything that you eat or drink, the amount that you eat, the time when you eat, and the circumstances of your eating. I call this your eating context. By this term, I mean describing the things that are going on when you eat. This includes things like snacking on high-fat foods to cope with stress or eating because you are bored or to pass the time while watching television. How does that sound?

Ida: Sounds like a lot of work.

Counselor: It is, but it will help us analyze the strengths and weaknesses of your diet.

Ida: Okay.

Counselor: The next thing I'd like to do is explain the DASH eating plan. DASH stands for Dietary Approaches to Stop Hypertension. This diet emphasizes eating foods low in saturated fat, total fat, and cholesterol, and lots of fruits, vegetables, and low-fat dairy foods. The DASH plan includes whole grains, poultry, fish, and nuts, which are high in protein and fiber. The diet allows for eating smaller amounts of fats, red meats, sweets, and drinks high in sugar. It provides lots of potassium, calcium, and magnesium, while lowering salt and sodium; this mix of nutrients can also reduce your blood pressure. It

was developed by the government to help people with hypertension eat in a way that helps them control their high blood pressure. Here, take a look at these charts [hands Ida **Table 9.8**]. What do you think of this plan?

Ida: It seems confusing, having to measure all of this stuff and keep track of things.

Counselor: It is a little confusing at first. I'd suggest you keep making the foods you currently make—just cut down on the portion sizes and substitute some of the low-fat and sugarless items. Why don't you try the diet this week, and next week we can talk about the success and any problems you are having?

Ida: Okay, I'll try it.

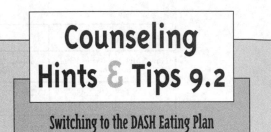

Counseling Hints & Tips 9.2

Switching to the DASH Eating Plan

The following tips are suggested to help clients convert their eating habits to the DASH plan:

1. Change gradually. Add a vegetable or fruit serving at lunch and dinner.
2. Use only half of the butter or margarine you do now.
3. If you have trouble digesting dairy products, try lactase enzyme pills or drops—they're available at drugstores and groceries. Alternatively, buy lactose-free milk or milk with lactase enzyme added to it.
4. Get added nutrients such as the B vitamins by choosing whole-grain foods, including whole-wheat bread or whole-grain cereals.
5. Spread out the servings. Have two servings of fruits or vegetables at each meal, or add fruits as snacks.
6. Treat meat as one part of the meal, instead of the focus. Try casseroles, pasta, and stir-fry dishes.
7. Have two or more meatless meals each week.
8. Use fruits or low-fat foods as desserts and snacks (NIH, 2000a).

————[**Table 9.8**]————

DASH Eating Plan

The DASH Eating Plan Shown Below Is Based on 2000 Calories per Day. The Number of Daily Servings in a Food Group May Vary from Those Listed, Depending on Your Caloric Needs.

Food Group	Daily Servings (except as noted)	Serving Sizes
Grains and grain products	7–8	1 slice bread 1 cup ready-to-eat cereal* $1/2$ cup cooked rice, pasta, or cereal
Vegetables	4–5	1 cup raw leafy vegetable $1/2$ cup cooked vegetable 6 ounces vegetable juice
Fruits	4–5	1 medium fruit $1/4$ cup dried fruit $1/2$ cup fresh, frozen, or canned fruit 6 ounces fruit juice
Low-fat or fat-free dairy foods	2–3	8 ounces milk 1 cup yogurt $1 1/2$ ounces cheese
Lean meats, poultry, and fish	2 or fewer	3 ounces cooked lean meat, skinless poultry, or fish
Nuts, seeds, and dry beans	4–5 per week	$1/3$ cup or $1 1/2$ ounces nuts 1 tablespoon or $1/2$ ounce seeds $1/2$ cup cooked dry beans
Fats and oils†	2–3	1 teaspoon soft margarine 1 tablespoon lowfat mayonnaise 2 tablespoons light salad dressing 1 teaspoon vegetable oil
Sweets	5 per week	1 tablespoon sugar 1 tablespoon jelly or jam $1/2$ ounce jelly beans 8 ounces lemonade

*Serving sizes vary between $1/2$ cup and $1 1/4$ cups. Check the product's nutrition label.
†Fat content changes serving counts for fats and oils. For example, 1 tablespoon of regular salad dressing equals one serving, 1 tablespoon of low-fat salad dressing equals one-half serving, and 1 tablespoon of fat-free salad dressing equals zero servings.

Directive 2: Be Physically Active

1. *Initial assessment.* Instruct clients to keep a daily physical activity log to assess physical activity and exercise patterns.
2. *Construction of a physical activity plan.* Teach clients how to increase their levels of physical activity using the U.S. Surgeon General's recommendations for increasing moderate physical activity.
3. *Ongoing assessment.* Instruct clients to continue keeping their physical activity logs and to note areas that are healthy as well as those that need improvement.

Logical Consequences of Being Physically Active

1. Clients will understand their current patterns of physical activity and exercise.
2. Clients will understand how to incorporate the Surgeon General's recommendations for physical activity into their lifestyles.
3. Clients will develop physical activity plans that are tailored to their particular needs.
4. Clients will comply with physical activity plans because they are tailored to their specific needs.
5. Clients will monitor their physical activity levels and understand their strengths and weaknesses.

Instructions for Being Physically Active

1. Clients are asked to keep a physical activity log. In it, they should log all physical activities performed. These activities could range from doing housework to going to the gym and lifting weights.
2. Instruct clients to bring their diaries to future sessions. Explain that you will go over the diary at the next visit to help them assess their current activity level.
3. Describe the Surgeon General's guidelines for moderate physical activity.
4. Set reasonable physical activity goals. Remember—you are not an exercise physiologist. You are trying to encourage clients to look for ways to incorporate 30 minutes of

moderate physical activity into their lives. Always advise clients to see their physicians for physical examinations before beginning any exercise program.

5. Help each client tailor a plan for incorporating 30 minutes of moderate physical activity into his or her daily schedule.

Example

Counselor: Ida, I'd like you to keep another diary, similar to the one you are keeping re-

---

[Table 9.9]

Moderate Activity Guidelines

Less Vigorous, Requires More Time
Washing and waxing a car for 45–60 minutes
Washing windows or floors for 45–60 minutes
Playing volleyball for 45 minutes
Playing touch football for 30–45 minutes
Gardening for 30–45 minutes
Wheeling self in wheelchair for 30–40 minutes
Walking 1³/₄ miles in 35 minutes (20 min/mile)
Basketball (shooting baskets) for 30 minutes
Bicycling 5 miles in 30 minutes
Dancing fast (social) for 30 minutes
Pushing a stroller 1¹/₂ miles in 30 minutes
Raking leaves for 30 minutes
Walking 2 miles in 30 minutes (15 min/mile)
Doing water aerobics for 30 minutes
Swimming laps for 20 minutes
Playing wheelchair basketball for 20 minutes
Playing basketball for 15–20 minutes
Bicycling 4 miles in 15 minutes
Jumping rope for 15 minutes
Running 1¹/₂ miles in 15 minutes (10 min/mile)
Shoveling snow for 15 minutes
Stairwalking for 15 minutes
More Vigorous, Requires Less Time

Source: Surgeon General's Report on Physical Activity. http://www.cdc.gov/nccdphp/sgr/ataglan.htm.

garding your diet. It is called a physical activity diary. It is almost the same as the diet diary, except that it monitors your physical activity level [hands Ida a sample, see **Figure 9.3**].

Ida: It looks almost like the diet diary.

Counselor: Exactly. It just logs your physical activity. I want you to keep track of everything you do that involves physical activity, from household chores to exercise classes to sporting activities. Bring the physical activity diary back next week, and we'll discuss it. Okay?

Ida: Okay.

Day 1	From ____ Until ____	Action	Duration	Description
	Example: 1:00 A.M. to 6:15 A.M.	Went for a hike	2 hours and 15 minutes	Enjoyed a good walk up and down mild hills in cool forest
			End of day 1 activity

Figure 9.3 Physical activity diary.

Counselor: Ida, take a look at this chart [hands Ida **Table 9.9**]. It is based on the 1999 Surgeon General's Report on Physical Activity and Health and recommends getting a moderate amount of physical activity each day. You can use common chores to get a moderate amount of physical activity every day. This is roughly the equivalent of physical activity that uses approximately 150 calories of energy per day. If you got 30 minutes of moderate exercise every day, it would add up to about 1000 calories per week. Do you see that?

Ida: Yes, I do a lot of these things already.

Counselor: Okay, that is good. More vigorous activities can help you use up the same amount of calories in a shorter time. If you do these activities for a longer period of time, you can burn even more calories. Which kinds of activities do you think you'd be interested in doing?

Ida: I like to walk and work in the garden. Both of these are hard for me to do in the winter.

Counselor: What is it about walking in the winter that you don't like?

Ida: I get home when it is dark, and I don't like walking outside in the cold and darkness.

Counselor: Have you ever thought about buying a treadmill to walk on indoors during the winter?

Ida: Yes, I just haven't been motivated enough to spend the money.

Counselor: You could even set it up in front of the TV and turn on a gardening show. That way, you can do the two things you like, even in the winter.

Ida: I have a spare TV with a DVD player in the den. I could put the treadmill there and buy a couple of gardening DVDs.

Counselor: Sounds like a plan. Why don't you research this possibility during the next week, and we'll work out a plan at our next session if you decide you want to do this?

Ida: Okay.

Counselor: Good. Next week, we'll talk about setting up what I call a "four-season activity plan," where you pick some physical activity you like to do each season. This will help you look forward to the changing seasons and ensure that your activities don't slack off when the season changes.

Ida: That sounds like a good idea.

Directive 3: Reducing Sodium in One's Diet

1. *Explain sodium and salt risks.* Teach clients how salt and sodium are related to hypertension.
2. *Choose foods low in salt.* Teach clients how to choose foods that are low in both salt and sodium.
3. *Use alternative spices.* Teach clients how to use spices, garlic, and onions to flavor foods without adding salt.

Logical Consequences of Reducing Sodium in One's Diet

1. Clients will understand how salt and sodium are related to each other and to high blood pressure.
2. Clients will understand how to choose foods low in salt and sodium.
3. Clients will learn how to use alternative seasonings and reduce their reliance on salt.

Specific Instructions for Reducing Sodium in One's Diet

1. Choose foods that are low in salt (sodium chloride) and other forms of sodium.
2. Before trying salt substitutes, clients should consult their doctors. These items contain potassium chloride and may be harmful for patients with certain medical conditions.
3. Experiment with herbs, spices, garlic, and onions to make food spicy without salt and sodium.
4. Minimize consumption of processed food.
5. Use food labels to help you choose products that are low in sodium.

Example

Counselor: Ida, an important part of keeping blood pressure at a healthy level is using less salt and sodium. Most of us use more salt than we really need, and it is already present in many of the foods we eat every day. We really should not eat more than 2.4 grams—2400 milligrams—of sodium, or about 1 teaspoon of table salt, per day. This amount includes all salt and sodium, both that already present in food and that added during cooking and at the table.

Ida: That doesn't seem possible. I put salt on everything.

Counselor: Most people do until they realize how important it is to cut back on it and they begin to pay attention to the amount used. Fortunately, there are a couple of things you can do, like using other spices and salt substitutes. Before you start using salt substitutes, however, check with your doctor because the substitutes contain potassium chloride and may affect other medical conditions you might have.

Ida: So what can I do? I like salt.

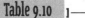

Table 9.10

Sodium Reduction Tips

Buy fresh, plain frozen, or canned "with no salt added" vegetables.

Use fresh poultry, fish, and lean meat, rather than canned or processed types.

Use herbs, spices, and salt-free seasoning blends in cooking and at the table.

Cook rice, pasta, and hot cereal without salt. Cut back on instant or flavored rice, pasta, and cereal mixes, which usually have added salt.

Choose "convenience" foods that are low in sodium. Cut back on frozen dinners, pizza, packaged mixes, canned soups or broths, and salad dressings—these often have a lot of sodium.

Rinse canned foods, such as tuna, to remove some sodium.

When available, buy low- and reduced-sodium or no-salt-added versions of foods.

Choose ready-to-eat breakfast cereals that are low in sodium.

Counselor: Here is a list of tips for reducing the amount of salt and sodium you consume [hands Ida **Table 9.10**]. Look at these and tell me which ones you think you can use.

Ida: Most of these things seem pretty reasonable. The hardest thing for me is to stop putting salt on my food.

Counselor: How about a compromise? Until you speak to your doctor about salt substitutes, try putting half of the amount of salt on your food that you currently use. Let me know how this strategy works when you come back next week.

Ida: That seems like a good idea. In the meantime, I'll call my doctor.

Counselor: Ida, another simple way to cut back on salt and sodium is to eat less processed food. Although sodium is found naturally in food, most of the salt and sodium that we consume come from processed foods.

Ida: What do you mean by "processed food"?

Counselor: Good question. Processed food includes things like regular canned vegetables and soups, frozen dinners, lunchmeats, instant and ready-to-eat cereals, and salty chips and other snacks. There is a good chance that anything that you don't make fresh has extra sodium in it unless it was intentionally left out. Many food manufacturers now offer low-sodium foods. They are usually found in a special place in your local supermarket. You might try looking for this section the next time you go shopping.

Ida: I will.

Counselor: The last thing you need to do is to start looking at food labels. Here is a chart that shows you where the sodium content is found on a food label [hands Ida **Figure 9.4**]. Do you see where the sodium is listed?

Ida: Yeah, look at the difference in the two labels.

Counselor: Frozen foods have much less sodium than a lot of canned foods. I'd like you to

Food labels can help you choose items lower in sodium as well as in calories, saturated fat, total fat, and cholesterol.

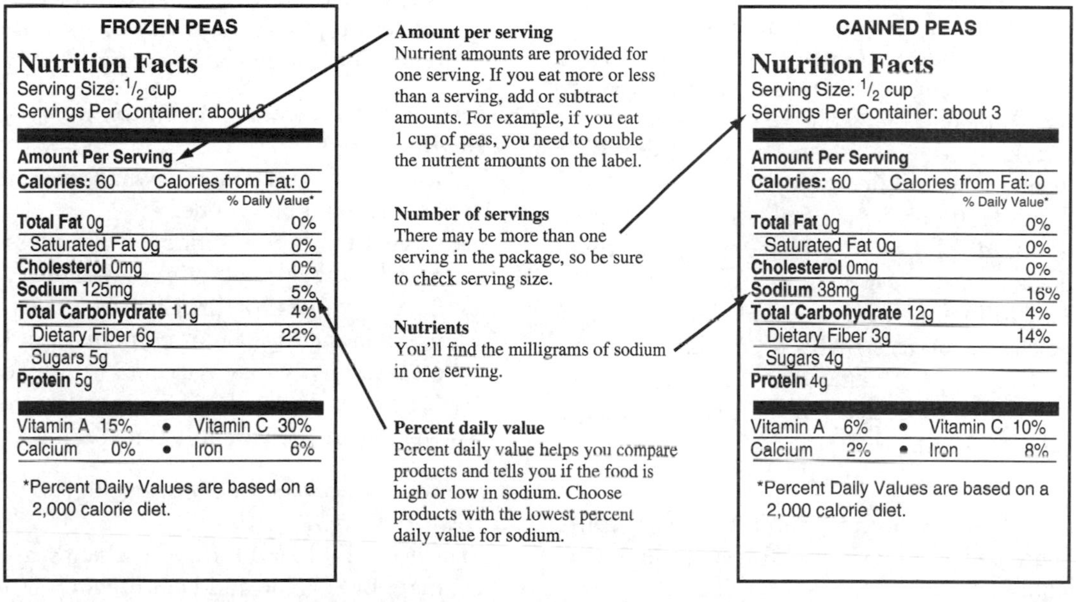

FROZEN PEAS

Nutrition Facts
Serving Size: $1/2$ cup
Servings Per Container: about 3

Amount Per Serving
Calories: 60   Calories from Fat: 0
                                    % Daily Value*
Total Fat 0g   0%
   Saturated Fat 0g   0%
Cholesterol 0mg   0%
Sodium 125mg   5%
Total Carbohydrate 11g   4%
   Dietary Fiber 6g   22%
   Sugars 5g
Protein 5g

Vitamin A 15%   •   Vitamin C 30%
Calcium   0%   •   Iron   6%

*Percent Daily Values are based on a 2,000 calorie diet.

Amount per serving
Nutrient amounts are provided for one serving. If you eat more or less than a serving, add or subtract amounts. For example, if you eat 1 cup of peas, you need to double the nutrient amounts on the label.

Number of servings
There may be more than one serving in the package, so be sure to check serving size.

Nutrients
You'll find the milligrams of sodium in one serving.

Percent daily value
Percent daily value helps you compare products and tells you if the food is high or low in sodium. Choose products with the lowest percent daily value for sodium.

CANNED PEAS

Nutrition Facts
Serving Size: $1/2$ cup
Servings Per Container: about 3

Amount Per Serving
Calories: 60   Calories from Fat: 0
                                    % Daily Value*
Total Fat 0g   0%
   Saturated Fat 0g   0%
Cholesterol 0mg   0%
Sodium 38mg   16%
Total Carbohydrate 12g   4%
   Dietary Fiber 3g   14%
   Sugars 4g
Protein 4g

Vitamin A 6%   •   Vitamin C 10%
Calcium   2%   •   Iron   8%

*Percent Daily Values are based on a 2,000 calorie diet.

? Which product is lower in sodium?
Answer: The frozen peas. The canned peas have three times more sodium than the frozen peas.

Figure 9.4 How to read food labels.

start reading labels like this one between now and next week.

Ida: Okay, I'll do this and we'll talk about it next week.

Directive 4: Drinking Alcohol in Moderation

1. Teach clients how alcohol is related to hypertension.
2. Describe what constitutes excess drinking behavior.
3. Teach clients the equivalencies of alcoholic beverages.

Logical Consequences of Drinking Alcohol in Moderation

1. Clients will understand how excess drinking contributes to obesity and hypertension.
2. Clients will understand what excess drinking levels are and set reasonable levels for their drinking.
3. Clients will understand how the different kinds of alcoholic beverages are related.

Specific Instructions for Drinking Alcohol in Moderation

1. Alcoholic drinks contain "empty calories," which means that they supply very few nutrients yet add extra calories to the diet. For this reason, it is easy to gain excess weight when consuming alcoholic beverages.
2. Drinking too much alcohol can harm the liver, brain, and heart.
3. A moderate amount of alcoholic beverages is one drink per day for women and two drinks per day for men.
4. The following beverages all count as one drink: 12 ounces of beer (regular or light, 150 calories), 5 ounces of wine (100 calories), or 1.5 ounces of 80-proof whiskey (100 calories).

Example

Counselor: Ida, another thing that can contribute to hypertension is drinking too much alcohol.

Ida: That is not a problem for me. I don't really drink much at all. Maybe I'll have a glass of wine with dinner.

Counselor: Good, because having more than one drink a day adds extra calories to your diet and makes it easy to gain weight and keep your blood pressure elevated.

Ida: What about beer? Every once in a while, I like to have a beer or two when we go out for Mexican food.

Counselor: Ida, the following alcoholic beverages all count as one drink: 12 ounces of beer, 5 ounces of wine, or 1.5 ounces of 80-proof whiskey. Just remember that if you have more than one of these beverages on any day, you should do something to compensate for the extra calories, such as cut back on the amount of food you eat or get some extra exercise.

Directive 5: Maintaining a Healthy Weight

1. *Do an assessment.* Instruct clients to calculate their healthy body weight based on BMI tables.
2. *Set reasonable weight-loss goals.* Help clients set reasonable weight-loss goals of around two pounds per week.
3. *Develop a program.* Help clients develop a weight-loss program based on combining moderate physical activity or exercise with reduced-calorie/healthy eating (DASH diet).

Logical Consequences of Maintaining a Healthy Weight

1. Clients will understand what their healthy body weight should be.
2. Clients will set reasonable weight-loss goals based on their healthy body weight.
3. Clients will tailor programs to their needs while adhering to a combination of increased physical activity and healthy eating.
4. Clients will reach/maintain their healthy weights in a reasonable time period.

Specific Instructions for Maintaining a Healthy Weight

1. Check Table 9.11 for the client's approximate BMI value and healthy body weight.
2. Compare the client's weight and BMI against the values for normal, overweight, and obese (overweight is defined as a BMI

of 25 to 29.9; obesity is defined as a BMI equal to or greater than 30).

3. Measure the client's waist. (A waist measurement of more than 35 inches in women and more than 40 inches in men is considered high.)

4. Use the figures to determine how much weight the client has to lose.

5. Set up a timeline to lose weight using a 2 pounds per week schedule.

6. Develop a weight-loss program combining the DASH eating plan and the physical activity plan.

Example

Counselor: Ida, the first step in developing a personal weight management program for you is to find your healthy weight and waist measurement and then to compare them to your current weight and waist measurement. Let's take a minute to look at charts developed by the government to help us assess these things [hands Ida **Table 9.11**].

Ida: According to the government chart, I should weigh 122 pounds and have a BMI of 21. My waist shouldn't be larger than 35 inches. What exactly is a BMI?

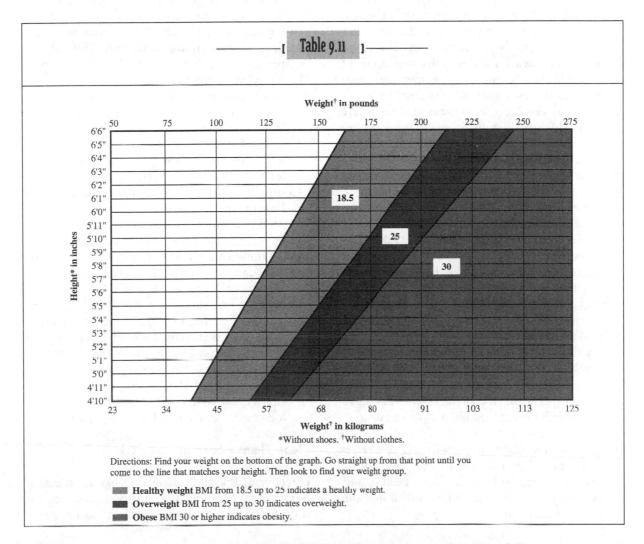

Table 9.11

Weight† in pounds

Height* in inches

Weight† in kilograms

*Without shoes. †Without clothes.

Directions: Find your weight on the bottom of the graph. Go straight up from that point until you come to the line that matches your height. Then look to find your weight group.

Healthy weight BMI from 18.5 up to 25 indicates a healthy weight.
Overweight BMI from 25 up to 30 indicates overweight.
Obese BMI 30 or higher indicates obesity.

Counselor: A BMI is a measure of your weight in relation to your height. It approximates your total body fat in relation to being overweight. The only problem with just using your BMI is that it is not 100% accurate for everyone. Someone who is very muscular, for example, will weigh more than someone who isn't as muscular, but muscle is actually lean tissue and doesn't pose the same risk as fat tissue. The BMI alone can't assess this difference. In such a case, the BMI can overestimate body fat. It can also underestimate body fat in older persons or those losing muscle. To account for this possibility, we combine the BMI with a waist measurement. Usually, people who are carrying excess fat will have too much body fat in the stomach. This shape increases disease risk. A waist measurement of more than 35 inches in women and more than 40 inches in men is considered high.

Ida: Okay, let me get on the scale and see where I am. [Ida goes behind a screen, takes off her clothes, and weighs herself.] Wow, do I really have to tell you what I weigh?

Counselor: It's okay, Ida. Remember, I've been there myself.

Ida: I weigh 170 pounds.

Counselor: That's okay, Ida. Get dressed and come around, and I'll take your waist measurement. [Ida does so.] Your waist is 37½ inches. Let's see, if we put the measurements together, you need to lose about 50 pounds and 3 inches around your waist. That should get your BMI down to 21, where it should be.

Ida: Wow, that seems like a lot to ask.

Counselor: Ida, I know it seems daunting but if we break this into trying to lose up to 2 pounds per week, in about five months you'll get there. If we started this week [it's January], you'll be there just in time for summer. I know you can do it.

Ida: You really think so?

Counselor: I know it. It is up to you. We've already talked about how to exercise and eat well according to DASH. All we need to add is how to cut calories while still doing the same healthy things.

Ida: How do we do that?

Counselor: You can also use the DASH eating plan to make it a lower-calorie diet. The whole idea is to continue to eat according to your healthy eating plan but to trim calories by making simple switches like eating smaller portions, using low-fat and fat-free dairy products, and cutting back on sugar wherever possible. What do you think about the ideas in the chart? [Counselor hands Ida **Table 9.12**.]

Ida: They are not too different from what we've already talked about. I think I can do this.

Counselor: Good, what you want to do is lose 1 to 2 pounds per week. One pound equals about 3500 calories. To lose 1 pound per week, you need to eat 500 fewer calories each day. Another option is to burn 500 calories per day more than you usually do by exercising. One of the best ways is to combine the two strategies and cut 250 calories by eating smarter and 250 calories by exercising more. What do you think?

Ida: The combination plan seems the best for me. It seems like the plan that involves the least sacrifice on my part.

Counselor: Okay, we've already talked about how to add the exercise part, so now you just need to combine the two. Where do you want to begin to cut back on the calories?

Ida: I think I'll start substituting low-fat and fat-free dairy products and sugar substitutes. That way I can eat foods I like but have lower-calorie substitutes. I'm already going to start walking for 45 minutes each morning.

Counselor: I want you to keep track of your diet and physical activity in the diaries we already discussed. Make sure to note the exact versions of the foods you've eaten to show these changes, and we'll go over your logs next week when I see you again. Good luck!

Ida: Thanks. See you next week.

Directive 6: Taking Prescribed Drugs as Directed
Nonmedical counselors do not prescribe medications for clients. Their sole role in this directive is

Table 9.12

How to Lose Weight on the DASH Eating Plan

The DASH eating plan was not designed to promote weight loss. But it is rich in low-calorie foods such as fruits and vegetables. You can make it lower in calories by replacing high-calorie foods with more fruits and vegetables—and that also will make it easier for you to reach your DASH eating plan goals. Here are some examples:

To increase fruits:
- Eat a medium apple instead of four shortbread cookies. You'll save 80 calories.
- Eat $1/4$ cup of dried apricots instead of a 2-ounce bag of pork rinds. You'll save 230 calories.

To increase vegetables:
- Have a hamburger that's 3 ounces Instead of 6 ounces. Add a $1/2$ cup serving of carrots and a $1/2$ cup serving of spinach. You'll save more than 200 calories.
- Instead of 5 ounces of chicken, have a stir fry with 2 ounces of chicken and $1\,1/2$ cups of raw vegetables. Use a small amount of vegetable oil. You'll save 50 calories.

To increase lowfat or fat free dairy products:
- Have a $1/2$ cup serving of lowfat frozen yogurt instead of a $1\,1/2$-ounce milk chocolate bar. You'll save about 110 calories.

And don't forget these calorie-saving tips:
- Use lowfat or fat-free condiments, such as fat-free salad dressings.
- Eat smaller portions—cut back gradually.
- Choose lowfat or fat-free dairy products to reduce total fat intake.
- Use food labels to compare fat content in packaged foods. Items marked lowfat or fat-free are not always lower in calories than their regular versions.
- Limit foods with lots of added sugar, such as pies, flavored yogurts, candy bars, ice cream, sherbet, regular soft drinks, and fruit drinks.
- Eat fruits canned in their own juice.
- Snack on fruit, vegetable sticks, unbuttered and unsalted popcorn, or bread sticks.
- Drink water or club soda.

Source: NIH (2003b).

to help clients achieve maximum compliance with the medications prescribed by their physicians. Counselors must be sure to make this role clear to clients and their physicians before discussing medication-taking instructions.

1. *Understand the relationship between lifestyle changes and drugs.* Sometimes lifestyle changes alone will not lower blood pressure

enough, and drugs must be prescribed. Even if clients need drugs, they still must make the lifestyle changes.
2. *Know the different categories of drugs.* Many drugs are available that can lower blood pressure. They work in various ways.
3. *Take drugs as prescribed.* It's important to take drugs exactly as the physician prescribed them.

4. *Be aware of side effects*. If you have side effects, tell your doctor so the drugs can be changed or the dosage adjusted.

5. *Recognize the potential need for multiple drugs*. Many people need to take two or more drugs to bring their blood pressure down to a healthy level.

6. *Be aware of polydrug interactions*. Clients must tell their doctors about any nonprescription drugs that they are taking and ask how these agents could potentially interact with their hypertension medications.

Logical Consequences of Taking Prescribed Drugs as Directed

1. Clients will understand that while they must make lifestyle modifications such as eating healthy and reducing sodium, these changes may not be enough to lower their blood pressure without drugs.

2. Clients will understand how the different categories of hypertension drugs work and that many different medication options are available.

3. Clients will know exactly how to take their drugs as prescribed.

4. Clients will know the possible side effects of their medications and what to do if they experience those adverse effects.

5. Clients will understand that sometimes they may need to take two or more drugs to bring their blood pressure down to a healthy level.

6. Clients will understand that other prescription and nonprescription drugs can affect the use of their hypertension medications and must inform their doctors of these other medications.

Specific Instructions for Taking Prescribed Drugs as Directed

Counselors need to go over the following set of specific instructions for *each* hypertension medication prescribed for the client.

1. *Categories of medications*. Clients need to know the different types of drugs that are currently available and how they work in controlling high blood pressure.

2. *Medication name*. Clients need to know the names of the medications they have been prescribed.

3. *Efficacy*. Clients need to believe that their medications are the best available choices for their particular problems, especially if the treatment is difficult to take or produces side effects.

4. *Dosage and schedule*. Clients need to know how many pills to take each day, how doses should be spaced out, and how long to take the drugs. Otherwise, they will not take the medications correctly.

5. *Side effects*. Clients need to know what side effects to expect or they will discontinue taking medications when these side effects occur.

6. *Contraindications*. Clients need to know what to avoid while taking their medications or they might experience unanticipated side effects or a reduction in efficacy.

7. *Symptom response*. Clients need to know that controlling hypertension through medication does not result in any noticeable changes even though the drug may be working.

8. *Missed doses*. Clients need to know what to do if they miss a dose or they might stop taking their medications completely.

9. *Polydrug interactions*. Clients need to know how their hypertension medication interacts with other drugs they are taking.

When counseling clients about medication taking, it is important to pay attention to the compliance-enhancing strategies discussed in Chapter 2.

Example

Counselor: Ida, let's go over the different categories of hypertension medications and see where the medications your doctor prescribed fit [hands Ida a copy of Table 9.7]. Can you find your medications on this chart?

Ida: Here are mine [Ida identifies her drugs].

Counselor: Your medication is called [drug name]. You are going to take [number] pills, [number] times a day for [number] days.

Continue to take your pills, even if you don't feel any different from when you were not taking them. The pills should be spaced about [number] hours apart. You can take your medication with [food or drink] or on an empty stomach.

It is the best medicine we can give you. It will moderate your blood pressure if you take it exactly as I tell you to.

Tell me what your daily schedule is like and when you think you can take each pill.

Ida: I get up about 5:30 A.M., jump in the shower, and spend about the next 30 minutes on my hair and make-up. Then I get dressed, make the kids and myself breakfast, and pack their lunches. We eat and I drop them off at school on my way to work. I drive to work and arrive at about 8:00 A.M. I work from 8:30 A.M. until noon, have a 30-minute lunch break, and then work until about 6:00 P.M. I drive home, get dinner ready, and eat at about 7:30 P.M. I clean up the kitchen, do a load of wash, and watch a little television. I usually go to sleep at about 11:00 P.M.

I guess I could take a pill at [time].

Counselor: Good. Here, I'll write this down on your pill envelope. Your medication is [name], and you'll take one pill at [time] and one pill at [time]. You'll take each pill with [food or drink] and continue taking them even though you will notice no changes in the way you feel. If you miss a dose, take it at [time]. (Tailoring, repetition, and written reinforcement)

Counseling Hints & Tips 9.3

Adhering to Medication Regimens

Hypertension medications work in a variety of ways to lower and moderate blood pressure. Many clients who are currently taking hypertension medication do not fully understand what they are taking or how to take their medication properly. Adherence to treatment regimens ensures that clients will moderate their hypertension and not develop complications associated with their diseases. Here are some helpful hints:

1. Put a favorite picture of yourself or a loved one on the refrigerator with a note that says, "Remember to take your high blood pressure drugs."
2. Keep your high blood pressure drugs on the nightstand next to your side of the bed.
3. Take your high blood pressure drugs right after you brush your teeth, and keep them with your toothbrush as a reminder.
4. Put "sticky" notes in visible places to remind yourself to take your high blood pressure drugs. You can put notes on the refrigerator, on the bathroom mirror, or on the front door.
5. Set up a buddy system with a friend who also is on daily medication and arrange to call each other every day with a reminder to "take your blood pressure drugs."
6. Ask your child or grandchild to call you every day with a quick reminder. It's a great way to stay in touch, and little ones love to help the grown-ups.
7. Place your drugs in a weekly pillbox (available at most pharmacies).
8. If you have a personal computer, program a start-up reminder to take your high blood pressure drugs, or sign up with a free service that will send you a reminder e-mail every day.
9. Remember to refill your prescription. Each time you pick up a refill, make a note on your calendar to order and pick up the next refill one week before the medication is due to run out (NIH, 2003b).

Ida, when taking these pills you might experience [side effects]. These are normal. Unless they worsen, continue to take your medication as directed. (Side effects)

[Drug name] can also have the following contraindications [list them], so while you are taking these pills try to avoid [activities]. (Contraindications)

Ida, I know this is a lot to remember, so why don't you just repeat these instructions back to me. (Patient quiz)

Ida: Okay, I take one pill at [time] and one pill at [time]. I continue taking them regardless of how I feel unless the side effects get worse. I should try to avoid [activities]. If I miss a pill, I should [new schedule]. I keep taking the pills and come see you in [number] weeks.

Counselor: Good. I expect you to follow this plan exactly as we developed it. When you come back in for follow-up tests, bring your pill envelope so I can check to make sure you took all of your pills. (Expectation citing)

Summary

This chapter discussed how to counsel someone with high blood pressure. It began with an overview of the physiology of blood pressure and an explanation of how to distinguish normal pressure from hypertension. It then moved into a discussion of the epidemiology of hypertension and a description of both controllable and noncontrollable risk factors for the disease. The chapter progressed to a discussion of control and prevention strategies, including strategies that revolve around lifestyle modifications and medication taking.

There are six goals for hypertension counseling: (1) follow a healthy eating plan, (2) be physically active, (3) reduce the amount of sodium in the diet, (4) drink alcohol only in moderation, (5) maintain a healthy weight, and (6) take prescribed drugs as directed. The microskills model can be applied to counseling hypertension patients, including use of adherence strategies for ensuring maximum compliance with hypertension medication.

Study Questions

1. Describe the epidemiologic trends of hypertension over the past 20 years.
2. Why is hypertension such a serious personal and public health problem?
3. What are the main goals of hypertension counseling?
4. How is high blood pressure similar to and different from at least two other chronic diseases?
5. List and describe the risk factors for hypertension.
6. How do the different categories of hypertension medications work in controlling high blood pressure?
7. How does the asymptomatic nature of hypertension affect the emotional responses of clients with the condition?
8. How can counselors with hypertension use self-disclosure to influence clients?
9. How does changing the focal point help clients view their hypertension differently?
10. What are the key directives and logical consequences for each of the hypertension counseling goals?

References

American Heart Association (AHA) (2003). *Heart Disease and Stroke Statistics—2004 Update*. Dallas, TX: American Heart Association.

Blonna R (2005). *Coping with Stress in a Changing World*, 3rd ed. Dubuque, IA: McGraw-Hill.

De le Varre C (2003). *Talking to Your Health Care Provider*. Chapel Hill, NC: School of Information and Library Science, University of North Carolina at Chapel Hill. www.ils.unc.edu.

Dosh SA (2001). The diagnosis of essential and secondary hypertension in adults. *Journal of Family Practice* August: 221–228.

Ivey AE, Ivey M (2003). *Intentional Interviewing and Counseling: Facilitating Client Development in a Multicultural Society*, 5th ed. Belmont, CA: Thomson/Brooks Cole.

Mayo Clinic (2003). *High Blood Pressure Risk Factors*. www.mayoclinic.com/invoke.cfm?objectid=D2F240ED-803D-4E1A-A692B907BFCFDD6D&dsection=4.

National Institutes of Health (NIH) (2003a). *The Seventh Report of the Joint National Committee on Prevention, Detection, Evaluation, and Treatment of High Blood Pressure.* NIH Publication no. 03–5233. National Heart, Lung, and Blood Institute, National High Blood Pressure Education Program. www.nhlbi.nih.gov/guidelines/hypertension/.

National Institutes of Health (NIH) (2003b). *Your Guide to Lowering Blood Pressure.* NIH Publication no. 03–5232. National Heart, Lung, and Blood Institute, National High Blood Pressure Education Program. www.nhlbi.nih.gov/health/public/heart/hbp/hbp_low/hbp_low.pdf.

Onusko E (2003). Diagnosing secondary hypertension. *American Family Physician* January (67):67–74.

United States Department of Health and Human Services (USDHHS), Office of Disease Prevention and Health Promotion (ODPHP) (2003). *Healthy People 2010: A Systematic Approach to Health Improvement.* www.healthypeople.gov/Document/html/uih/uih_bw/uih_2.htm#obj.

Chapter 10

Counseling Persons with Chlamydia and Other Sexually Transmitted Diseases

Learning Objectives

By the end of the chapter students will:

1. Understand the nature and extent of the sexually transmitted disease (STD) problem in the United States

2. Describe the four goals of STD counseling

3. Compare and contrast *Chlamydia trachomatis* infection to a variety of other STDs

4. Explain how the pyramid of risk model assesses personal STD risk

5. Compare and contrast the use of introductory skills with clients infected with *Chlamydia* and clients having non-STD health problems

6. Explain how body language is related to judgmentalism and nonjudgmentalism when counseling STD clients

7. Discuss the relevance of neutral sexual language when using introductory, attending, and responding skills with clients infected with *Chlamydia*

8. Describe how to use self-disclosure effectively

9. Discuss how changing the focal point can help clients understand and negotiate proper sex partner evaluation

10. List and describe the key directives and logical consequences for each of the STD counseling goals

Introduction

Sexually transmitted diseases (STDs), also known as sexually transmitted infections (STIs), are infections that are almost always contracted through sexual contact. We will use the descriptor STDs for these diseases, because it is the term of choice used by the Centers for Disease Control and Prevention (CDC), the lead agency in the United States for the control of infectious diseases. Although in theory STDs can be transmitted through any form of sexual contact, vaginal and anal intercourse are much more *efficient* modes of transmission than is oral-genital sexual contact. Some STDs, such as human immunodeficiency virus (HIV) infection and hepatitis B, also are transmitted by contaminated blood through needle sharing associated with injection drug use (Eng & Butler, 1997).

More than 65 million people in the United States are currently infected with an incurable STD, and each year an additional 15 million people develop new cases of one or more of the 25 diseases categorized as STDs. Of these new cases, roughly half are incurable, lifelong infections (DSTD, 2000; Cates et al., 1999). STDs represent 87% of all cases of infectious disease reported to the CDC. Five of the top ten most frequently reported diseases in the United States are STDs (DSTD, 2002). The STD epidemic is really a series of epidemics because such CDC-reportable diseases actually include more than two dozen different types of infections, many of which are asymptomatic (without symptoms). Because of the asymptomatic nature of many STDs, many people who are infected go undiagnosed. This issue has led public health officials to refer to the problem as the "hidden epidemic" (DSTD, 2000).

Counseling persons with STDs presents a unique challenge because of the hidden nature of the conditions, the diversity of diseases, and the personal, sexual nature of the problem. Some STDs, such as gonorrhea, chlamydia, and syphilis, are well known, are easily diagnosed through clinical examination and laboratory tests, and can be cured using a variety of broad-spectrum antibiotics and/or penicillin. Other STDs, such as genital warts and genital herpes, are chronic in nature, are not as easily diagnosed through clinical examination and laboratory testing, and are not curable. Treatment of these infections is often **palliative**—that is, designed to remove or lessen the symptoms and minimize the likelihood of recurrence. Still

other STDs such as HIV/AIDS, while easily diagnosed, are so feared by clients that testing alone poses formidable obstacles unlike any associated with the other STDs.

Patients whose sexually transmitted infections were detected through positive screening tests often require a different counseling approach from those who volunteered for treatment because they were symptomatic or who came in with an infected sex partner. The latter types of patients are usually highly motivated and cooperate more fully with therapeutic regimens. Clients whose infections were uncovered through routine screening tests often do not believe they are infected and can prove more resistant to counseling.

Overall Goals of STD Counseling

There are four major overall goals of counseling clients with STDs:

1. Reduce overall STD morbidity and mortality
2. Ensure that the client's current infection is treated/managed properly
3. Prevent spread of the infection to exposed sex partners
4. Prevent reinfection of the client (DSTD, 2000)

As the lead agency in the United States for monitoring STD-associated morbidity and mortality, the CDC's Division of Sexually Transmitted Disease (DSTD) participates in the Healthy People 2010 project and has set targets for STD morbidity and mortality rates. We will refer to these target rates as we discuss the individual STDs.

Ensuring that clients adhere to their therapeutic plans is essential to treating them and reducing overall morbidity and mortality. If patients do not adhere to their treatment plans and remain infected, they may spread their infections or develop complications that make further treatment more difficult. Tailoring treatment plans to individual clients and their particular diseases is essential to success. We will discuss strategies for optimizing adherence to therapeutic regimens as we discuss individual STDs.

Preventing the spread of STDs is a two-pronged effort: (1) making sure that infected clients adhere to their treatment regimens and (2) ensuring that exposed sexual partners are examined and given treatment to prevent disease from developing in these individuals. We will discuss specific strategies used to prevent the spread of infections.

Preventing reinfection also hinges on ensuring that patients comply fully with their treatment regimens. Research shows that more than half of all STD patients who become reinfected within the first month of treatment have either been re-exposed to an initial sex partner (from the first episode) before that person received preventive treatment or failed to take all of their medication as indicated (Cates & Stone, 1992). Preventing reinfection therefore starts with counseling for maximum compliance with treatment regimens. In addition, counselors must spend time discussing a variety of primary prevention strategies, ranging from consistent and correct condom use to having clients reduce their overall numbers of sex partners (CDC 2002a, 2002b).

Overview of *Chlamydia trachomatis*

Epidemiology

Chlamydia trachomatis is the most prevalent sexually transmitted bacterial pathogen in the United States. In 2000, 702,093 cases of chlamydia were reported to the CDC from 50 states and the District of Columbia (DSTD, 2001). In 2000, the chlamydia rate was 257.5 cases per 100,000 persons. This represents an increase of 2.3% from the rate of 251.6 cases per 100,000 persons in 1999. The reported number of chlamydia cases was approximately double the 358,995 reported cases of gonorrhea (DSTD, 2001).

Between 1987 and 2000, the chlamydia rate in the United States increased from 50.8 to 257.5 cases per 100,000 persons (DSTD, 2001). Most experts agree that the continuing increase in reported cases of chlamydia is due to increased screening for this infection as well as the development and use of more-sensitive screening tests

(DSTD, 2001). **Figure 10.1** shows the rapid climb in rates during the years 1984–2000.

Although the current estimated incidence is about 3 million cases annually (down from estimates of 4 to 5 million), chlamydia rates continue to rise. This infection represents a serious disease threat because of its asymptomatic nature. Seventy-five percent of affected women and 50% of affected men usually have no symptoms for chlamydia. As a consequence, screening sexually active women and their sex partners for chlamydia in a variety of healthcare facilities is the heart of the government's prevention program. Most public STD and family planning clinics routinely screen all gonorrhea patients for infection with *Chlamydia trachomatis,* recognizing that roughly 50% of all gonorrhea patients have coexistent infection with *Chlamydia* (Cates et al., 1999).

Reported chlamydia rates in women are much higher than in men **(Figure 10.2)** because traditionally screening programs have been directed mostly at women. Chlamydia exists at **endemic** levels in certain populations of young women. More than 40% of all cases of chlamydia are among 15- to 19-year-olds, for example. In studies of adolescents, approximately 10% of all girls and 5% of all boys tested positive for the disease (DSTD, 2000).

Nongonoccal urethritis (NGU) is a urethral infection in men that is not due to gonorrhea. This catch-all diagnosis is often made when a man with clinical symptoms of **urethritis** tests negative for gonorrhea. Rather than take additional urethral

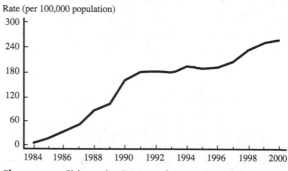

Figure 10.1 Chlamydia: Reported rates: United States, 1984–2000. (*Source:* DSTD (2002).)

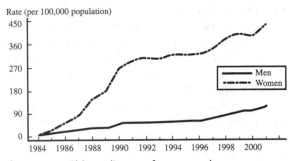

Rate (per 100,000 population)

Figure 10.2 Chlamydia rates for men and women. (*Source:* DSTD (2002).)

specimens and order laboratory tests for other possible causative organisms, the clinician will opt for a diagnosis of NGU knowing that prescribing a regimen of broad-spectrum antibiotics will likely kill the organism causing the problem. Most cases of NGU are attributed to infection with *Chlamydia trachomatis* (Cates et al., 1999).

Figure 10.3 shows the number of visits to physician offices prompted by NGU. Visits to physicians for NGU peaked in 1990 and, except for a slight increase in 1999, have declined steadily in recent years (DSTD, 2002). Annual incidence of NGU is estimated at approximately 3 million cases annually in the United States (DSTD, 2000).

Chlamydia rates by race/ethnicity show a slightly lower rate of infection among whites than among other racial/ethnic groups. As with many

STDs, rates are highest in the southern part of the United States than in the other regions (DSTD, 2002; Guaschino & DeSeta, 2000).

Diagnosis

Chlamydia is a sexually transmitted disease caused by infection with the *Chlamydia trachomatis* organism. *Chlamydia trachomatis* is transmitted through contact with infected semen or cervical mucus. It also can be passed through oral contact (usually **fellatio**) with infected mucous patches in the throat.

During sexual contact, the organisms are passed by person-to-person contact with the infected ejaculate or mucus. Incubation is from 1 to 30 days. The initial symptoms of chlamydia in men are a scanty, clear to milky-white discharge from the penis, and burning upon urination. Some women notice a scanty, clear to milky-white discharge and irritation of the vulva. As noted earlier, 75% of women and 50% of men fail to show any symptoms for chlamydia. For this reason, the government's prevention program for the disease focuses on screening sexually active women (and their sex partners) for chlamydia in a variety of healthcare facilities.

In the 1960s and 1970s, chlamydia was believed to be a relatively minor problem. Men with the infection were often referred to as having "nonspecific urethritis" and were not counseled extensively regarding the necessity of having their sexual partners examined. Chlamydia, however, was discovered to be a major source of pelvic inflammatory disease (PID). As many as 20% of all women with *Chlamydia trachomatis* infection will develop PID. PID can result in chronic pain, **ectopic pregnancy,** and sterility, and in rare instances is fatal. More than half of all PID is caused by chlamydia. In contrast, infection in men rarely leads to major complications. Fewer than 1% of men infected with *Chlamydia trachomatis* develop **epididymitis** (Morse, Moreland, & Thompson, 1990).

A recent advance in chlamydia and gonorrhea testing is the Nucleic Acid Amplification Test

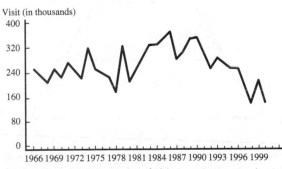

Visit (in thousands)

Figure 10.3 Nonspecific urethritis: initial visits to physicians' offices by men: United States, 1966–2000. (*Source:* DSTD (2002).)

(NAAT). This test detects the presence of *Chlamydia* through DNA testing. It actually identifies nucleic acid sequences that are specific to the *Chlamydia* organism. Unlike smear or culture tests, the NAAT does not require viable organisms to diagnose the disease. Specimens are easily obtained through urine samples. Patients do not need to be symptomatic to obtain specimens, and samples can be obtained anywhere urine collection can be performed. The beauty of the NAAT is that it reduces dependence on invasive tests and allows public health programs to expand testing into locations such as schools, where other means of testing were unacceptable (Blonna & Levitan, 2005). A recent study in a Philadelphia school-based clinic setting demonstrated a yield of more than 20% among students tested (Bertrami, 2002).

Another advantage of the NAAT is its ability to test for gonorrhea infection at the same time using the same specimen. The Philadelphia study found that almost half of the students infected with *Chlamydia* had coexisting gonorrhea. These gonorrhea cases would often go undetected with traditional tests that checked for only chlamydia. The ability to test for both infections simultaneously using a simple, easy-to-obtain urine specimen represents a major breakthrough in STD testing and is a valuable tool in the prevention of gonorrhea and chlamydia (CDC, 2002b).

Treatment

Chlamydia trachomatis infection is relatively easy to treat. Azithromycin 1 g, taken orally in a single dose, or doxycycline 100 mg, taken orally twice a day for seven days, are the two recommended treatments. The organism is destroyed by a number of antibiotics (CDC, 2002a).

Prevention: A Pyramid of Risk for STDs

Blonna and Levitan (2005) have developed a new way to conceptualize community and personal STD risks. Their "pyramid of risk" consists of various public and personal factors that build upon one another. **Figure 10.4** illustrates this model.

The foundation of the pyramid is made up of **demographic** variables that influence STD (including HIV) risk. These factors are generally beyond clients' control.

The second level of risk focuses on the sexual and medical histories of clients and their partners. Because these risks are part of the past, they also cannot be changed. They represent the histories that clients bring to any sexual encounter. It is beyond the scope of this book to describe these levels of risk in any detail. Essentially these factors cannot be changed in the lives of clients and their sex partners, yet can still increase risk for acquiring STDs. For a thorough discussion of these levels of risk, see Blonna and Levitan (2005, Chapter 15).

The third level of risk represents clients' current sexual relationships. The fourth, and final, level of risk is the one on which most educators focus: personal sexual behavior. Both the third and fourth levels represent risk factors that can be modified. We will discuss these variables and how they impact counseling someone with chlamydia or another STD.

Although the four levels in the pyramid influence STD risk independently, the interaction of

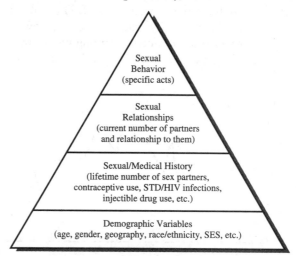

Figure 10.4 There are four levels of STD risk. (*Source:* Richard Blonna and Jean Levitan, *Healthy Sexuality*, © 2005 by Thomson-Wadsworth. Reprinted by permission of the publisher.)

levels can have a synergistic effect that can increase or reduce an individual's personal risk dramatically.

Sexual Relationships

Sexual relationships refer to the connections between people rather than to the specific sexual behaviors in which they engage. In general, the risk for STDs decreases as sexual relationships move away from multiple, anonymous, sexual encounters and toward monogamous (with uninfected partners), trusting partnerships. STD risks associated with sexual relationships are specifically related to the overall number of partners and the quality of the relationship (trust, understanding, and knowledge of one's partner). **Figure 10.5** shows the continuum of risks for sexual relationships.

Two lifestyle dimensions that influence "partner risk" are *familiarity risk* and *exclusivity risk*. Familiarity risk is synonymous with *anonymity*. Laumann et al. (1994) operationally defined the extent of familiarity along a continuum that measured how long the study subjects knew their partners before having sex with them. Their findings confirmed that the less familiar one is with the sex partner (the greater the anonymity), the greater the risk is. Anonymity is a risk factor because it influences the ability to make an informed choice about the risk for acquiring an STD.

Laumann et al. (1994) defined exclusivity as being the quality of the sexual relationship. Ex-

clusivity, they said, must be examined for *both* partners. If one partner is monogamous but the other is not, the benefits of exclusivity are lost. Further, if an uninfected person is monogamous with someone who has an STD, exclusivity can actually increase the risk by increasing the extent of exposure. For exclusivity to work, both partners have to be uninfected and monogamous. Subjects (and partners) who are not sexually exclusive have been found to be at increased risk for acquiring an STD (Laumann et al., 1994).

The highest risks are associated with the "interaction of risky partners" (lack of exclusivity and familiarity) and many partners. This sexual lifestyle, which combines multiple partners with anonymous sexual encounters, creates a deadly synergy that increases the risk exponentially (Laumann et al., 1994).

Sexual Behavior

At the top of the pyramid of risk is sexual behavior. In general, the risks increase as behaviors incorporate unprotected insertion and ejaculation (see **Figure 10.6**). Lower-risk behaviors are nonpenetrative and do not involve an exchange of bodily fluids. Moving along the continuum of risk, the behaviors reflect attempts to utilize barrier protection against infectious agents. The highest-risk behavior is receptive anal penetration including ejaculation, which consists of unprotected ejaculation of semen into the delicate, nonlubricated tissue of

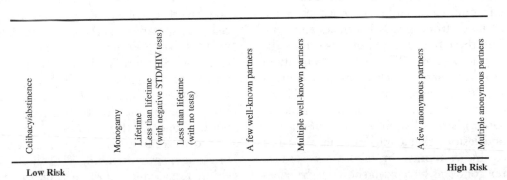

Figure 10.5 Multiple, anonymous sexual partners pose the greatest STD risk. (*Source:* Richard Blonna and Jean Levitan, *Healthy Sexuality,* © 2005 by Thomson-Wadsworth. Reprinted by permission of the publisher.)

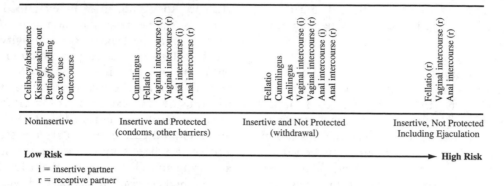

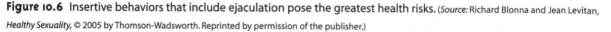

Noninsertive	Insertive and Protected (condoms, other barriers)	Insertive and Not Protected (withdrawal)	Insertive, Not Protected Including Ejaculation
Celibacy/abstinence	Cunnilingus	Fellatio	Fellatio (r)
Kissing/making out	Fellatio	Cunnilingus	Vaginal intercourse (r)
Petting/fondling	Vaginal intercourse (i)	Anilingus	Anal intercourse (r)
Sex toy use	Vaginal intercourse (r)	Vaginal intercourse (i)	
Outercourse	Anal intercourse (i)	Vaginal intercourse (r)	
	Anal intercourse (r)	Anal intercourse (i)	
		Anal intercourse (r)	

Low Risk ⟶ High Risk

i = insertive partner
r = receptive partner

Figure 10.6 Insertive behaviors that include ejaculation pose the greatest health risks. (*Source:* Richard Blonna and Jean Levitan, *Healthy Sexuality,* © 2005 by Thomson-Wadsworth. Reprinted by permission of the publisher.)

the rectum. This behavior gives infectious agents direct access to the bloodstream. Theoretically, the risk for acquiring an STD is greater for the receptive partner of any sexual activity.

Ample evidence supports the notion that condoms (both male and female), if worn properly and used consistently, help protect the wearer against some STDs by preventing direct contact between the penis and cervical, vaginal, rectal, or pharyngeal secretions or lesions. They also protect against exposure to penile lesions, discharges, and infected semen. Proper use for preventing STDs requires putting the condom on prior to any sexual contact, and it must remain intact throughout sexual activity.

Condoms are more effective against sexually transmitted infections such as gonorrhea, chlamydia, trichomoniasis, and HIV, which are transmitted by fluids from mucosal surfaces and from semen (and therefore captured or blocked by the condom), than against STDs that are transmitted by skin-to-skin contact such as human papillomavirus (HPV), herpes simplex virus (HSV), syphilis, and chancroid. The causative organisms for the latter diseases live in outcrops of blisters, warts, and lesions that could exist in areas not protected by condoms. In laboratory studies, male latex condoms have been shown to be effective in preventing the passage of bacterial pathogens (gonorrhea and chlamydia) and viral organisms (such as HIV, HSV, and HPV) (Grimes & Cates, 1990; Conant, Hardy, Sernatinger, et al., 1986; Minuk, Bohme, & Bowen, 1986). Similar findings have not been found for natural membrane condoms. Although they block the passage of sperm and are similar in their ability to prevent pregnancy, their pores are large enough to allow the passage of some STD causative organisms. Male condoms made of natural membrane tissue from sheep should not be the first choice for the prevention of STDs if one is allergic to latex. Male and female condoms made of polyurethane are a better choice (CDC, 2002a).

In human studies, condoms also have been shown to be effective in reducing the risks for contracting STDs. Studies from all over the world, with diverse populations of users, have consistently documented that condoms reduce the risks for spreading STDs. Research dating as far back as the 1940s has examined the use of condoms by troops in World War II and the Korean and Vietnam conflicts. In all three wars, soldiers and seamen using condoms had significantly lower rates of infection than their peers who did not use condoms (Hart, 1974).

More recent studies of male college students, men and women attending STD clinics, sex workers in Kenya and Zaire, and many others have documented that condoms provide some protection against a host of STDs (Darrow, 1989;

Cameron et al., 1991; Mann, Quinn, Piot, et al., 1987). Although use of condoms does not provide 100% protection against STDs, studies show that they have reduced risk by 50%–80% in actual users (Cates & Stone, 1992).

Although the male condom is the most reliable form of barrier protection against the infectious organisms causing STDs, studies show that the women who stand to benefit the most do not use them consistently and correctly. The least consistent users of the male condom are adolescent women, women with a history of STDs, and lower-socioeconomic-status (SES) women (who generally have less power and equality in their sexual relationships with men and have weaker negotiating skills) (Rosenberg & Gollub, 1992). This need not be a problem if more women were to use female barriers consistently and correctly.

Clinical studies of the effectiveness of female condoms in preventing STDs are very limited. Laboratory studies have demonstrated the effectiveness of these contraceptives in blocking viruses. Female condoms are recommended for use when male condoms cannot be used properly (CDC, 2002a).

In both laboratory and STD clinic studies, the following data have been reported for the sponge, diaphragm, and spermicides in relation to STD prevention:

- An overall reduced STD infection rate among barrier users compared to nonbarrier users
- Lower STD infection rates (87% less) for women using barrier contraceptives and receiving care at a health maintenance organization (HMO) than for nonusers
- Lower STD infection rates (61% less than for nonusers) for women attending STD clinics who used barrier contraceptives
- Up to 70% effectiveness against gonorrhea when using barrier contraceptives
- Up to 40% effectiveness against chlamydia when using barrier contraceptives (Rosenberg & Gollub, 1992)

In a study of 5681 STD patients focusing on the effectiveness of various contraceptive methods in protecting against STDs, not only was there a lower rate of infection among barrier users, but the lowest rates of infection were among sponge and diaphragm users. These rates were stable across all types of subjects, forms of sexual behavior, and STDs (Rosenberg & Gollub, 1992).

Even though condoms have a higher rate of theoretical effectiveness against STDs, the women who need them the most tend to use them less consistently and correctly. Woman-centered barrier contraceptives, although theoretically less effective against STDs, have provided greater actual effectiveness for women who used them instead of the male condom.

The effectiveness of nonpenetrative sexual activity in preventing STDs is extrapolated from the hypothesized ability of these methods to prevent unintended pregnancy by preventing the deposit of live sperm into the vagina. Because these methods exclude penetration and ejaculation, their ability to prevent pregnancy is very high (theoretically close to 100%).

Methods such as masturbation, use of sex toys, and even oral-genital sexual contact in preventing the transmission of STDs have not been scientifically studied and documented. Do these methods offer the same protection as other nonpenetrative sexual activities against STDs? No one knows for sure. When theorizing about their ability to prevent STDs, one can say that, because they do not involve penetration and ejaculation, they must offer a high level of protection against STDs as well. We are not as totally convinced of this relationship as some other safer sex educators are.

The major difference in the ability of these activities to prevent STDs would be the presence or absence of genital symptoms that could potentially spread pathogens even in the absence of penile penetration and ejaculation. Also, STD organisms, in rare instances, could be passed from genital ulcers to the eyes via contaminated fingers. For instance, if a person who had genital lesions associated with herpes were to engage in mutual masturbation with his or her partner, and then rubbed the eyes, HSV could be spread to this site.

Lillie's Risk

Lillie is 43, divorced, and heterosexual; she identifies as Mexican American. A continuing student, she made these comments in class:

> Thank you! Finally, someone has said what I believed all along: It's not just sexual behavior that's the risk. It's the behavior in the context of a relationship that determines risk. I was always so annoyed and insulted when sex educators told me that I should always insist that my partner wear a condom and that any woman who is sexually active is at equal risk of becoming infected. I always felt that as long as I had one uninfected partner, and the two of us were monogamous, I was at low risk. It's funny because even though I'm not married, my boyfriend (of three years) is less of a threat to me than my husband used to be. My ex-husband was always cheating on me, and I was worried that even though I was monogamous, he'd bring something home to me.
>
> I fully trust my current boyfriend. We've been monogamous (though unmarried) for three years, and I've never felt safer. We spent a lot of time building the trust and commitment in our relationship. I have great sex with him because I can fully relax and trust him, even though I've never gone down the list of things I need to know about his sexual past. We did talk about whether either of us ever had a viral STD, because viruses are forever.

Source: Richard Blonna and Jean Levitan, *Healthy Sexuality,* © 2005 by Thomson-Wadsworth. Reprinted by permission of the publisher.

This possibility explains why we present sexual behaviors on a continuum of risk from low to high. No behavior except celibacy is completely risk free. Viewing sexual activity in this way will allow you to examine the risk of specific behaviors in the context of other sexual activities. You must also evaluate any behavior within the context of the relationship you have with your partner. The less you know about your partner, the more risky any behavior becomes.

Counseling Clients with Chlamydia Using Microskills

Counseling clients with STDs presents unique challenges because of the sexual nature of the infection. Counseling clients with chlamydia poses some interesting problems because clients are often asymptomatic and their infections are discovered through screening tests. Many times these tests are performed as part of routine examinations for other health issues. For example, many women who attend family planning clinics for birth control services will be screened for chlamydia as part of their annual examination.

Healthy People 2010 Leading Health Indicators

Responsible Sexual Behavior (STDs)
Health Implications of Irresponsible Sexual Behavior
Unintended pregnancies and sexually transmitted diseases, including infection with the human immunodeficiency virus that causes AIDS, can result from unprotected sexual behaviors. Abstinence is the only method of complete protection. Condoms, if used correctly and consistently, can help prevent both unintended pregnancy and STDs.

In 1999, 85% of adolescents abstained from sexual intercourse or used condoms if they were sexually active. In 1995, 23% of sexually active women reported that their partners used condoms (USDHHS, 2003).

More than 20 diseases are capable of being transmitted sexually. An estimated 15 million new cases of STDs are reported each year, with about 4 million occurring in adolescents. As mentioned earlier, women generally suffer more serious STD complications than men, including pelvic inflammatory disease, ectopic pregnancy, infertility, chronic pelvic pain, and cervical cancer from the human papillomavirus. The economic cost of STDs and their complications is conservatively estimated at $17 billion annually (USDHHS, 2003).

Objectives for the Nation
* Increase the proportion of adolescents who abstain from sexual intercourse or use condoms if currently sexually active
* Increase the proportion of sexually active persons who use condoms

Cindy is a 30-year-old single bisexual female who identifies as Caucasian. Cindy is an editor for a major publisher, and has two steady sex partners, Marissa and Roger. Cindy recently went for her annual ob/gyn examination at a local family planning clinic. Her chlamydia test came back positive. It was repeated and came back positive a second time. Cindy was treated and counseled at the clinic. The remainder of the chapter will use

Cindy as the example as we work through the microskills model used in counseling her.

Introductory Skills

Counselors must pay particular attention to the introduction when working with STD patients, because it is critical in establishing trust and setting a nonjudgmental tone that is essential to success. Clients such as Cindy are often reluctant to discuss their infections and must be won over early in the interview.

Counseling Hints & Tips 10.1

Guidelines for STD Counseling

The following general tips are useful in STD counseling:

1. *Assure and demonstrate confidentiality.* In addition to telling clients that everything you discuss will be kept in confidence, show that you mean it. Don't talk about previous clients in the presence of your current client. Don't keep client records on your desk for new clients to see. Don't talk about other clients on the phone in the presence of your current client.
2. *Never assume anything.* Just because your client "looks" a certain way (has a wedding band on/doesn't have one on, dresses neat/messy, is clean/dirty, is timid/aggressive) doesn't mean his or her sexual behavior will fit this stereotype. Let clients tell you about their sexual lives.
3. *Be able to justify all questions.* You are on solid ground if you have logical reasons to ask clients about the details of their sexual lives. If you don't have a good reason to delve into certain sexual issues, don't go there.
4. *Be nonjudgmental.* STD patients will often behave in ways that go against your moral/ethical codes. Your job is not to provide moral education, but rather to help them by working within their personal constructs and assisting them in understanding how sexual lifestyle relates to risk.

5. *Avoid STD jargon.* Health care is rife with acronyms for tests, treatments, diagnoses, and so on. Stay away from this jargon when talking to clients. Use plain English to explain things.
6. *Use appropriate language.* Try to use sexual health terms that clients understand. Using a word such as "coitus" instead of the more commonplace "intercourse," for instance, can create distance between you and the client.
7. *Offer options based on clients' lifestyles.* In a perfect world, everyone would have one, uninfected partner for life or would be blissfully celibate on a voluntary basis. In the real world, clients may have sex with multiple, anonymous partners, often while under the influence of psychoactive substances. Work within these parameters, and you'll have a greater likelihood of being able to offer your clients something to help them lower their risk.
8. *Adding risk-reduction behaviors is easier than taking away risky behaviors.* It is very difficult to extinguish a behavior that has been reinforced with pleasure over time (such as sexual intercourse with multiple partners). It is easier to add on occasional condom use (use condoms with partners you don't know well) than to reduce the numbers of partners.

Identify Yourself and Explain Your Role

Counseling people with STDs requires that counselors explore clients' sexual/medical histories in great detail. This point needs to be explained to clients up front so they have no misconceptions about what will be brought up and why it needs to be discussed. Counselors should be able to justify asking any questions of a sexual nature as long as they relate to helping clients manage their STDs. Try writing a script for this part of the introduction and practice it until it becomes second nature to you. When introducing yourself, it is very important to make a concerted effort to establish a skin-to-skin human connection with the client. A firm handshake (ungloved) is a good way to do so. Extend your hand, make eye contact, and smile as you give the client a firm (but not crushing) handshake.

Example

Counselor: (Extending hand, smiling) Hi, I'm _____. I'm one of the counselors at the clinic. My job is to make sure you understand why you are here, what disease you have been diagnosed with having, how you got it, how to get rid of it, how to prevent getting infected again in the future, and what to do if you think you might be infected in the future.

You have chlamydia. Because it is a sexually transmitted disease, I must talk to you about some very personal issues related to your sex life. I will ask you about all of the people you have had sex with over the past couple of months and the kinds of sexual activities you've had with them. I am not here to judge you. My job is to help you make the best decisions for yourself regarding how to manage your infection. Together, we will work out a plan for making sure that your chlamydia is cured and reducing your risks for becoming infected again.

I want you to understand that everything we say is confidential and that your name and anything we talk about cannot be shared with anyone else.

Clarify the Client's Name

A simple way to verify the client's name is to use an open-ended statement following your introduction. Do so while you are still standing and immediately following your handshake and self-identification.

Example

Counselor: (Before sitting and explaining his role) And your name is . . . ?

Explain the Client's Role

After exchanging names and describing your role, start to explain the client's role. A simple explanation should include the three key elements of the client role discussed in Chapter 3: (1) active participation, (2) self-responsibility, and (3) honesty.

Example

Counselor: Cindy, your role in this process is to be as open and honest as possible when talking to me. The only way I can help you is if you tell me exactly what is going on with you and your sex partners. You'll have to take an active role in this process and take responsibility for getting better. Together, we can work out a treatment plan that will work best for you in getting better and preventing you from becoming infected again in the future.

Set Goals for the Session(s)

As an STD counselor, you have five specific, primary goals for your clients:

1. Ensuring treatment adherence
2. Scheduling follow-up visits and contingencies for missed visits
3. Developing a plan to get all sex partners evaluated
4. Developing a plan for reducing future risk of infection
5. Describing proper sick role behavior in response to future disease suspicion (Blonna & Levitan, 2005)

In addition to these primary goals, counselors must assess clients' goals regarding their infections. The best way to deal with this issue is to describe your goals and assess clients' needs.

Example

Counselor: Cindy, there are five things I *must* discuss with you today regarding your *Chlamydia* infection. First, I must explain how to follow your treatment regimen. Second, I must set up a follow-up appointment for you. Third, both of us must develop a plan to get all of your sex partners evaluated. Fourth, we must work out a plan to reduce your risks for becoming infected again in the future. Fifth, we must discuss what you need to do if you think you have been exposed to this infection again in the future. What goals do you have for our session(s)?

Give the client time to think this through before moving into the next part of their session.

Transition to the Client's Story

A good way to make the transition from the introduction to getting clients to tell their stories is to use open-ended statements regarding what happened. Here are a few examples:

"Cindy, why don't you tell me what led to you being here today."
"Cindy, tell me a little bit about what you know about chlamydia."
"Cindy, tell me a little bit about your sex life for the past month."
"Cindy, tell me how you think you got infected."

The idea in using these open-ended statements is to get clients talking about their current *Chlamydia* infections as well as their sexual lifestyles. You can start with either topic, but understanding both of these two components of the overall story is essential to meeting your five goals for counseling.

Attending Skills

One of the most interesting (and challenging) things about counseling STD patients is the diversity of their stories. Listening to their stories will give you insights into the nature of their sexual lifestyles in general as well as how they relate to their current infections. At the heart of all of the stories are sexual themes involving various combinations of settings, partners, and behaviors. It is essential that you set a nonjudgmental tone from the start while attending. Counseling Hints 10.1 describes a few key things to consider when attending to STD clients' stories.

Nonverbal Skills

As an STD counselor, there is a good chance you will hear stories that at times clash with your personal sexual attitudes, values, and behaviors. Some of these stories might make you feel uncomfortable. It is important not to show this discomfort through nonverbal cues related to your body language and eye contact.

Often, when confronted with stories (sexual and other) that make us uncomfortable, we will inadvertently tense individual body parts or major areas or avert eye contact. For instance, clenching and unclenching the hands signals the client that something about his or her story is making you uncomfortable (see **Figure 10.7**). More obvious is tension across the chest and shoulders and facial tension (e.g., tight jaw muscles, furrowed brow).

Averting eye contact because dealing with the client makes you feel uncomfortable is another behavior to guard against. While it is normal to look away and periodically break eye contact (especially when *you* are talking), averting eye contact with clients when *they* are talking shows them that something is wrong (e.g., you are uncomfortable, disapproving, or bored).

Verbal Following

A key aspect of verbal following in chlamydia (and all STD- and other sexuality-related) stories is paying particular attention to sexual orientation issues. Clients will often give you clues to their sexual orientation by using neutral words to test your acceptance level. For instance, they

My First S&M Client

Karen, 40, is a married white female masochist. Karen was Dr. Blonna's first STD client who was a masochist. She had come into the STD clinic because she was named as a sexual partner to another case of syphilis. Her examination and blood tests showed that she was infected with secondary syphilis. Karen was tall, muscular, and attractive in a cold, intimidating way.

When Dr. Blonna explained to Karen that she was named as a sexual contact to someone diagnosed with a case of syphilis, she seemed hardly surprised and almost amused—a very unusual response pattern. When confronted about this attitude by Dr. Blonna, she said, "I'm not surprised. I always knew that eventually my lifestyle would catch up to me."

"Tell me a little about your lifestyle," Dr. Blonna said.

Karen looked Dr. Blonna in the eye and said, "I like to have sex with lots of different people. I like it when men treat me rough."

Dr. Blonna, trying to maintain a cool, professional manner, said, "Okay, please explain." (You could also say something else.)

"Well," Karen continued, "I like men to tie me up and hurt me."

"Hurt you," Dr. Blonna responded (squirming in his seat a little, averting eye contact with Karen).

"Yeah, you know," Karen said, "slap me around a little, pinch my nipples real hard, stuff like that. Last week I celebrated my fortieth birthday by having sex with 40 different men in the same night at my party."

"In the same night?" Dr. Blonna asked.

At this point Dr. Blonna, who had never talked to a masochist in such detail, was beginning to feel a little uncomfortable. He realized that he was clenching and unclenching his right fist as Karen detailed her sexual exploits. He saw Karen look at his hand, smile, and go into even more detail.

"Yeah, it was all planned. I invited 40 friends, rented a place that caters to such parties, and had a nonstop orgy all night. It got a little hairy at times. I passed out a couple of times due to a combination of fatigue and pain. I was sleepy for a full day following the party, and I woke up with a bunch of bruises and a bad taste in my mouth."

At this juncture, Karen paused, crossed her legs (showing a lot of flesh), and lit a cigarette (smoking was allowed in the clinic at that time).

Dr. Blonna excused himself from the interview at this point, stepped outside to compose himself, and spoke with his supervisor regarding his discomfort with the story. He wondered whether he could continue in an effective manner because it was obvious the client was enjoying his discomfort and essentially playing with him.

After a short discussion Dr. Blonna went back in, finished the interview, and wrote up a list of about 30 of the sex partners who were locatable and in the area.

Postscript: This incident led Dr. Blonna to pursue additional training in human sexuality, so he could become more comfortable dealing with clients with a wide variety of sexual interests and **paraphilias**.

---

might use words like "partner" or "lover" instead of "boyfriend" or "girlfriend," or "husband" or "wife," when referring to people they have had sex with recently.

Examples

Cindy: To tell you the truth, there were only two people with whom I've had sex in the past month.

Cindy: To be honest, I've had only two lovers over the past month.

Such subtle nuances in language are rarely coincidental. If you are not listening carefully, and follow up her references to partners or lovers with statements such as "Cindy, tell me more about these guys" (which implies that Cindy is heterosexual), you will begin to create barriers between the two of you. Besides making an inaccurate assumption, this kind of verbal following shows Cindy that you are not listening carefully to her story. Do not assume anything about your clients' sexual orientation,

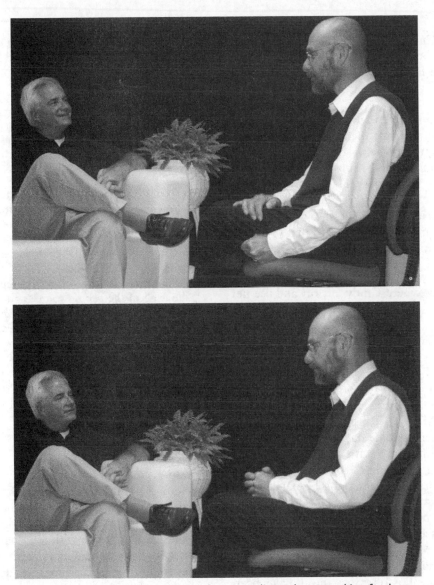

Figure 10.7 Clenched hands and other signs of discomfort warn clients about speaking freely. (Photos by Michael Blonna)

but rather let them tell you about the specifics of their relationships.

The same can be said of their sexual behavior. Don't assume anything about what clients do sexually, regardless of their sexual orientation, their physical appearance, their age, or any other variables that factor into your views and expectations regarding clients' sexual rela-

tions. Once again, be careful about the words you use to pursue and clarify sexual behavior. For example, if Cindy told you she has had two lovers in the past two months, and you want to know how often they had sex and what kinds of sexual activities they engaged in, the best way to do so would be to use more open sexual language.

Example

Counselor: Cindy, you just mentioned that you've had two lovers in the past month. Tell me a little bit about how often you had sex with them and the kinds of things you did.

This is much more open and nonjudgmental than saying, "Cindy, you just mentioned that you had sex with two guys in the past month. How often did you have intercourse with them?" The latter statement shows Cindy that you assume she is straight and she had vaginal intercourse with her lovers. The former statement shows Cindy that you are not assuming anything and that you want her to tell you about what went on.

Example

Pick up exactly where Cindy left off and use her terminology.

Counselor: Cindy, tell me more about these two lovers.

Cindy: Sure. I'm not certain where I got this infection, but it had to come from one of the two people I've had sex with in the past year, Roger or Marissa. Roger and I go way back to our undergraduate days at Boston College. We shared a house with three other people, two guys and another woman. Roger and I were exploring our emerging bisexuality and became best of friends as well as lovers. After college we moved into a two-bedroom condo that we lease together in the Back Bay section of Boston. Marissa is a woman I have worked with for the past year at a major publishing company in Boston. She and I have been lovers for about six months.

Because Cindy sensed the counselor's nonjudgmental tone, she felt comfortable going into more detail regarding her story.

Vocal Tone

Try to match the pace and tone of clients' stories. STD patients experience a range of emotions regarding their infections, and they express these

Counseling Hints & Tips 10.2

Using Neutral Sexual Language in Your Introduction

A good way to set the stage for acceptance of all partner variations and sexual activities is to use similar language in the introduction. For instance, instead of talking about boyfriends/girlfriends, husbands/wives, and sexual intercourse, you can adopt more neutral language.

For example, say, "Cindy, I must talk to you about all of the *people* you've had *sex* with in the past month," instead of "Cindy, I must talk to you about all of the *men* you've had *sexual intercourse* with in the past month." The latter statement signals to Cindy that you assume she is heterosexual and engaging in only vaginal intercourse. The former statement shows Cindy that you are open to however she defines her sexual orientation and behavior.

emotions in the way they tell their stories. Cindy's tone is very matter-of-fact with little emotion. Her pace is conversational and her vocal tone is even. She is not rushing through her story, nor is she drawing it out with long pauses. Her voice is occasionally animated as she makes a point or tries to illustrate something. She does not seem to be upset about having to tell her story.

Other clients might respond to being infected with *Chlamydia* entirely differently, and their stories might be told with more emotion. Such emotional involvement might show through in the pace of the storytelling. Clients who are emotionally upset might pause more frequently to compose themselves or get the courage to discuss such painful issues. They also might speak more softly and adopt a more submissive tone, implying embarrassment, guilt, or shame.

Don't respond to their stories with your own tone and pace. Let their emotions and style dictate yours.

Responding Skills

Nonverbal Minimal Encouragers

As illustrated in Diverse Perspectives 10.2, when you are uncomfortable with certain issues, your body language and eye contact will often give you away. In Dr. Blonna's case, it was obvious to Karen that he was uncomfortable and this fact influenced how she communicated with him from that point on. Other clients might have reacted differently. Another client might have backed off from revealing some of the details and withheld information because of the way the counselor reacted. In either case, the nature of the story changed because the counselor sent out nonverbal messages that he was uncomfortable with the story.

In dealing with chlamydia and other STD patients, it is crucial that your body language and nonverbal feedback come across to the client as nonjudgmental. Discomfort about being judged is a major barrier when working with STD patients.

Try to maintain a relaxed posture, and periodically scan your own body for signs of any tension that might be transmitted to clients. Chapter 3 showed what open and closed body language look like. Try especially hard to avoid judgmental poses such as folding your arms over your chest or looking "down" at clients (see **Figure 10.8**).

Clients also send out nonverbal messages about how they feel about telling certain parts of their stories. Pay attention to the same attributes in your clients that you might notice in yourself. Aversion of eye contact, tension, and closed body posture all might indicate unspoken problems that you may need to address at the appropriate time. These reactions could also represent discrepancies between *what* is being said and *how* it is being said.

Verbal Minimal Encouragers

Simple "uh huhs," key words, and mirroring can be used to get clients to continue their stories. These tools are especially helpful when dealing with sensitive sexual subjects because they demonstrate acceptance and assist in keeping clients talking. In Diverse Perspectives 10.2, Dr. Blonna illustrates the use of verbal minimal en-

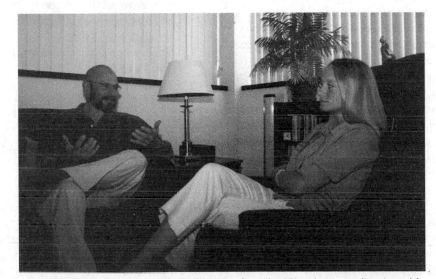

Figure 10.8 A judgmental body posture (arms folded across chest, looking down at client) could put STD patients on the defensive. (Photo by Michael Blonna)

couragers when Karen mentions that she likes to be tied up and "have people hurt me." He follows this remark with "hurt you?" Here he repeats the key word in the sentence to show that he is following Karen's story and wants her to continue. As a result, Karen goes into greater detail. Dr. Blonna also could have mirrored that statement by saying, "You like to be tied up and have people hurt you." If repeated in a nonjudgmental tone, at the appropriate time, mirroring is a powerful way to acknowledge important parts of the story without having to ask questions.

Open Invitation to Talk

Using questions to clarify sexual information is very important because intimate relationships and behaviors are often quite confusing. Being sure you understand who is doing what with whom on what occasions requires a skillful, nonjudgmental use of questioning skills.

Open-Ended Statements and Questions

One helpful way to clarify sensitive sexual information with chlamydia patients is to use open-ended statements liberally to create a more relaxed, conversational tone. It is better to obtain the answers to a series of individual sexual questions through one or two open-ended statements than by asking clients a slew of yes/no questions. Try to close your eyes and visualize the difference in the two approaches. Think of the series of closed questions as coming from a counselor in a white lab coat, looking very clinical, standing over the client with a clipboard and a checklist of items. As each question is answered, the "professional" checks off each answer. Now visualize a counselor, sitting comfortably in a chair facing the client, talking about these same issues but in a more conversational manner, just listening to the story.

When counseling clients with STDs, such as Cindy who has chlamydia, it is important to understand exactly which sexual behaviors they engaged in so you can ensure that they receive the correct examinations and tests and that you help them develop risk-reduction plans appropriate to

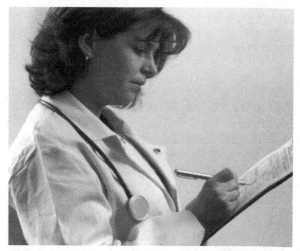

Figure 10.9 Taking a medical history by checking items off a list can be very threatening. (© Photos.com)

their needs. The way you uncover this information, however, can vary drastically. For instance, here is a short list (there are many more) of closed sexual questions that could be used with Cindy:

"Cindy, when you have sex with Roger, do you have vaginal intercourse?"

"Cindy, when you have sex with Roger, do you have anal intercourse?"

"Cindy, when you have sex with Roger, do you have oral sex?"

"Cindy, when you have sex with Marissa, do you have oral sex?"

"Cindy, do you ever have sex with Marissa and Roger at the same time?"

"Cindy, when you have sex with Roger, do you use condoms?"

"How many times have you had sex in the past month?"

"When was the last time you had sex?"

You can get the answers to these questions by asking each question directly, or you can ask one or two indirect, open-ended questions and listen to clients describe their sexual behavior. If they miss one or two questions, you can follow up your open-ended question with one or two closed questions.

Example: Open-Ended Statements

Counselor: Cindy, tell me about your sex life with Roger and Marissa.

Counselor: Cindy, tell me about what you, Roger, and Marissa do sexually.

Counselor: Cindy, tell me what body parts you use during sex and what you like to do.

Cindy: It's kind of embarrassing to talk about the details, but here goes. I really like sex and trying out different kinds of things—positions, toys, sexy clothing, fantasy themes. You know, stuff like that. Nothing too kinky, but just fun. Roger has always been into that kind of stuff, and we've had sex in some interesting places over the years and done some wild things, like having sex on the infield grass at Fenway Park when it was closed. Marissa is a lot of fun, too. She's into strap-ons and likes to play a real dominant role while I play the submissive partner. We're all really into oral sex, too.

Using open-ended questions to get the same needed sexual information is a less intrusive way to gather the data. It also allows you to listen more and observe how the client comes across. Rather than focusing on which closed question to ask next, you can sit back and listen to the client. You can always use closed questions to go back and clarify any missing information.

Example

Counselor: Cindy, you mentioned that you like having oral sex with Marissa and Roger. Do you like to give or receive it?

Counselor: Cindy, you mentioned the phrase "strap-on." Do you mean Marissa uses a strap-on dildo to penetrate you?

Paraphrasing, Reflection of Feelings, and Summarizing

Paraphrasing and reflection of feelings work similarly for chlamydia patients as they do for other counseling clients. The major difference is the wide range of emotions associated with sexually transmitted diseases. Because the diseases always involve at least one other person, infection with an STD such as chlamydia often evokes strong emotions related to the partner.

Chlamydia patients experience a range of partner-related emotions, with the exact responses depending on whether they feel at fault for infecting their partners or perceive themselves as victims. Emotions ranging from concern and fear to embarrassment over potentially infecting sex partners are common. Feelings of anger and hostility are common toward partners who are blamed for being the source of their infections.

Paraphrasing judiciously throughout clients' stories will help you clarify how clients view their infection and its relationship to their sex partner(s). This practice will also aid you in reflecting clients' feelings toward themselves and their partners. Getting to the feelings associated with being infected and dealing with sex partners is important because they can serve as barriers to effective sick role behavior.

Once clients' thoughts and feelings about being infected are expressed, summarization helps clarify what each client is thinking and feeling. It is an opportunity for clients to hear their stories again and decide whether anything needs to be added, deleted, or clarified. It also shows them how well you are following and your assessment of the situation.

Example: Paraphrase

Counselor: Cindy, let me make sure I understand your story. In the past two months, you've had two sex partners, Roger and Marissa. You know both of them very well and enjoy a variety of sexual activities with them, particularly oral sex. Is that right?

Cindy: Yeah, that's right.

Example: Reflection of Feelings

Counselor: Cindy, you seem a little embarrassed to talk about your sex life with Roger and Marissa.

Cindy: Not really. It's just discussing the details that is a little embarrassing. I really don't want to come off as some kind of a sex freak or anything to you.

Example: Summary

Counselor: Let me see if I get this right, Cindy. You've have had two sex partners this past month, Roger and Marissa. You know them both very well and like to engage in a variety of sexual activities with them, particularly oral sex. You seem to be okay talking to me about this but are a little embarrassed because I might get the impression that you are some kind of sex freak. Is that accurate?

Cindy: Pretty much. I really live kind of a boring life. I mean, I work about 60 hours a week and really don't spend 24 hours a day having sex. We really have sex only two or three times a week. It's just that when we do, we sometimes get kind of carried away.

Influencing Skills

As mentioned earlier, the five primary issues that must be covered with all STD patients are: (1) treatment adherence, (2) follow-up, (3) sex partner evaluation, (4) response to future disease suspicion, and (5) reduction of risk for future infection (Blonna & Levitan, 2005). Many of the influencing skills can be used to achieve these goals.

Self-disclosure

As mentioned in Chapter 5, self-disclosure is an excellent technique for building confidence in clients regarding their perceived ability to change. Self-disclosing to clients that you, the counselor, know what they are going through because you have had an STD in the past is one way to do so. You do not need to go into details, nor do you need to identify the exact disease. A nonspecific reference will suffice.

Example

Counselor: Cindy, I kind of know what you are going through. I had an STD myself, and it was tough dealing with it and having to talk to my sex partners about it. I got through it okay, and I know you can, too.

Be careful that clients don't use your self-disclosure as an opportunity to shift the discussion to you. By self-disclosing, you are merely trying to establish a connection with clients and empower them by showing them that if you could deal with this issue, so can they.

Confrontation

Confrontation will come into play extensively, especially when responding to incongruities related to sexual history, use of risk-reduction methods, and sex partner evaluation. While other issues may present opportunities for confrontation among some counseling clients, most have conflicting stories or mixed messages regarding these three topics.

Clients will usually present different stories related to their overall sexual lifestyle and their immediate sexual behavior during the critical period necessary for sex partner follow-up. Chlamydia (and other STD) patients will behave in this way for a variety of reasons. Sometimes they honestly can't recall information regarding prior sex partners or the details of past encounters. In some cases, this failure could be due to the anonymous nature of the partner. Often STD patients don't know their partners well (or at all) before having sex with them. It could also be related to their overall level of sexual activity. Clients who are very sexually active with multiple partners often lose track of the details of their relationships with specific people. They will start out with one version of their story, then tell a different version later in the session.

Clients may intentionally tell discrepant stories for a variety of reasons. Many mistrust community health professionals and do not want to discuss personal sexual information with them. Sometimes clients are afraid that their confidentiality will not be maintained. Other times they simply do not trust any public officials and will give a version of the story that doesn't match a later variation. Clients who are embarrassed about their sexual activities will sometimes discuss only parts of their stories and withhold other parts, especially if they sense any judgment on the part of the counselor.

Many clients whose stories contain discrepancies are trying to hide some facet of the story that is either too difficult for them to deal with or they feel will lead to too many problems if discussed. These issues range from ethical issues, such as extramarital or extra-relationship sexual encounters, to involvement in illegal sexual behavior, such as prostitution. Often these discrepancies are uncovered because clients forget the original, contrived story and at a later point omit some key aspect of the story or change the story slightly.

Confronting any discrepancies is essential to meet the goals of the counseling session.

Example

Counselor: Cindy, although you say that you are okay discussing your sex life, you don't seem real comfortable. You look kind of tense and you've been avoiding looking at me when discussing your two sex partners. What is going on?

Counselor: Cindy, although you say you are having sex with only two people, you seem to be holding something back. By the way you are sitting and avoiding looking me in the eyes, I sense that there is more to this story. What else is there?

Changing the Focal Point

Changing the focal point is an excellent way to help clients develop plans to accomplish the five goals of STD counseling, particularly sex partner evaluation. Asking clients to think about how their partners would feel about having chlamydia or react to their (the clients') infections is a good way to start developing a plan.

Example

Counselor: Cindy, because we are going to have to talk to both Marissa and Roger, I'd like you to put yourself in their shoes and think about how they'd react to being exposed to chlamydia. How do you think each of them would react?

Cindy: I think Roger will be pretty cool about it. We've been together for a long time and have kind of an open relationship. We're both into girls, and he allows me to date women. I extend him the same freedom, only asking that he try not to fall in love with someone else. I really do love him but also want to enjoy my attraction to women. Because of this unique relationship, I know he has slept around a little and chances are he probably gave this disease to me. I think he'd be glad that I told him about it before he develops any complications.

Counselor: What about Marissa?

Cindy: I'm not sure about Marissa. She and I just recently became lovers, but we've known and worked with each other for a while. She is kind of kinky but in a very reserved, proper way, if you know what I mean.

Counselor: What do you mean?

Cindy: Well, for instance, she'll come into work in a very conservative business suit but slip me a note that she has her mini-egg vibrator inserted in her vagina and she is thinking about my vagina. Crazy stuff like that. She was raised in a very conservative Midwestern family, and her dad was a Baptist minister, but she has a wild side that I love. She has had only a couple of lovers besides me. I'm afraid she might get grossed out by my being infected and possibly spreading this disease to her. I don't want to jeopardize our relationship.

Counselor: What do you think you could say to soften the blow?

Cindy: I guess I could be honest with her, tell her how much I care about her and that she is my only lover other than Roger, who she doesn't view as a threat. I think she'll believe me, but she might get mad at Roger.

Directives and Logical Consequences

For each of the five key goals in an STD counseling session, several directives and logical consequences must be discussed. The logical consequences will vary depending on how the counselor and client work together to negotiate the directives. For instance, ensuring that all sex partners are examined and receive **prophylactic treatment** can be done three ways: (1) the counselor can do it, (2) the client can do it, or (3) the counselor and client can do it together. Each option has a different set of directives and logical consequences associated with those directives. We will go over each goal and discuss the specific directives, logical consequences, and adherence concerns associated with it.

Directive 1: Ensuring Treatment Adherence

Ensuring treatment adherence is essential to both primary and secondary disease prevention activities. Adherence to treatment regimens ensures that clients will get treated properly and not develop complications associated with their diseases. To ensure adherence to treatment regimens, the following key directives must be discussed:

1. *Medication name.* Clients need to know the names of their medications so they can discuss their treatment, look up additional information about the medication, and so on.
2. *Efficacy.* Clients need to believe that their medications are the best options available for their particular problems, especially if the treatment is difficult to take or produces side effects.
3. *Dosage and schedule.* Clients need to know how many pills to take each day, how to space doses, and how long to take the medications, or they will not take their medications properly.
4. *Side effects.* Clients need to know what side effects to expect or they will discontinue taking their medications when these side effects occur.
5. *Contraindications.* Clients need to know what to avoid while taking their medications or they might experience unanticipated side effects or reduction in efficacy.
6. *Symptom resolution.* Clients need to know when symptoms will begin to subside and what to do when that happens.

7. *Missed doses.* Clients need to know what to do if they miss a dose or they might stop taking their medications completely (CDC, 2002a).

Logical Consequences of Ensuring Treatment Adherence

1. If you take your medication as indicated, your infection will be cured.
2. If you take your medication as indicated, your symptoms will begin to lessen or disappear after a few days.
3. If you do not take your medication as indicated, you will not be fully cured and may develop a drug-resistant variant of your infection.
4. If you do not take your medication as indicated, you have a greater chance of developing some of the medication's side effects.
5. If you do not avoid the contraindications, you have a greater chance of developing some of the side effects associated with them, which might reduce the effectiveness of your medication.

Specific Instructions for Ensuring Treatment Adherence

1. *Medication name.* Tell clients the name of their medication (both the prescribed name and the generic name). Be sure to write this information down for them.
2. *Efficacy.* Tell clients "this is the *best* medicine for you." Sell them on the effectiveness of the medication.
3. *Dosage and schedule.* Tell clients how many pills to take each day, when to take them during the day, and when to stop.
4. *Side effects.* Tell clients what the most common side effects of the medication are and what to do if they experience them.
5. *Contraindications.* Tell clients what to avoid while taking their medications.
6. *Symptom resolution.* Tell clients when they should expect to see their symptoms begin to lessen. Tell them what to do once this begins to happen.

7. *Missed doses.* Tell clients how to take the medication if they miss a dose.

Example: Giving Instructions

Counselor: Cindy, let's go over how to take your medication.

Your medication is called doxycycline.

You are going to take one pill, twice a day, for seven days. Take all of the pills, even if you feel better and you think your chlamydia has gone away.

The pills should be spaced about 10 to 12 hours apart. You can take a pill with food or on an empty stomach.

This option is the best medicine we can give you, and it will cure your chlamydia if you take it exactly as I tell you to. [Logical consequences]

Tell me what your daily schedule is like and when you think you can take each pill.

Cindy: I get up about 6:00 A.M., run on my treadmill for 30 minutes, shower, eat, get dressed, and walk to work at about 8:00 A.M. I work from 8:30 A.M. until noon, have a 30-minute lunch break, and then work until about 6:00 P.M. I walk back home and eat dinner at about 7:00 P.M. I usually go to sleep at about 11:00 P.M. I guess I could take a pill with breakfast at 7:00 A.M. and dinner at 7:00 P.M.

Counselor: Good. Here, I'll write this down on your pill envelope. Your medication is doxycycline. You'll take one pill at 7:00 A.M. and one pill at 7:00 P.M. You'll take each pill with a meal and continue taking them until all are finished after seven days. If you miss a dose, take it about five hours before your next regularly scheduled pill. [Tailoring, repetition, written reinforcement]

Cindy, when taking these pills, you might experience some mild nausea or diarrhea, mild chest pains, and swelling in the face, lips, tongue, and throat. These side effects are normal. Unless they worsen, continue to take your medication as directed. [Side effects]

Doxycycline can also make people more sensitive to the sun's rays and result in burning your skin or developing a rash [logical consequences]. While you are taking these pills, try to avoid being in direct sunlight for any length of time. Use a hat and wear long sleeves and pants if you must go out in the sun while taking the medication. [Contraindications]

Cindy, I know this is a lot to remember, so why don't you just repeat these instructions back to me. [Patient quiz]

Cindy: Okay, I take one pill at 7 A.M. and one pill at 7 P.M. with meals. I continue taking them regardless of how I feel, unless the side effects get worse. I should try to stay out of the sun or cover up if I do go out. If I miss a pill, I take it about five hours before the next pill. I keep taking them for seven days.

Counselor: Good. I expect you to follow this plan exactly as we developed it. When you come back in for follow-up tests, bring your pill envelope so I can check to make sure you took all of your pills. [Expectation citing]

Directive 2: Return for Follow-up

It is important for patients to return for follow-up for several reasons. The follow-up visit allows clinicians to reexamine patients to ensure that their symptoms have resolved, administer repeat tests to assess for cure, discuss other test results that may have come back (either positive, negative, or inconclusive), and answer any questions that might have arisen since the patients' initial visits.

Follow-up visits also provide counselors with an opportunity to assess the progress made in getting sex partners examined and treated. Likewise, they can check for discrepancies with issues discussed during the first meeting and report on any problems that may have arisen since the first visit. These and other issues must be discussed with clients when setting up follow-up appointments.

1. *When to return for follow-up tests.* Follow-up tests are generally scheduled for the week following the completion of treatment.

2. *What to do if the follow-up appointment has to be cancelled.* Clients should call the counselor to reschedule their appointments so their time slots can be reassigned to other patients (CDC, 2002a; Blonna et al., 1987).

Logical Consequences of Returning for Follow-up

1. If you return for follow-up, we can make sure your medication worked properly and help you ensure that all of your sex partners have been examined and treated.
2. If you return for follow-up, we can perform additional tests if necessary.
3. If you don't return for follow-up, we may not be able to provide these services for you and ensure that your disease has been taken care of properly.

Specific Instructions for Returning for Follow-up

1. Tell clients that they need to return for follow-up tests after they finish their medication.
2. Explain to them why follow-up is important.
3. Work with clients to tailor follow-up appointments that are convenient for them.
4. Tell clients what to do if they cannot make a scheduled appointment.

Example: Giving Information and Instructions

Counselor: Cindy, it is important for you to return in about 7 to 14 days for follow-up. At that time, we'll reexamine you to make sure your chlamydia is completely gone [logical consequence], verify that you took all of your medication, conduct follow-up tests, and check to see how your sex partner evaluation is going. I remember your schedule, and it seems pretty tight. We have evening hours on Tuesday and Thursday in addition to our regular hours. When can you come back? [Tailoring]

Cindy: I would prefer to take some time off of work and come back at the same time as today's visit [Monday at 9:00 A.M.].

Counselor: Okay, I'll write down an appointment for you on Monday, two weeks from today, at 9:00 A.M. If you can't make it, please call the number on the card [points to number] the day before so we can give your time slot to someone else. If I don't hear from you otherwise, I'll expect to see you two weeks from today at 9:00 A.M. [tailoring, expectation citing, repetition, written reinforcement]. If you don't return or call, I'll have to come out to your house or call you at work [logical consequence].

Directive 3: Sex Partner Evaluation

The timely follow-up, examination, and preventive treatment of all sex partners is important for several reasons. It is essential for preventing clients from getting reinfected by their original sex partners. The majority of repeat STDs are linked to sex partners named during the initial examinations who failed to be examined and treated. Sex partner examination and treatment are also necessary to stop the spread of infection to other persons. Lastly, sex partner follow-up and treatment are necessary because of the asymptomatic nature of many cases of chlamydia. We cannot assume that sex partners who become infected will develop symptoms and seek prompt treatment. It is important to treat all sex partners regardless of their test results because they may be incubating the disease. It is better to treat them prophylactically and prevent them from developing the disease than to allow them to incubate the infectious organism, develop infection, and risk spreading the disease.

1. All sex partners within a disease's "critical time period" must be examined, tested, and given prophylactic treatment. This critical time period will vary according to the disease. For chlamydia, all sex partners within the past 60 days (60 days from diagnosis of the first onset of symptoms) must be examined and treated.
2. All sex partners in the past 60 days must receive a test for chlamydia.

3. All sex partners in the past 60 days must receive treatment for chlamydia and not wait until the test results return, regardless of their test results.
4. There are three ways to persuade sex partners to be evaluated: (1) the counselor can do it, (2) the client can do it, or (3) the counselor and client can do it together.

Logical Consequences of Sex Partner Evaluation

1. Expect resistance from your sex partners, and be prepared to convince them of the necessity for preventive treatment.
2. Explain that if all sex partners are treated properly, the chances of reinfection are greatly reduced.
3. If you comply with the instructions for sex partner examination and treatment, you can be sure that your partners will be treated properly.
4. If you follow these instructions, you are taking the first step toward reducing your risk for future reinfection.
5. If you don't follow these instructions, you cannot be sure that your partners were treated properly and no longer pose a risk for reinfecting you (DSTD, 2002).

Specific Instructions for Sex Partner Evaluation

1. Tell clients that all sex partners within 30 days prior to their chlamydia tests must be examined, tested, and given preventive treatment.
2. Tell clients that their sex partners can come into the clinic or go to any doctor as long as they meet the criteria in instruction 1.
3. Obtain the names and addresses of the sex partners.
4. Work out a plan for having each one be examined and treated.
5. Explain to clients why it is critical that every partner be examined and treated.
6. Tell clients that there are three ways to persuade sex partners to be evaluated: (1) the counselor can do it, (2) the client can do it, or (3) the counselor and client can do it together.

Example: Giving Information and Instructions

Counselor: Cindy, as we discussed, both Roger and Marissa will need to be examined and treated because they are the only two people you have had sex with in the past two months. You realize that by saying this you are telling me that one of them gave you chlamydia, because it is unlikely that you caught this STD from the last sex partner before them. There are three ways to take care of them: You can do it, I can do it, or we can do it together. What do you prefer? [Tailoring]

Cindy: I guess I'll tell them myself.

Counselor: I need to know where they will go for their examination and treatment.

Cindy: I'll bring them both here for Wednesday night's clinic.

Counselor: Okay, I'll expect to see you here then [expectation citing]. If either one of them wants to go somewhere else, I need to call their clinician and make sure they get both tested and treated preventively, because private doctors and other clinics often do not have that as their protocol for treating chlamydia patients [logical consequence].

Cindy: Okay, I'll be sure to tell them that.

Counselor: Cindy, which one of them do you think gave you chlamydia?

Cindy: I'm not sure, although I know Roger has sex with other women occasionally. I will have to talk to him about it. I don't think Marissa has had sex with anyone else in about a year.

Counselor: If you feel it would be helpful, I could role-play with you so you can practice what you have to say to them and prepare for dealing with whatever resistance they might have.

Cindy: No, that won't be necessary.

Directive 4: Response to Disease Suspicion

As discussed in Chapter 2, proper sick role behavior is essential for preventing the spread of infectious diseases. Waiting even a few days and continuing to have sex can result in spreading an STD to

When clients decide to take responsibility for sex partner evaluation, they often underestimate how difficult it actually is. Besides dealing with the emotional aspects involved in telling their partners, they must ensure that it is done promptly and that the partners' healthcare providers are called to alert them. Sometimes role-playing can help clients visualize the process and practice what they will actually say to their partners.

Example

Counselor: Cindy, let's role-play this scenario so you can get a sense of what you will say to Roger and Marissa when you speak to them. I'll be Roger. Let's imagine it is tonight and you are going to talk to him, okay?

Cindy: Okay, let's give it a shot.

Counselor (as Roger): Hi, Cindy. How was your day?

Cindy: I actually didn't go straight to work today. I went to the doctor. Let's have a glass of wine. I've got something important I need to talk to you about.

Counselor (as Roger): The doctor? What is going on?

Cindy: (Handing counselor a glass of wine) Well, as you know, I had my annual visit to my doctor two weeks ago. When I was there, they took a chlamydia test and it came back positive.

Counselor (as Roger): Chlamydia—isn't that an STD?

Cindy: Yeah, I'm afraid so. You're going to need to have a test and get some treatment.

Counselor (as Roger): Treatment? How do you know I have anything? I feel fine.

Cindy: Roger, you can have this disease, feel fine, and still be infected. Listen, I don't know where it came from. Let's worry about that after we are both finished getting treated, okay?

Counselor (as Roger): Okay, but that means anybody I have been with might also be infected, right?

Cindy: I'm afraid so Roger. I'm sorry!

Counselor (as Roger): Hey, it's not your fault. I could have just as easily given this to you.

Counselor: That went pretty well. Just remember, if he doesn't come down here to get examined and treated, you or I will have to call his doctor to make sure he gets prophylactic treatment. Okay?

Cindy: Okay. I don't think we need to role-play Marissa. I can handle it.

When clients role-play these scenarios, they can get a feel for what the actual experience will be like. The role-plays also allow counselors opportunities to correct improper information or techniques.

---

other people and increasing the number of cases within a community. If clients notice any STD symptoms in themselves or in their partners, or if they have changed their sexual behavior/lifestyle in any way that has increased their risk of infection, they need to do the following things:

1. Stop having any sex with their partner(s).
2. Come into the clinic or see a doctor immediately.
3. If possible, bring their sex partner(s) with them (DSTD, 2002).

Logical Consequences of Proper Response to Disease Suspicion

1. If you do these three things, you will increase the likelihood that your infection can be diagnosed and treated promptly, thereby reducing your risks for developing any complications.
2. If you do these three things, you can help us stop the spread of this disease.
3. If you do not follow these three guidelines, you run the risk of developing complications and having the infection spread to others unnecessarily.

Specific Instructions for Proper Response to Disease Suspicion

1. Explain to clients that anything that makes them suspicious that they might have an STD is reason enough to go to the clinic.
2. Explain to clients that some of the common suspicions are symptoms in themselves or in their partners, changes in their sexual behavior/lifestyle, and changes in their partners' sexual lifestyles.
3. Tell clients that the two most critical components of the proper response to disease suspicion are to stop having all forms of sex with their partner(s) and to come into the clinic or see a doctor immediately.

Example: Giving Information and Instructions

Counselor: Cindy, if you ever think you might have chlamydia or have been exposed to it or any STD in the future, I'd like you to do the following things. First, stop having any sex with your partners. Second, come into the clinic or see a doctor immediately. Third, if possible, bring your sex partners with you. If you do this, we can treat you and make sure you don't suffer any complications from this infection. [Logical consequence]

Cindy: Okay, but why can't I just wait and see if I develop any problem?

Counselor: I think you can see from your present infection that you can have chlamydia and not even know it. I'd prefer that you not wait to develop symptoms or complications, but rather come in if you are suspicious for any reason. It never hurts to get examined and have a test taken.

Cindy: I guess you are right.

Directive 5: Preventing Future Infection

Earlier in the chapter, we discussed the pyramid of risk for STDs. Counseling clients infected with STDs such as chlamydia involves educating them about things they can't change but need to be aware of in their partners (demographic variables and sexual/medical history) and helping them reduce risks associated with things they can change (sexual lifestyles and sexual behavior). Focusing on just one set of factors and ignoring the others isn't enough. Clients must develop personal risk-reduction plans based on their (and their partners') pyramids. These plans will vary according to the individuals involved. Although reducing risk in this way takes a little more thought, it also respects individuality.

Counselors can facilitate these plans by limiting their scope based on what clients tell them about their sexual lifestyles, behavior, past history, and present demographics. Counselors can use this information to help clients home in on strategies that seem more feasible for them based on their needs. Counselors need to focus on two key points:

1. Do not have sex with your current partners until you are sure they have been examined and given preventive treatment.
2. Develop a personal plan for reducing your risk of acquiring STDs based on your present sexual lifestyle (DSTD, 2002).

Logical Consequences of Preventing Future Infection

1. If you develop and follow a personal risk-reduction plan, you will greatly reduce the likelihood that you will contract chlamydia or another STD.
2. If you develop and follow a personal risk-reduction plan, you will greatly increase your chances of early detection and prompt treatment of any future infections.

Specific Instructions for Preventing Future Infection

1. Tell clients that their greatest risk of reinfection (especially in the first month following treatment) is from their current partners who have not gotten examined and treated.
2. Make sure they have a plan to get their sex partners evaluated.
3. Use your knowledge of their sexual lifestyles and behaviors to give them four or five options for reducing their risk of future infection that you think will fit their current sexual lifestyles.

4. Use forced-choice questions to get clients to pick three things they can do to prevent getting infected again.

Example: Giving Information and Instructions

Counselor: Cindy, based on what you've told me about your sex life and other factors, there are a few things that might work for you in reducing your risk of future infection. Your greatest risks are associated with Roger's sexual activities with other women. Assuming you want to continue this type of open relationship with Marissa and Roger, you need to consider the following strategies:

- Make sure Marissa and Roger get examined and treated before you have any kind of sex with them.
- Try to get Roger to limit his activities with other women. In general, the more exclusive he is with his other partners, the lower your risk.
- If Roger plans to continue to have sex with other women, start using a condom when having intercourse with him. You could use either a male or female condom.
- If condoms are not acceptable, consider using a diaphragm. Although it isn't perfect, it will reduce your risk and prevent unintended pregnancy.
- Make a habit of coming in more frequently for STD check-ups. If you do get infected again with any STD, frequent check-ups will lower your risk for developing complications.

In addition to not having sex with your partners until they get examined and treated, which three additional strategies would you be willing to adopt?

Cindy: I really don't like condoms, so the other three strategies seem best for me. I definitely need to talk to Roger about the nature and extent of his relationships with other women. Come to think of it, I need to ask Marissa the same kinds of things. The other strategies will be easy for me to try.

Counselor: Okay. Let's work on the other three. I'll talk to you about how things went with your discussions with Roger and Marissa when you return for your follow-up tests in a couple of weeks. What else can I help you with today?

Cindy: I can't think of anything else. I guess I'll see you in a couple of weeks. Goodbye.

Counselor: Goodbye, Cindy.

Summary

Chlamydia is one of more than 25 infections capable of being transmitted sexually. Because it is a bacterial infection, chlamydia, unlike some other STDs, can be cured by broad-spectrum antibiotics. This and certain other characteristics, such as its asymptomatic nature, present specific challenges to counselors. Blonna and Levitan's (2005) pyramid of risk describes the interaction of personal and community STD risk factors. This model can be used when counseling persons infected with *Chlamydia*.

The microskills model can also be used when counseling someone infected with *Chlamydia*. Using Cindy as a case study, the authors worked through the application of introductory, attending, responding, and listening skills to someone with chlamydia.

Study Questions

1. Describe the extent of the STD problem in the United States.
2. What does the phrase "capable of being transmitted sexually" mean?
3. List and describe the five goals of STD counseling.
4. How is *Chlamydia trachomatis* infection similar to and different from gonorrhea, HIV/AIDS, and syphilis?
5. How does the nature of a particular STD influence how one counsels someone with it?
6. Describe the four levels of the pyramid of risk model.

7. How can the pyramid of risk model be used to counsel someone with chlamydia?
8. How would the use of introductory skills differ when working with clients infected with *Chlamydia* compared with clients who have non-STD health problems?
9. Describe how body language influenced the nature of the counseling session discussed in Diverse Perspectives 10.2.
10. What is "neutral sexual language" (related to sexual orientation), and how does it affect introductory, attending, and responding skills when counseling clients infected with *Chlamydia*?
11. Describe the appropriate use of self-disclosure when counseling STD clients.
12. How does changing the focal point from the client or the disease to the sex partners help clients understand and negotiate proper sex partner evaluation?
13. List and describe the key directives and logical consequences for each of the five chlamydia counseling goals.

References

Bertrami R (2002). Chlamydia screening in the Philadelphia public schools. Presentation at the annual Meeting of the American Public Health Association, Philadelphia, November 2002.

Blonna R, Legos P, Burlak P (1989). The effects of an STD educational intervention on patient compliance. *Sexually Transmitted Diseases* 16:198–200.

Blonna R, Levitan J (2005). *Healthy Sexuality*. Pacific Grove, CA: Thomson Learning/Wadsworth.

Cameron DW, et al. (1991). Condom use prevents genital ulcers in women working as prostitutes: influences of human immunodeficiency virus infection. *Sexually Transmitted Diseases* 18:188–194.

Cates W, et al. (1999). Estimates of the incidence and prevalence of sexually transmitted diseases in the United States. *Sexually Transmitted Diseases* 26(suppl):S2–S7.

Cates W, Stone KM (1992). Family planning, sexually transmitted diseases and contraceptive choice: a literature update part I. *Family Planning Perspectives* 24:75–84.

Centers for Disease Control and Prevention (CDC) (2002a). 2002 Sexually Transmitted Disease: Treatment Guidelines. *Mortality and Morbidity Weekly Report* 51:RR-6.

Centers for Disease Control and Prevention (CDC) (2002b). Screening tests to detect chlamydia and gonorrhea infections. *Morbidity and Mortality Weekly Report* 51:RR-15.

Conant M, Hardy D, Sernatinger J, et al. (1986). Condoms prevent transmission of AIDS-associated retrovirus. *Journal of the American Medical Association* 255:1706.

Darrow WW (1989). Condom use and use-effectiveness in high-risk populations. *Sexually Transmitted Diseases* 16:157–162.

Division of STD Prevention (DSTD) (2000). *Tracking the Hidden Epidemics: Trends in STDs in the United States 2000*. Atlanta, GA: Centers for Disease Control and Prevention, Division of STD Prevention, Public Health Service.

Division of STD Prevention (DSTD) (2001). *Sexually Transmitted Disease Surveillance Report 2000*. Atlanta, GA: Centers for Disease Control and Prevention, Public Health Service.

Division of STD Prevention (DSTD) (2002). *Sexually Transmitted Disease Surveillance Report 2001*. Atlanta, GA: Centers for Disease Control and Prevention, Public Health Service.

Eng TR, Butler WT (Eds.) (1997). *The Hidden Epidemic: Confronting STDs*. Washington, DC: Academy Press, Institute of Medicine.

Grimes DA, Cates W (1990). Family planning and sexually transmitted diseases. In Holmes KK, Mardh PA, Sparling PF, et al. (Eds.) *Sexually Transmitted Diseases*, 2nd ed., pp. 1087–1094. New York: McGraw Hill.

Guaschino S, DeSeta F (2000). Update on *Chlamydia trachomatis* [review]. *Annals of NY Academy of Science* 900:293–300.

Hart G (1974). Factors influencing venereal infection in a war environment. *British Journal of Venereal Disease* 50:68–72.

Laumann EO, Gagnon JH, Michael RY, Michaels S (1994). *The Social Organization of Sexuality: Sexual Practices in the United States*. Chicago: University of Chicago Press.

Mann J, Quinn T, Piot P, et al. (1987). Condom use and HIV infection among prostitutes in Zaire [letter]. *New England Journal of Medicine* 316:345.

Minuk G, Bohme G, Bowen T (1986). Condoms and hepatitis B virus infection. *Annals of Internal Medicine* 104:584.

Morse S, Moreland A, Thompson S (1990). *Sexually Transmitted Diseases*. New York: Gower Medical Publishing.

Rosenberg MJ, Gollub EL (1992). Commentary: methods women can use that may prevent sexually transmitted disease, including HIV. *American Journal of Public Health* 82:1473–1478.

United States Department of Health and Human Services (USDHHS), Office of Disease Prevention and Health Promotion (ODPHP) (2003). *Healthy People 2010: A Systematic Approach to Health Improvement*. www.healthypeople.gov/Document/html/uih/uih_bw/uih_2.htm#obj.

254

Chapter 11

Injury Counseling: Torn Anterior Cruciate Ligaments

Learning Objectives

By the end of the chapter students will:

1. Understand the nature and extent of anterior cruciate ligament (ACL) injuries in the United States

2. Understand how ACL injuries vary by gender

3. Describe the goals of ACL injury counseling

4. Compare and contrast ACL counseling with other health counseling

5. Describe the risk factors for ACL tears

6. Discuss some common emotional responses to ACL injuries

7. Describe how counselors with a history of ACL injuries can use self-disclosure effectively

8. Discuss how changing the focal point can help clients view their ACL injuries differently

9. List and describe the key directives and logical consequences for each of the ACL injury counseling goals

Health Counseling for Tertiary Prevention

Chapters 11 and 12 focus on health counseling for tertiary prevention. As discussed in Chapter 1, health counseling, like health promotion and health education, can target any of the three levels of prevention: primary, secondary, or tertiary. Health counseling for tertiary prevention focuses on two issues:

limiting disability and premature death of clients who are suffering from disabilities and complications associated with specific injuries and health problems and rehabilitating clients to restore functioning to the highest level possible.

As in secondary prevention counseling, health counselors for tertiary prevention work with clients who already have the problem.

The major difference is that tertiary prevention clients not only have health problems, but are also suffering from complications and loss of functioning associated with their illnesses. Counseling them focuses on achieving adherence with both treatment and rehabilitative therapeutic regimens. Tertiary prevention clients have a host of emotional issues related to their disabilities. To halt the progression of their disabilities, teach them new skills, and restore functioning, counselors must work through these emotional issues (Mausner & Kramer, 1985).

Overview and Epidemiology of ACL Injuries

An estimated 70,000 to 80,000 cases of anterior cruciate ligament (ACL) tears occur each year in the United States. The highest incidence is in individuals 15 to 25 years old who participate in pivoting sports, and the costs associated with these injuries amount to almost $500 million per year. Seventy percent of ACL injuries occur in noncontact situations (Griffin, Agel, Albohm, et al., 2000; Hewett, 2000). These tears, which may be partial or complete, usually occur during athletic activity when a person stops suddenly and then changes direction, such as when running, pivoting, or landing after a jump. Sudden impact to the knee may also result in a torn ACL (HSS, 2003).

Diagnosis

The knee is essentially a modified hinge joint located where the end of the **femur** (thigh bone)

---

diverse perspectives 11.1

Gender Differences in ACL Tears

To the average person, a knee is just a knee, whether it is attached to a man or a woman. For the most part this is true: The ACL in men and women is essentially the same structure. Sports medicine professionals have found, however, that not all injuries to the knee are created equal.

More than 2.5 million high school girls and 145,000 college women participate in at least one competitive sport (Smith, 2000). Add at least that many who participate in recreational sports ranging from skiing to mountain biking, and you get a sense of the number of women participating in activities that put the knee at risk for sprains, strains, and tears.

Normally, one would expect that as more girls and women participate in competitive and high-impact sports and recreational activities, the incidence of knee injuries would increase. While this is true, what makes the data interesting is the disproportionate amount of knee injuries among women compared to men. It is estimated that females are much more likely than their male peers to suffer ACL tears. Untrained females had a 3.6 times higher incidence of knee injury than trained female athletes and a 4.8 times higher incidence than male athletes (Hewett, Lindenfeld, Riccobene, & Noyes, 1999). A leading professional sports medicine institution estimates that women in general have a four to eight times higher incidence of knee injuries than their male counterparts. Women also have a greater risk of suffering noncontact ACL tears than their male peers (Cincinnati Sports Medicine Research and Education Foundation, 2000). A noncontact tear occurs without contact with another person or object and is typically associated with landing after jumping, twisting, or turning. A survey completed by athletes who competed in the 1988 U.S. Olympic trials showed that 13 out of 64 females suffered an ACL tear compared to only 3 out of 80 males. In addition, there was a greater need for surgery with the female ACL tears (Ireland, Gaudette, & Crook, 1997; Ireland, 2002). It is estimated that each year, 1% of high school female athletes and 10% of college female athletes experience an ACL injury (Adams, 2002; Griffin et al., 2000; Woolston, 2000).

(Continued)

Gender Differences in ACL Tears (Continued)

The costs associated with reconstructive surgery and rehabilitation for these female athletes likely exceed $100 million annually (Brock, 2001).

Four main factors account for the increased risk for ACL tears among women: (1) anatomical characteristics, (2) hormonal patterns, (3) flexibility and strength levels, and (4) training issues.

A number of anatomical characteristics of women may account for their increased ACL tear risk compared to men. Women have a wider pelvis, which leads to a greater angle of the femur (thigh bone). That is, the femur angles inward from hip to knee, which leads to greater internal rotation forces of the knee joint and an internally facing patella (knee cap). Women also have a smaller notch at the end of the femur where it meets the tibia (shin bone). This impinges on the ACL, placing it under greater stress. Lastly, women have increased foot pronation (turning outward), which also places internal rotation forces on the knee. These anatomical characteristics collectively result in a biomechanical predisposition for an internal rotation of the knee resulting in a vulnerable ACL position (Brandon, 2004).

Women have a cyclic hormonal release pattern, such that key hormone levels vary according to where they are in their menstrual cycle. For instance, in midcycle, levels of estrogen, luteinizing hormone, and follicle-stimulating hormone peak just prior to ovulation and then drop off dramatically. Levels of progesterone, the hormone associated with the viability of the uterine lining, remain low through midcycle. Researchers have found a greater than expected level of ACL tears during the ovulatory phase (midcycle) of the menstrual cycle. Women who used oral contraceptives (which keep hormone levels constant) did not have a similar midcycle ACL injury pattern. This finding suggests that the increased risk is somehow associated with fluctuating hormone levels at midcycle (Wojtys, Huston, Boynton, et al., 2002; Andrews, 2000). Researchers are currently investigating whether changes in hormone levels during women's menstrual cycles affect the laxity (stretchiness) and strength of ligaments.

In general, women have less muscular development in their legs, hips, and trunk than men, which plays a crucial role in patella alignment. Women also have greater knee flexibility, which may decrease joint stability. This combination may predispose women to having less control and more internal rotation forces at the knee, rendering them more vulnerable to ACL tears. It might also explain their increased risk for noncontact ACL tears incurred during landing and cutting movements (Brandon, 2004).

Strength, flexibility, and coordination training are essential in reducing the risks associated with ACL tears. Noncontact ACL tears almost always involve a rapid deceleration of the knee joint. This can happen during a landing from a jump or during a leg plant in a cutting movement (side-step) (Cross, 1998). Athletes must be capable of performing a controlled and stable rapid deceleration of the knee in all directions—forward, diagonally, and sideways. Sometimes the knee is not stable during a rapid deceleration owing to forces from the hip and ankle placing the knee in a weak position. In this situation, a noncontact ACL tear can occur (Cross, 1998).

Training programs that enhance body control may decrease ACL injuries in women (Griffin et al., 2000). One way to improve body control is to include plyometric training into existing programs for strength and flexibility. Plyometric training involves hops, jumps, and bounds that force rapid eccentric (muscles lengthen while producing tension) contractions. Hewett (2000) found that plyometric training led to a decreased incidence of knee injury in female athletes.

As women continue to participate in greater numbers of competitive sports programs, trainers, coaches, and managers need to adapt their training programs to the special needs of female athletes so as to reduce their risks of incurring ACL injuries. To help prevent injuries, women athletes should make sure they are strong in the quadriceps, hamstrings, hip abductors, hip external rotators, abdominal muscles, and oblique muscles. The neuromuscular coordination of the knee joint deceleration movement should be trained with landing, cutting, and hopping drills. The correct techniques for landing and cutting should be practiced, and the correct shoes should always be worn (Brandon, 2004).

meets the top of the **tibia** (shin bone) (see **Figure 11.1**). This joint is responsible for controlling the movement of the knee. Four main ligaments connect these two bones. The **medial collateral ligament (MCL)** runs along the inner part of the knee and prevents the knee from bending inward. The **lateral collateral ligament (LCL)** runs along the outer part of the knee and prevents the knee from bending outward. The **anterior cruciate ligament (ACL)** lies in the middle of the knee. It prevents the tibia from sliding out in front of the femur and provides stability to the knee as it rotates. The **posterior cruciate ligament (PCL)** works in concert with the ACL in preventing the tibia from sliding backward under the femur. The ACL and PCL cross each other inside the knee, forming an "X." This is why they are called the **"cruciate"** (cross-like) ligaments.

ACL injuries are often associated with other injuries. A classic example is where the ACL is torn at the same time as the MCL and the **medial meniscus** (one of the shock-absorbing cartilages in the knee). This type of injury is most often seen in football players and skiers. Adults who tear their ACL usually do so in the middle of the ligament or pull the ligament off the femur bone. These injuries do not heal by themselves. In contrast, children are more likely to pull off their ACL with a piece of bone still attached. These ACL injuries may heal on their own, or they may require the bone to be fixed (HSS, 2003).

The diagnosis of an ACL tear relies on a combination of the patient's history, clinical examination, and laboratory tests. The physician will take a thorough history, addressing how the injury occurred and assessing when and how the pain first appeared. The classic ACL injury history involves a patient report of cutting, side-stepping, or landing from a jump; the knee giving way; and immediate pain and swelling following. It is also common for patients to report hearing a "snap" or "pop," which is followed by rapid swelling of the knee area (Cross, 1998).

The physician can assess damage to the ACL by conducting a special ligament stability test called the **Lachman's test** (see **Figure 11.2**). This test starts with the knee bent to 30 degrees. The physician gently pulls on the tibia to check the forward motion of the lower leg in relation to the upper leg. A

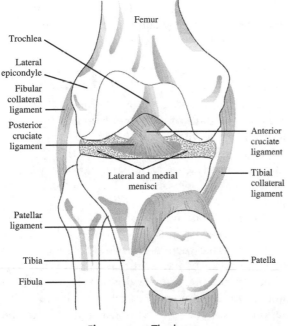

Figure 11.1 The knee.

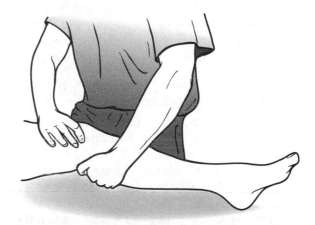

Figure 11.2 Lachman's test is commonly used to diagnose ACL injuries.

normal knee will have less than 2 to 4 mm of forward movement, and will come to a firm stop when no further movement is observed. A knee with an ACL tear will have increased forward motion and a soft feel at the end of the movement because of the loss of restraint of the forward movement of the tibia due to the torn ACL (yourmedicalsource.com, 2004).

A similar test, the **anterior drawer test,** starts with the knee bent to 90 degrees. A third test, the **pivot shift test,** puts greater stress on the knee as it is straightened by the physician from a bent and inwardly rotated position. The physician can feel the knee "give," an indication that other stabilizing structures within the knee besides the ACL may be torn (yourmedicalsource.com, 2004).

Most physical examinations are augmented with x-ray films to evaluate the possible tearing away of bone where the ligaments are attached. Also, x-rays may show any loose bone fragments or other fractures if they are present. Magnetic resonance imaging (MRI) tests are also used to provide images of all parts of the knee. An MRI uses powerful magnets to generate signals from inside the knee. These signals are then converted into a computer image that clearly shows any damage to the structures inside the joint (yourmedicalsource.com, 2004).

One additional test is performed with an instrument called the KT 1000. This device provides information about the integrity of the ACL by allowing the doctor or therapist to measure the amount of forward motion of the lower leg in relation to the upper leg (yourmedicalsource.com, 2004).

Treatment and Management

An ACL tear is an acute injury that results in pain, swelling, and stiffness. Most people are unable to walk without pain following such an injury. When the immediate swelling subsides, the knee is unstable, resulting in a sudden sense of shifting or buckling. Individuals with partial or complete ACL tears cannot jump and land on the knee, accelerate and then change directions, or rapidly pivot on the knee (Griffin et al., 2000).

The immediate treatment for all ACL injuries is to immobilize the knee with a splint, apply ice, elevate the joint (above the level of the heart), and administer pain relievers such as nonsteroidal anti-inflammatory drugs (e.g., ibuprofen). The patient should not put any demands on the knee until evaluation and treatment have taken place (HSS, 2003). Some people may need crutches to walk until the swelling and pain have improved. Physical therapy may help patients regain joint motion and leg strength. If instability continues even after leg strength and knee motion have been regained, most orthopedists will recommend a reconstruction of the ACL.

In most nonathletes, sudden movements such as changing direction, acceleration and deceleration, and jumping are rare and can be controlled for without an extraordinary loss of quality of life (HSS, 2003). The long-term outcomes for people treated nonsurgically vary. Those who try to return to their previous pattern of unrestricted activity are likely to experience some instability and pain. Pain may be associated with the physical therapy regimen as well. However, most people complain that their knee is unstable and tends to "give out" with attempted physical activity (HSS, 2003). Most athletes who do not have surgery find they are unable to return to their previous level of play.

Evidence suggests that nonsurgical treatment of ACL tears increases the risk of other forms of knee injuries (Griffin et al., 2000). Damage to the ACL, even in the absence of other injury, puts the menisci (the pads of cartilage that cushion the femur and tibia where they meet at the knee joint) at greater risk of tearing themselves (HSS, 2003). Once the menisci are torn, pain and swelling may ensue, and the person has an increased risk for developing osteoarthritis (HSS, 2003).

Because of the nature of ligaments, once they are torn, they usually do not mend like other forms of tissue such as muscle. Once an ACL is torn, it cannot be fixed. Instead, a new one needs to be constructed. Surgery does not just repair the injured ACL; in most cases, surgery plus rehabilitation makes the knee stronger and reduces the risk of injury to the meniscus.

Injuries and Violence

Health Implications of Injuries and Violence

While athletic injuries are used to illustrate how to counsel someone for tertiary prevention in this book, motor vehicle crashes are actually the most common cause of serious injury, with about 15.6 deaths per 100,000 persons occurring annually. More than 150,000 Americans die each year from injuries associated with motor vehicle crashes, firearms, poisonings, suffocation, falls, fires, and drowning. More than 90% of the U.S. population sustains a significant injury at some time during their lives (USDHHS, 2003).

Homicide is the most accurate indicator of the level of violent crime in the United States. Homicide rates in the 2000s have been the lowest reported in the past 20 years. Nevertheless, homicide remains a leading cause of death among young, inner-city, minority men.

The combined economic costs of injury and violence in the United States are estimated at more than $224 billion per year. These costs include direct medical care and rehabilitation as well as productivity losses among the U.S. work force. The economic costs associated with motor vehicle crashes alone exceed $150 billion annually (USDHHS, 2003).

Objectives for the Nation

- Reduce deaths caused by motor vehicle crashes
- Reduce homicides

In the surgery, part of the patellar tendon and bone from the knee and surrounding leg bones are grafted to the ACL. Grafts from cadavers may also be used to reconstruct the ACL. The surgery involves drilling holes in the leg bones and inserting the new bone and tendon grafts, which are anchored in place with screws. Over time, the graft attaches itself to the body naturally and becomes a fully functioning part of the knee.

Weight bearing is encouraged as soon as possible after surgery (depending on the doctor). Rehabilitative physiotherapy begins in the hospital or at a rehabilitation facility three to four days after the operation. Rehabilitation continues for several months and is broken down into six phases:

Phase 1: decreasing pain and swelling following surgery. Improve the range of motion and promote muscle activity and strength.

Phase 2: joint protection. Bend the knee zero to 100 degrees.

Phase 3: bend the knee from zero to 130 degrees.

Phase 4: full range of motion of the knee. Weight may be added to gradually increase resistance to existing exercises.

Phase 5: lunges, stepping exercises.

Phase 6: return to activity using a functional brace for athletic activities and work situations, jogging on a treadmill, and using other activities to maintain strength and flexibility (HSS, 2003).

Serious and Career-Ending Injuries

An offshoot of the tremendous interest in sport in America at the youth, high school, college, and professional levels is the attention given to career-ending injuries. Often, career-ending athletic injuries are perceived as life-threatening and disabling conditions. In fact, only a small percentage of athletic injuries are severe and result in subsequent permanent disability. Kujala et al. (2003) found that of 54,186 sports injuries reported to a major insurance company, only 102 (0.02%) resulted in permanent disability. While the number and percentage of career-ending and permanently disabling athletic injuries are small compared to the overall number of injuries, the effects of these events on individual athletes are potentially devastating.

Wiese-Bjornstal et al. (1998) proposed a three-part appraisal model for understanding how athletes respond to serious injuries: (1) cognitive appraisal, (2) emotional response, and (3) behavioral outcomes. The meaning of the injury and its subsequent psychological effects are the result of the combination of the three dimensions of appraisal. Additionally, their appraisal and response will change as the duration of the injury and the rehabilitation process proceed.

The cognitive dimension includes such factors as the perceived severity of the injury, the sense of loss or relief associated with the injury, and the attribution associated with it. Athletes vary in the accuracy of the perceived seriousness of their injuries. Sometimes this perception is based on not fully understanding the injury; at other times it is the result of wishful thinking or denial regarding the seriousness. Most athletes usually respond to injury with a sense of loss because participation in their chosen sport has been so consuming and has represented a major part of their lives and self-identity. For some athletes, however, a potentially career-ending injury may represent a way out of a commitment to a sport or lifestyle that is no longer attractive. These athletes feel relief rather than regret or loss regarding the potential career-ending aspect of their injuries. Lastly, the way athletes perceive their injuries is influenced by what they attribute the injury to. For instance, their appraisal will differ if they think the injury was the result of a freak accident beyond their control or the result of something they (or the team) did wrong or could have prevented.

The emotional response consists of the predominant emotions experienced by athletes following injury and during rehabilitation. It can be positive and result in feeling challenged and motivated to get back to normal as soon as possible. Such a response will facilitate rehabilitative and readjustment efforts. Alternatively, the emotional response can be negative and involve such emotions as fear, anger, and frustration. Such emotions can make rehabilitation and readjustment difficult. Negative emotions can cause setbacks in the rehabilitation process.

Behavioral outcomes refer to things such as adherence to rehabilitation regimens, use of coping resources and strategies, and use of social support. Athletes who admit they need help and seek out coping and social supports will have a different perspective on the long road through surgery and rehabilitation than athletes who do not seek out and accept help or for whom these resources do not exist. Behavioral outcomes also encompass the response to the progression of the injury and the way this evolution affects coping and continued rehabilitation. Often, the rehabilitation process is not smooth and athletes suffer setbacks. How athletes respond to these setbacks and continue to cope and use social support will influence their response to their injuries.

Hobfoll's (1988) conservation of resources theory proposes that athletes have a number of resources available, including physical health, finances, mobility/independence, self-perception, achievements, and social roles. All of these resources are affected by injury, but some are affected more than others, thereby affecting the perception of the injury. Further, Hobfoll (1988) suggests that resources that are lost or diminished due to injuries can be somewhat offset by social support involving encouragement, reassurance, advice, personal and financial assistance, and the triggering of other latent personality resources within the injured athletes themselves.

Ford and Gordon (1999) reviewed several theories regarding the losses suffered by athletes who experience severe or career-ending injuries. They propose that loss occurs across four dimensions: (1) loss of a significant or valued person, (2) loss of some aspect of self, (3) loss of external objects, and (4) developmental loss. The most common loss, according to Ford and Gordon, is the loss of some aspect of the self—most notably, self-identity or sense of importance. For many athletes, their predominant self-identity is as an athlete and participant in their sport. Losing the ability to participate involves losing a part of the self. Additionally, many athletes view their self-worth and importance within the context of their athleticism. Being injured, especially if it is to the extent that they may no longer be able to perform at the high level to which they are accustomed, means having to reexamine and reestablish their worth. Ford and Gordon (1999) also found that athletes experienced loss across the other three dimensions, which manifested itself as lost mobility, independence, sense of control, self-confidence, virility, daily activity patterns and social ties, status, attention, and opportunities for income and financial rewards.

Applying Kübler-Ross's Model to Career-Ending Injuries

The loss experienced by athletes who suffer career-ending injuries can actually mimic the loss experienced by those who lose a loved one. Such loss can be understood using Kübler-Ross's (1975) stages of death and dying.

> *Stage 1: Denial.* In this stage, the athlete does not admit the reality of the situation. "No, I'll be back playing again in [number] months."
>
> *Stage 2: Anger.* Athletes in this stage vent their anger at the situation, coaches, the opposition, and other things related to the injury. "Why me, why did this have to happen to me? If it wasn't for [target], I'd have never gotten injured."
>
> *Stage 3: Bargaining.* In this stage, the athlete bargains with God, the doctor, the surgeon —anyone who can get the athlete back to where he or she was before the injury. "God, if you just get me through this and back on the field I'll . . . ."
>
> *Stage 4: Depression.* During this stage, the realization that the career is over takes hold and the athlete begins to grieve for the anticipated loss of his or her career. "There is nothing left for me to do. My life as I know it is over."
>
> *Stage 5: Acceptance.* In this final stage, athletes accept their fate and are psychologically ready for the loss. Unlike being prepared for physical death, as Kübler-Ross (1975) envisioned, it is acceptance of the end of life as they once knew it.

When counseling someone who has experienced a serious or career-ending injury, it is important for counselors to assess what the injury means to the athlete. Many issues factor into the appraisal process, so one should always treat athletes as individuals when assessing the meaning of their injuries.

Goals for Counseling Someone with a Torn ACL

As a rehabilitation counselor working with clients with knee injuries, you have four primary goals: (1) assessment of the client's goals for rehabilitation, (2) development of a rehabilitation plan based on the client's goals and lifestyle, (3) teaching the client how to perform rehabilitative exercises to build strength, flexibility, and endurance in the knee, and (4) teaching the client procedures for pain management and dealing with swelling.

Counseling Clients with ACL Injuries Using Microskills

Counseling clients with torn ACLs and similar injuries will vary according to the nature of the injury, its meaning to the client, and the treatment plan in which the client is engaged. Counseling big-time athletes or professionals will differ from working with clients who are "weekend warriors" or are not athletic at all. Setting realistic counseling goals is totally dependent upon the client's lifestyle.

Case Study 11.1
Tanisha

Tanisha is 20 years old, single, and a college sophomore, and she identifies as an African American. She attends a major private university in the southern United States on a full athletic scholarship for soccer. She was one of the most sought-after high school soccer players in the country and chose to go to her university so as to follow in her parents' footsteps. Both of her parents are alumni of the same institution. During the first game of the national college soccer championships, Tanisha was involved in a three-player collision at the mouth of the opposing team's goal. Tanisha, a striker, suffered a devastating knee injury while trying to score on the play. She was carried off the field and rushed to the university hospital's Sports Medicine Clinic, one of the best facilities in the country. After a day in the hospital, she met with her doctors and trainers associated with the clinic's rehabilitation facility.

Introductory Skills

As discussed in Chapter 3, a good introduction is essential to establishing trust, which is essential for effective counseling. It is important when working in rehabilitation settings to clearly articulate your role and explain how it fits into the treatment team consisting of primary physicians, orthopedic/sports medicine specialists, nurses, and rehabilitation personnel.

Identify Yourself and Explain Your Role

As suggested in prior chapters, writing a script for your introduction and practicing it until it becomes second nature will help you use this skill effectively. When introducing yourself, it is very important to make a concerted effort to establish a skin-to-skin human connection with the client. A firm handshake is a good way to do so. Extend your hand, make eye contact, and smile as you give the client a firm (but not crushing) handshake. Be careful with handshakes when dealing with clients who have hand, arm, and shoulder injuries. A gentle touch on the shoulder may be more appropriate with these clients.

Example

Counselor: (Extending hand, smiling) Hi, I'm [name]. I'm one of the rehabilitation counselors at the clinic. My job is to help you understand the nature of your injury, to explain your options regarding treatment and reha-

bilitation, and to work with you in whatever therapeutic capacity you and your doctors agree upon. I will help you develop a rehabilitation plan based on your needs and lifestyle. To do so, I'll need you to be honest in discussing your injury and its effects on your lifestyle and your future plans. Please feel free to discuss any issue related to your injury, the rehabilitation process, or anything going on in your life that concerns you. My job is to help you make the best decisions for yourself regarding how to manage your injury. I want you to understand that everything we say is confidential and that your name and anything we talk about cannot be shared with anyone else.

Clarify the Client's Name

A simple way to verify the client's name is to use an open-ended statement following your introduction. Do so while you are still standing and immediately following your handshake and self-identification.

Example

Counselor: (Before sitting and explaining his role) And your name is . . . ?
Tanisha: My name is Tanisha.
Counselor: Nice to meet you, Tanisha.

Explain the Client's Role

After exchanging names and describing your role, start to explain the client's role. A simple explanation should include the three key elements of the client role discussed in Chapter 3: (1) active participation, (2) self-responsibility, and (3) honesty.

Example

Counselor: Tanisha, your role in this process is to be as open and honest as possible when talking to me. The only way I can help you is if you tell me exactly what is going on in your mind regarding your injury. I promise to not make any assumptions about your injury and what it means to you. Although I can empathize with you and what you are going through, you'll have to take an active role in describing your experience and take responsibility for getting better. If you are open and honest with me, together we can work out a rehabilitation plan that will help you get to where you want to be regarding your knee and the other issues surrounding it.

Set Goals for the Session(s)

The four primary goals when working with clients with knee injuries are: (1) assessment of the client's goals for rehabilitation, (2) development of a rehabilitation plan based on the client's goals and lifestyle, (3) teaching the client how to perform rehabilitative exercises to build strength, flexibility, and endurance in the knee, and (4) teaching the client procedures for pain management and dealing with swelling. In addition to these primary goals, counselors must assess clients' other goals regarding their rehabilitation process. The best way to do so is to describe your goals and assess clients' needs.

Example

Counselor: Tanisha, my work with you will revolve around four primary goals. First, I will help you develop a set of goals to guide your rehab. Second, I will help you develop a rehabilitation plan based on your choices and lifestyle. Third, I will teach you how to perform the various rehabilitative exercises to strengthen your knee and restore flexibility and endurance. Fourth, I will teach you procedures for managing your pain and dealing with swelling. What other goals do you have for our time together?

It is important for counselors to give clients time to think this through before moving into the next part of the session.

Transition to the Client's Story

A good way to make the transition from the introduction to getting clients to tell their stories is to use open-ended statements. The idea in using these open-ended statements is to get clients talking about their current injuries and how those injuries affect their lifestyles and relationships.

Example

Counselor: Tanisha, why don't you tell me a little about yourself.

Counselor: Tanisha, tell me a little bit about what you know about knee injuries.

Counselor: Tanisha, tell me a little bit about what happened to your knee.

Tanisha: I am a second-semester college sophomore. I went to a prep school for a year after high school to bring up my grades a little and then transferred to the university. It gave me a full scholarship to play soccer and attend class.

Counselor: Um, hum.

Tanisha: Everything was going great. I really like the university and am doing well in class and on the team. When I was a freshman, our team went all the way to the NCAA finals. I actually got to start one of the playoff games. I was doing great this year, before my injury. I was just named as a first-team All American at my position. Then this happened.

Attending Skills

Listening to clients discuss their injuries will give you insights not only into the nature of their injuries, but also how these injuries relate to their current lifestyles and future plans. Counselors need to be careful about assuming to know what injuries mean to clients. It is better to set a nonjudgmental tone while attending and let clients tell you what they mean. A major part of helping clients rehabilitate their injured bodies and minds is determining whether they perceive their injuries in logical/rational or illogical/irrational ways. The best way to do so is to listen to their stories and observe how they tell them.

There is a good chance that the way clients appraise their injuries will differ markedly from the way counselors perceive them. It is important to remember that the meaning of injuries for clients will vary tremendously depending on a number of variables. For instance, there is a good chance that a sedentary, 52-year-old businessman who tears his ACL will view the significance of the injury differently than a 20-year-old All American soccer player. Also, two 52-year-old sedentary businessmen will view the same injury differently, as would two 20-year-old All American soccer players. Lastly, the same knee injury will mean different things to the same client depending on when it occurs in the course of his or her life. If the 52-year-old businessman had torn his ACL when he was 20, it would probably mean something entirely different to him than it does at age 52.

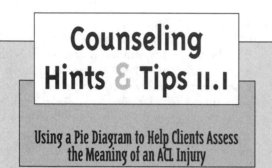

Counseling Hints & Tips 11.1

Using a Pie Diagram to Help Clients Assess the Meaning of an ACL Injury

Sometimes using a visual aid can help clients assess what their ACL injuries mean to them. A simple pie chart, similar to the ones used to illustrate data and statistics, can be very helpful.

1. Have clients draw a medium-sized (5-inch diameter) circle.
2. Ask them to think about the various facets of their self-identity or personality.
3. Give them examples such as athlete, mother, sister, and student.
4. Ask them to divide their pie into segments representing these facets.
5. Have them decide what percentage (or slice) of the pie is represented by each facet.
6. Ask them to describe how their ACL injury affects each segment now.
7. Repeat step 6 and ask them how their injury will affect each segment six months from now.

Their pies will give you a sense of how they perceive their injury and assist you in proceeding with their counseling.

Nonverbal Skills

It is important to appear relaxed and open when listening to clients' stories. The best way to do so is to assume a comfortable body position, with shoulders square to the client. Be sure to use culturally appropriate eye contact when attending.

Verbal Following

As with stress counseling, a key aspect of verbally following injury stories is paying particular attention to logical versus illogical thinking. This consideration is crucial in helping clients set reasonable goals for rehabilitating their torn knee ligaments. Illogical thinking can manifest itself at either extreme of the rehabilitation continuum: Clients may feel that they will never get better or that they will be back to 100% in an unreasonably short period of time with minimal work. A major aspect of the rehabilitation process is setting reasonable goals and helping clients deal with the setbacks associated with achieving these goals. Counselors' initial verbal following will often set the stage for understanding how clients perceive this issue.

Example

Tanisha: (Continuing with her story) Yeah, so this injury ruined everything. Not only did I get hurt, but I also messed up my chance to help my team win the championship. Even though we won the first game, we go up against the reigning national champs tomorrow and I won't be able to play. If we lose, I may never get a chance to be a national champion again. This will really kill my chances of a professional career. Oh, why did this have to happen to me?

Vocal Tone

Try to match the pace and tone of clients' stories. Clients with torn knee ligaments such as Tanisha experience a range of emotions regarding their injuries, and they express these emotions in the way they tell their stories. Some will be very animated and go into gory detail regarding their injuries and the events leading up to them. Others will be very reserved and sketchy in their descriptions, almost as if retelling their story is too painful to deal with. Don't respond to clients' stories with your own tone and pace, but rather let their emotions and style dictate yours.

Responding Skills

Nonverbal Minimal Encouragers
As noted throughout the text, using encouraging body language will help keep clients talking. Be sure that your body language and nonverbal feedback come across as nonjudgmental and unassuming. Let clients tell you what their injuries mean to them. Try to maintain a relaxed posture, and periodically scan your own body for signs of any tension that might be transmitted to clients. Use simple gestures such as head nods, hand circles, and facial expressions (e.g., smiling, raising the eyebrows) to keep clients talking.

Verbal Minimal Encouragers
Simple acknowledgments such as "uh huhs," key words, and mirroring are very important tools to get clients to continue their stories. They are especially helpful in encouraging clients to explain how they perceive their injuries.

Example

Counselor: Go on.

Tanisha: I just feel so . . . devastated, like everything in my world is falling apart.

Counselor: Devastated? (Key word)

Tanisha: Yeah. In one split second, everything I've worked so hard for the last 10 years has just fallen apart. I just feel like I've lost everything.

Counselor: Uh, humm. (Simple acknowledgment)

Tanisha: I'm just so afraid. My whole life up to this point has revolved around soccer, and now I am afraid that it will all just disappear.

Counselor: It will all disappear. (Mirroring)

Tanisha: Yeah. I'm in school on a soccer scholarship. I know that I am still supposed to get my money even if I get hurt, but I just worry about it. Plus, I really want to play. I want to finish out my college career and play pro soccer in Europe for a few years, then come back and go to law school. I have the rest of my whole life figured out and now this.

Counselor: I see. (Simple acknowledgment)

Open Invitation to Talk
Careful use of questioning to clarify how clients view their injuries is very important because of the many ways people perceive them. Clearly, Tanisha views her injury as the end of the world as she has known it for the past decade. A skillful, nonjudgmental use of questions will help her counselor clarify how she views her injury and its effect on her life.

Open-Ended Statements and Questions
The liberal use of open-ended statements can create a more relaxed, conversational tone. Asking a couple of open-ended statements and then sitting back and listening to clients' stories is much more efficient than asking a string of closed questions. It is better to use the closed questions to tease out information not covered by clients' responses to open-ended queries.

Example

Instead of asking multiple questions like

"Tanisha, do you think your injuries will end your career?"

"Tanisha, do you think you'll ever be able to play soccer again?"

"Tanisha, do you think you will ever be able to play soccer at the same level that you are now playing?"

"Tanisha, do you think you'll lose your place on your team because of this injury?"

ask

"Tanisha, how do you think this injury will affect your future with the team?"

"Tanisha, how do you think this injury will affect your future ability to play soccer?"

Tanisha: I'm really worried about two things: being able to come back and play soccer again at the same competitive level, and losing my starting spot on the varsity to another woman. I guess I'm also worried that because of this injury I might not reach my dream of playing professional soccer. I really don't know who to believe about these things. I've talked to other players who have had ACL tears, and they tell me it is really rough to rehab them, but a person can come back stronger than ever after having the surgery and rehab. I talked to my parents, however, and they told me not to get my hopes up—that there is always my college degree to fall back on and not to worry about playing professional soccer.

Counselor: What do your coaches say?

Tanisha: I really haven't had a long talk with them. They are on the road right now, playing in the NCAA tournament. I got a couple of phone calls and some nice gifts from them, but they basically told me to relax and just focus on getting better. I really can't read them.

Paraphrasing

As described in Chapter 4, effective paraphrases have three elements: (1) a short restatement of the client's story in your own words, (2) use of a key word or phrase, and (3) a check-out phrase. It is important to use paraphrasing extensively with clients with knee injuries to be sure that you fully understand their stories and what their injuries mean to them.

Example

Counselor: Tanisha, before we move on, let me be sure I understand your story so far. You've worked hard to earn a starting spot on the varsity team. In the most important game of the year—maybe even your life—you tear your ACL and are forced to miss the rest of the game and the postseason. You're really afraid because you're not sure if your soccer career is over. Is that right?

Tanisha: Yes and no. I think I'll be able to go back and play soccer someday. I'm just not sure I'll be able to play at the same level and win my spot back.

Because the counselor "checked out" his paraphrase, he found that the key element of Tanisha's story revolves around her ability not only to play soccer, but also to play at the same high level she attained prior to her injury.

Reflection of Feelings

Accurate reflection of feelings and emotions is crucial when counseling clients with knee and other injuries because of the fears they have related to reinjury, pain, and self-doubts. To successfully rehabilitate her knee, Tanisha will have to put up with an extraordinary amount of pain and torturous workouts to rebuild her strength, flexibility, speed, and stamina. She will have to work through her doubts and fears to regain full use of her knee. She will also have to understand the difference between good and bad pain associated with the healing process.

Example

Counselor: Tanisha, it seems to me that the greatest emotion you are feeling right now is fear. You are afraid of the unknown related to your injury. Is that accurate?

Tanisha: Exactly. I'm kind of a control freak, and not being in control of this situation and its influence on my future has me scared to death. I don't doubt my ability to work hard and rehab this knee. I'm just afraid that even if I work my way back and regain 100% of my strength, flexibility, and endurance, I'll lose some edge. I mean, I have not stopped working out in three or four years. There hasn't been any "off" season. I have been playing and training nonstop since my sophomore year in high school. I am scared to death of doing nothing for the next six to nine months.

Counselor: Tanisha, trust me, you won't be doing "nothing" over the next several months.

You'll be training as hard as you ever did. It's just that it will be different.

Summarizing

Summarizing helps clarify clients' thoughts and feelings about their knee injuries and put them into context. It offers an opportunity for them to hear their stories again and decide whether anything needs to be added, deleted, or clarified. It also shows them how well counselors are following the story. Remember, summaries include both the cognitive (thoughts, facts) and affective (feelings and emotions) dimensions of clients' stories. In Tanisha's case, it is clear that the major issue isn't whether she wants or can manage rehabilitation of her knee; the major issue relates to the *outcome* of this rehabilitation.

Example

Counselor: Tanisha, before we move on, let's make sure I understand exactly what is going on regarding your knee injury. I actually should call it "injuries," because you have damage to two different ligaments. The sense I have is that you are afraid, but it isn't fear related to the injury and the work involved in rehabbing it. You seem to understand and accept the work involved. You also seem like a very hard-working young woman. Your biggest concerns focus on the results of this rehabilitation. You are very afraid that everything that you've worked so hard to get—your scholarship, starting spot on the varsity, and potential pro career—is in jeopardy. Is this accurate?

Tanisha: Yeah. The other thing is the newness of this entire experience to me. I've never had a serious injury before. I really hate hospitals, and the idea of being in a hospital and undergoing surgery is kind of scary. Again, I feel out of control. Hospitals to me represent places where I give up control and am putting my life and self in the hands of others. I don't like this.

Counselor: You've mentioned the issue of control a couple of times. It seems that you like to be in control and are afraid to relinquish it.

Tanisha: You can say that again. I like to be in the center of the action and in control.

Influencing Skills

As mentioned earlier in this chapter, the four primary goals when working with clients with knee injuries are (1) assessment of the client's goals for rehabilitation, (2) development of a rehabilitation plan based on the client's goals and lifestyle, (3) teaching the client how to perform rehabilitative exercises to build strength, flexibility, and endurance in the knee, and (4) teaching the client procedures for pain management and dealing with swelling.

Self-disclosure

As mentioned in Chapter 5, self-disclosure is an excellent technique for building confidence in clients regarding their perceived ability to change. It is an even stronger influencing skill when it relates to knee injuries, because the counselor is literally "walking proof" that the rehabilitation works. When counselors disclose to clients that they can empathize with what they are feeling because they had the same fears and doubts, clients feel connected to them in a deeper way. There is no need to go into great detail regarding the counselor's surgery and rehab. The crucial issue is to establish a real connection based on the shared injury and rehab experience and the emotions associated with both.

Example

Counselor: Tanisha, I know what you are experiencing. I had a promising career in baseball that was interrupted by a torn ACL in my senior year of college. I worked my way back to the same level I had attained prior to the injury but decided that I really didn't want to pursue a professional baseball career. I was more interested in going to physical therapy school.

Tanisha: Really, you did all that work and then called it quits?

Counselor: I think I was really on the fence all along. The injury and rehab just helped me make up my mind.

Tanisha: Yeah, I guess I'd have no problem just finishing school and going on to law school.

Case Study 11.2
Joe

Joe, 58, is married, and identifies as Italian American. Joe is a friend of Dr. Blonna. His story is typical of athletes who experienced ACL tears in the 1960s when the level of technology was entirely different.

Joe: I injured my knee playing high school football in 1966. At that time we were very unsophisticated regarding off-season training. All potential players came to tryouts at the end of August. If you made the team you were expected to "get into shape" prior to the first game of the season, which took place around the third week of September.

Dr. Blonna: That is very different than today.

Joe: I know. My son played high school football and he was *recruited* out of the Pee Wee league. He was required to work out all year long and *report* to tryouts in the best shape possible.

Dr. Blonna: What does this have to do with your injury?

Joe: I was always about 30 pounds overweight and lost 10 to 15 pounds during the first month of the season. I was a good player and the coach cut me some slack. I think, however, that this contributed to my injury in my senior year of high school.

Dr. Blonna: How so?

Joe: I came to camp in my senior year at 35 pounds over my playing weight. I had discovered girls that summer, got my driver's license, and had just relaxed and screwed around all summer. I was a good student, had good grades, and just wanted to have some

fun going into my senior year. I didn't work out at all for the six months leading into football season. Anyway, I reported to tryouts overweight and out of shape. I made the team with no problem.

Dr. Blonna: What happened then?

Joe: I never really lost the weight I needed to and was carrying about 25 extra pounds over my normal playing weight of 220 pounds on a 5′10″ frame. We were scrimmaging another team in between our second and third games of the season. I went to make a cut to throw a block, and when I twisted I heard a loud pop. I went down in agonizing pain. My knee instantly started to swell, and I could not put any pressure on it. I don't remember how long it took, but they finally were able to get me some ice. I wound up in the hospital about two hours later. I vaguely remember the next couple of days but basically they told me to ice it and rest and have x-rays.

Dr. Blonna: Go on.

Joe: My dad was pissed. We had no medical insurance to cover any fancy surgery, and my dad didn't want me to play football anymore anyway. I kept working on him to convince him to let me get the surgery and I'd find some way to pay him back. He never wavered, though, and I didn't have the surgery. I really don't remember too many details but I was on crutches for a long time. My doctors gave me some exercises to do but I never really did them. Physical therapy wasn't an option for me. We had no insurance for it and were pretty poor.

Dr. Blonna: What happened next?

Joe: Needless to say, I missed the whole season and I was on crutches for a good part of my senior year. My knee healed to a certain extent, but it was very wobbly and gave out a lot. I had to give up football and all other sports. I tried wearing a brace to play but it was too unstable. I never got a chance to play any more football. Years later, after my dad died and after I was married and became a teacher, I took one summer and had arthroscopic surgery to repair the knee correctly. I took a long time to rehabilitate it because of my age and the lapse in time since the original injury, but I am now able to live a normal life. I even play golf and can use an exercise bike to stay in shape.

Confrontation

Confrontation will come into play extensively, especially when responding to incongruities related to clients' injuries. Chapter 5 described how confrontation is a skill that respectfully and gently makes clients aware of incongruities and discrepancies in their lives and their stories. Most clients have conflicting stories or mixed messages about their injuries and what they mean to them.

Sometimes clients will intentionally tell discrepant stories to hide parts of their stories that are either too difficult for them to deal with or they feel will lead to too many problems if discussed. These issues range from fear of the unknown to involvement in activities that they (the clients) would rather not share with anyone. Confronting clients' discrepancies, regardless of their origin, is essential to meet the goals of the counseling session. Using Ivey and Ivey's (2003) one hand, other hand approach is most helpful when employing this skill.

Example

Counselor: Tanisha, on the one hand, you mentioned how your whole life revolves around soccer and your immediate goals involve playing pro soccer. On the other hand, you just said you'd have no problem not playing anymore, finishing school and going to law school. I'm confused.

Tanisha: Well, I guess I really don't mean no problem.

Counselor: Uh humm.

Tanisha: I don't know. It is too scary to think about, okay.

Counselor: It is scary.

Tanisha: Yeah, I know, in my mind, that I have options and plans beyond soccer to fall back

on. I guess I'm trying to convince myself that they would really be enough if I couldn't go back to playing.

Changing the Focal Point

Changing the focal point is an excellent way to help clients gain a new perspective on their injuries. In viewing their problem through the eyes of others involved in their story, they often gain insights that change the way they view their situation and influence their future behavior.

Example

Counselor: Tanisha, let's step back from the problem for a minute and try to look at what is going on from another perspective. It might help you understand your problem a little better. Take a couple of minutes and try to think about how your parents view your injury. When you can visualize this, share your thoughts with me.

Tanisha: (A couple of minutes later) I think both my mom and dad are on the same page with this. I think they see this injury as a wake-up call for me.

Counselor: Wake-up call?

Tanisha: Ever since my success with soccer early on, they have told me to view the sport as something wonderful but temporary in my life. They have never put pressure on me to depend on it for anything. They saved money for me for college, and I always had good grades and excellent college board test scores. They've always deemphasized the importance of soccer.

Counselor: Go on.

Tanisha: Both have said many times that athletes can have their whole world turned upside down with a simple twist, turn, or fall and that the smart ones always have a plan B, to use their words.

Counselor: Plan B?

Tanisha: A fall-back plan. Mine has always been college and law school. Both of my parents are professionals. My dad is a lawyer, and my mom is a certified financial planner with an M.B.A. in finance. They played sports but always took school seriously. I guess they always knew that something like this could happen at any time and they wanted me to be prepared for life beyond soccer.

Counselor: Do you think you are?

Tanisha: To tell you the truth, I'm not sure. I have been doing what they said, taking my school seriously, but have never really thought about a life without soccer.

Counselor: Tanisha, I'm not convinced that your life without soccer has to happen just yet, but maybe knowing that your parents are there for you and that there *is* a life beyond soccer can help you deal with the next few months while this all sorts itself out.

Tanisha: Yeah, I guess that is a helpful way to look at it.

Eliciting and Reflecting Meaning

The last few chapters have included many examples showing how eliciting and reflecting meaning helps influence clients by giving them insights into the meaning of their health problems. The examples have illustrated how important it is for counselors to be sure that they understand the meaning of their clients' injuries before moving on to giving directives and instructions for their rehabilitation. As mentioned earlier, a good way to elicit meaning is to ask clients to make sense of the meaning of their stories.

Example

Counselor: Tanisha, we've been talking a lot about your injury and how it might affect your future. Why don't you try to put it into perspective for me. At this point, what would you say this injury means to you?

Tanisha: All right, I'll try. I guess I am feeling that my life as I know it is over. When I actually stop and hear myself saying that, it sounds crazy because I really haven't suffered a life-threatening or career-ending injury. It just seems to be that way for me. I wish I

could just settle down, but all I think about is this injury and what it might mean to my future. I guess I'm not really sure what it means because I'm not 100% sure if I can come back from it.

Counselor: Okay, we'll start from there.

Interpretation of Meaning and Reframing

Counselors use interpretation of meaning to make sense of what health problems mean to clients. This process is very similar to eliciting and reflecting feelings, but is counselor directed. Interpretation of meaning differs from eliciting and reflecting meaning in that it comes from counselors and includes their perspectives on the meaning of clients' stories. After interpreting the meaning of clients' stories, counselors can reframe the stories and present different versions for clients to ponder. As mentioned in Chapter 5, these alternative ways of viewing their problems provide new options to consider for dealing with the problems and allow clients to see their problems in new and different ways.

Clients like Tanisha who have never been injured tend to have fear and think the worst regarding their injuries. In rehabilitation counseling for athletic injuries, counselors can draw on their experiences with similar clients from the past to help put their current clients' stories into their proper perspective.

Example

Counselor: Tanisha, I know that you are feeling that your world has fallen apart. Your dreams of winning the NCAA championship just came to a screeching halt, and you are thinking that your career and future plans are over. Perhaps everything looks very grim, and it is hard to draw anything positive out of this experience. Let me try to create a different way of looking at your injury for you to consider.

Tanisha, think about your contributions to the team throughout this season, even to the point of getting injured. You played a key role in getting the team to this point. Their success is derived in large part from your efforts. Even in the game during which you were injured, you scored the go-ahead goal that proved to be the game winner. If the team wins the NCAA championship, you are still a big part of their success. It is still your championship as well as theirs.

In addition, try thinking about your injury slightly differently. Most athletes who suffer the same injury can return to their previous level of health prior to the injury. In fact, many come back even stronger. The surgical procedure you will undergo has been performed routinely now for several years with a very high success rate. The biggest variable associated with full recovery is the commitment and hard work of the client. I have no doubts that you will commit yourself 100% to your rehabilitation and will come away stronger than ever. Try not to even look at this experience as anything other than a chance to get in the best shape of your life for next season.

Lastly, put yourself in your coach's position. In you he has an All American, a hard worker, an excellent role model for the younger women on the team. You know his system, and you are a proven performer and the heart of his team. If you come back, better than ever, he'd be a fool not to give you your starting job back, if for nothing else than to inspire the other women. What do you think about this?

Tanisha: I hadn't really thought about all of that. I guess you're right. I do feel that this title run is also my championship, even if I didn't play at the end. I do have two more years of eligibility left and the coach has always liked me. He's the one who recruited me as a freshman in high school. I guess I need to start thinking more positively about my chances to return.

Counselor: I agree. I haven't once heard you complain or wonder about the effort rehabbing your knee will entail, so I know you are not afraid of a little hard work.

Directives and Logical Consequences

Several potential directives, instructions, and logical consequences are associated with each of the four goals of injury counseling: (1) assessment of the client's goals for rehabilitation, (2) development of a rehabilitation plan based on the client's goals and lifestyle, (3) teaching the client how to perform rehabilitative exercises to build strength, flexibility, and endurance in the knee, and (4) teaching the client procedures for pain management and dealing with swelling.

Directive 1: Assessing the Client's Goals for Rehabilitation

Help the client assess his or her goals for rehabilitation by choosing surgery and rehabilitation or rehabilitation alone.

Logical Consequences of Assessing the Client's Goals for Rehabilitation

1. Clients will tailor a therapeutic plan to fit their needs.
2. Clients are more likely to comply with plans they develop and that meet their needs.

Specific Instructions for Assessing the Client's Goals for Rehabilitation

1. Review with clients the material provided by physicians regarding the outcomes associated with the two options (rehabilitation alone or surgery plus rehabilitation).
2. Ask clients to describe the pros and cons of both options.
3. Ask clients to explain which option they think meets their needs.
4. Assess whether you agree and explain your interpretation.

Example

Counselor: Tanisha, I want to discuss the material given to you by your doctor regarding the two options for dealing with your knee injury: surgery plus rehabilitation or rehabilitation alone. Did you get a chance to look it over?

Tanisha: Yes, it seems that my chances of getting back to 100% are best if I combine surgery plus rehabilitation.

Counselor: Yes, you must consider the following things if you choose the nonsurgery option:

- You will have to give up all high-demand activities, such as basketball, football, and skiing, that include cutting, jumping, and decelerating.
- You will have to undergo a two- to three-month progressive rehabilitation program that will take place in the physical therapy clinic.
- This process is physically demanding, and you may feel pain and fatigue.
- There is a chance that physical therapy will not heal you and you will still have to go for surgery and rehab again to fix the problem (HSS, 2003).

Tanisha: I understand. I really never considered the nonsurgery route, because it seemed that if I went that way I'd never be able to play competitive soccer again.

Counselor: Okay, but before you make your final decision, let me go over a few points about surgery plus rehabilitation option. You must consider the following things before you choose this option:

- Having surgery will definitely reduce your chance of reinjuring your ACL.
- Surgery will make your knee stronger, and you will be less likely to injure your meniscus.
- The surgery involves taking part of the patellar tendon and bone from your knee and surrounding leg bones to graft to your ACL.
- The surgeons will actually drill holes in your leg bones and insert the new bone and tendon grafts, which will be anchored in place with screws.
- In time, the graft will attach itself to your body naturally and become a fully functioning part of your knee.
- Weight bearing is allowed as soon as possible (depending on the doctor).

- Physiotherapy is started in the hospital or at a rehabilitation facility three to four days after the operation. It will last for about one month.
- Physical therapy then shifts to a clinic, where it continues for the next three to four months.
- Return to sports with a brace is allowed at four to six months post-op. The brace is used only for the first season after injury.
- Eventually you should not require the brace to play sports over the long term.
- The surgery/rehabilitation process will cause some pain and swelling, which we will teach you how to manage.
- It is normal to experience frustration and doubt during the rehab process.
- While complications are minimal, the following outcomes are experienced by a small percentage of clients. First, blood clots may cause the leg to swell, grow warm to the touch, and become painful. Second, infection is a possibility, though the chances are low because antibiotics are given intravenously before and after surgery. Third, stiffness may be caused by excessive scarring inside the knee joint after ACL reconstruction. Performing range-of-motion exercises immediately following surgery is important to prevent knee stiffness. Fourth, graft impingement is possible. If the drilled holes in the knee are not placed correctly, the graft may press against the bone as the knee bends and straightens.

Tanisha, outpatient physical therapy and rehabilitation for your injury has six phases:

Phase 1: decreasing pain and swelling following surgery. The goal is to improve the range of motion and promote muscle activity and strength.

Phase 2: joint protection. Exercises seek to bend the knee zero to 100 degrees.

Phase 3: bend the knee from zero to 130 degrees.

Phase 4: full range of motion of the knee. Weight may be added to gradually increase resistance to existing exercises.

Phase 5: lunges and stepping exercises.

Phase 6: return to full activity. A functional brace may be required for athletic activities and work situations, and you may need to jog on a treadmill and undergo isokinetic testing.

Your schedule for returning to work and school activities following surgery is as follows:

1. Most patients use crutches for the first 7 to 14 days to help them walk. You will be instructed to follow up at our office to monitor your recovery from surgery.
2. If your job involves sitting down, some doctors may want you to return to work as soon as a week after surgery.
3. If your job requires standing, it may be four to six weeks before you return to work.
4. If your job requires lifting moderate loads or climbing activities, your recovery time may be anywhere from two to four months (yourmedicalsource.com, 2004).

Because you are a student who will be sitting most of the day, I would imagine that your doctor should clear you to return to class within one to two weeks following surgery. Make sure you check with him about this schedule. You should be able to drive a car within weeks after surgery. Do you understand these aspects of the surgery and rehabilitation plan?

Tanisha: Yes, I do and still want to proceed this way.

Counselor: Okay, we'll get in contact with your doctor to schedule the surgery. Let me go over the rest of our goals.

Directive 2: Helping the Client Develop a Rehabilitation Plan Based on His or Her Goals and Lifestyle

Help the client develop a rehabilitation plan based on his or her goals and lifestyle.

Logical Consequences of Developing a Rehabilitation Plan Based on the Client's Goals and Lifestyle

1. Clients will have a plan that is consistent with their needs and lifestyle.
2. Clients will be more likely to comply with the plan because it is tailored to their needs and lifestyle.

Specific Instructions for Developing a Rehabilitation Plan Based on the Client's Goals and Lifestyle

1. Reinforce the presurgery icing and exercise instructions given to clients by their physicians.
2. Set up a schedule for postsurgery in-hospital and outpatient rehabilitation.

Example

Counselor: Tanisha, let's make sure you understand what you have to do between now and when you have your surgery. The primary goals of treatment immediately after injury are (1) to reduce your pain and swelling and (2) to regain your range of motion and strength. Achieving these goals can help reduce complications after surgery. As soon as an ACL injury has occurred, the R.I.C.E. treatment is recommended until you have your surgery. You need to do the following things to reduce your pain and swelling:

- *Rest.* Rest the knee by not putting weight on the knee.
- *Ice.* Put ice on the knee to help decrease inflammation and pain.
- *Compression.* Using an ace bandage for compression around the knee is beneficial to control the swelling.
- *Elevation.* Lying down with the leg elevated higher than the level of the chest will help reduce the swelling.

Also, take pain medication as prescribed by your doctor. It may include anti-inflammatory as well as pain medication.

A simple exercise will help get your knee ready for surgery and postsurgery rehabilitation. It will help increase your strength and range of motion, and avoid joint stiffness and muscle tightness without further damage to your ACL. This exercise is called the quadriceps isometrics **(Figure 11.3)**. Position the knee about 10 degrees from being straight, with a small towel roll being placed directly behind the knee. Push in a downward direction into the towel roll for a count of 6 to 10 seconds. Repeat this exercise 10 times. You should practice it throughout the course of the day.

I know this is confusing, so can you please describe to me the instructions I have just given you?

Tanisha: Yes. You want me to use the R.I.C.E. formula for keeping the swelling down. I'm familiar with it, because I've used it before with a couple of minor sprains. I even have little cups of ice frozen in my freezer at home from the season. I am to use rest, ice, compression, and elevation a couple of times a day until I go to the hospital. In the meantime, I should take the medication that the doctor has prescribed for me exactly like he told me to. Right now, he has me on Tylenol with codeine every six hours. I am to start with the quad exercises. You want me to roll a small towel up and put it directly under my knee,

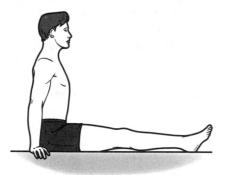

Figure 11.3 Quadriceps isometrics: Sit on a flat surface with legs out straight. Tighten the knee without moving the leg out of position. (To get the idea of this exercise, have someone place his or her hand behind your knee.)

then gently push down and hold it for 10 seconds. I'll do this exercise a few times a day.

Counselor: Good.

Tanisha: What if it hurts?

Counselor: It probably will hurt, but you are in no danger of making your ACL injury worse by doing this.

Tanisha: Okay.

Counselor: We must also talk about a schedule for you coming in to do your physical therapy exercises once you leave the hospital. The hospital staff will take care of you while you are an inpatient, but when you are released you'll need to come in to the rehab clinic three times a week to work on your knee. Tell me what your schedule will be like.

Tanisha: I imagine I won't be playing soccer, so I'll just have my classes to worry about. I'm in class on Monday through Thursday from 8:00 until about 12:30. After that I used to eat lunch, study, and head off to practice at 2:00 P.M. I'd be tied up with soccer until 6:00 and then come back to my room, go out with my roommates to eat at the cafeteria, have soccer meetings from 8:00 to 9:00 P.M., and be back in my room by 10:00 P.M. Weekends varied depending on whether the team was traveling.

Counselor: Would you prefer to come in for rehab during the afternoon after 2:00 P.M. or at night after 6:00 P.M.? Either case would kind of take the place of soccer.

Tanisha: I think I'll come over at 2:00 P.M. I can take the campus shuttle to the University Medical Center and this way have my evenings free.

Counselor: Okay, I'll put you in the book for 2:00 P.M. as soon as everything is settled with your surgery and hospital stay.

Directive 3: Teach the Client to Perform Rehabilitation Exercises

Teach the client how to perform rehabilitative exercises to build strength, flexibility, and endurance in the injured knee.

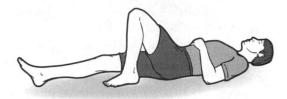

Figure 11.4 Heel slides: (1) Lie on your back and bend the knee, ensuring that the foot stays in contact with the floor. (2) Repeat 10 to 20 times. Slight discomfort may be felt, but not pain.

Logical Consequences of Teaching the Client to Perform Rehabilitation Exercises

1. Clients will perform exercises properly.
2. Clients will regain strength, range of motion, and increased endurance.

Specific Instructions for Teaching the Client to Perform Rehabilitation Exercises

1. Patients cannot take part in any of the other exercises until they have reduced swelling and are able to stand with equal weight on both legs.

2. The following instructions apply to five commonly prescribed rehabilitative exercises associated with ACL tears.

Heel Slide

Sit on a firm surface with your legs straight in front of you. Slowly slide the heel of your injured leg toward your buttocks by pulling your knee to your chest as you slide. Return to the starting position. Do three sets of 10 **(Figure 11.4)**.

Heel Raises

1. Balance yourself while standing behind a chair or counter.
2. Raise your body up onto your toes and hold it for 5 seconds, then slowly lower yourself down. Repeat 10 times. Do three sets of 10 **(Figure 11.5)**.

Elastic Tubing Hamstring Curls

1. Stand facing a door (about 3 feet from the door).
2. Loop and tie one end of the tubing around the ankle of your injured leg. Tie a knot in the other end of the tubing and shut the knot in the door **(Figure 11.6)**.

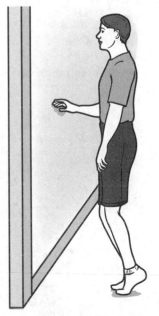

Figure 11.5 Heel raises.

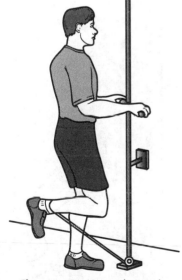

Figure 11.6 Hamstring curls.

3. Bend your knee so that your foot slides along the floor and moves back underneath your knee, stretching the tubing.

4. Slowly let your foot slide forward again. Do three sets of 10. You can challenge yourself by moving the chair farther away from the door and increasing the resistance of the tubing. To further challenge yourself, stand only on your injured leg and rise up on your toes, lifting your heel off the floor. Do three sets of 10.

Wall Squats

1. Stand with your back, shoulders, and head against a wall and look straight ahead. Keep your shoulders relaxed and your feet 1 foot away from the wall and a shoulder's width apart.

2. Place a rolled-up pillow or a soccer-sized ball between your thighs.

3. Keeping your head against the wall, slowly squat while squeezing the pillow or ball at the same time. Squat down until you are al-

most in a sitting position. Your thighs will not yet be parallel to the floor.

4. Hold this position for 10 seconds and then slowly slide back up the wall. Make sure you keep squeezing the pillow or ball throughout this exercise. Repeat 10 times. Build up to three sets of 10 **(Figure 11.7).**

Resisted Knee Extension

1. Make a loop from a piece of elastic tubing by tying it around the leg of a table or other fixed object.

2. Step into the loop so that the tubing is around the back of your injured leg. Lift your uninjured foot off the ground. Hold onto a chair for balance, if needed.

3. Bend your knee about 45 degrees.

4. Slowly straighten your leg, keeping your thigh muscle tight as you do so.

5. Do three sets of 10. An easier way to do this exercise is while standing on both legs **(Figure 11.8).**

At the end of the exercise treatment, ice the knee to help with pain and reduce swelling. Continue to take whatever medications were prescribed by the doctor (HSS, 2003).

Directive 4: Teach the Client Procedures for Pain Management

Teach clients procedures for managing pain and dealing with swelling.

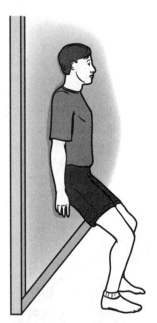

Figure 11.7 Wall squats.

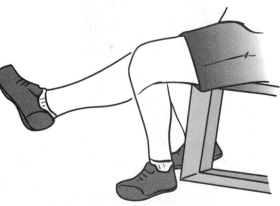

Figure 11.8 Knee extensions.

Logical Consequences of Teaching the Client Procedures for Pain Management

1. Clients will be able to distinguish good pain from bad pain.
2. Clients will be able to exert some control over their level of pain.
3. Clients are more likely to comply with their therapeutic plans if they understand and can manage their pain.

Specific Instructions for Teaching the Client Procedures for Pain Management

1. Pain from a torn ACL usually comes from swelling. Three methods can be used to help reduce pain: icing, elevation, and medications.
2. It is normal to experience some mild pain and throbbing after surgery and throughout your rehabilitation plan. It does not mean you have reinjured your knee.
3. Normal pain will respond to icing, rest, elevation, and use of medication.
4. Abnormal pain will not get better following the use of these strategies. If your pain continues or intensifies after trying these strategies, you should call your doctor immediately.
5. Apply ice to your knee for 20 minutes three to four times a day, and elevate your leg above your heart to reduce swelling.
6. Many different medications can be used to reduce swelling and control pain. It may take anywhere from three to six weeks for swelling and pain to go away and to get full motion back into the knee (HSS, 2003).

Summary

Most anterior cruciate ligament (ACL) injuries are caused by sudden motions involving twisting, cutting, changing speed and direction, or landing on the knee. A marked discrepancy in ACL tears is apparent between men and women, with several theories having been proposed to account for the higher incidence in women.

This chapter described the criteria used in diagnosing ACL tears, as well as treatment and management issues related to ACL injuries. It then moved into a discussion of how to counsel clients with ACL injuries. The primary goal of such counseling is to help clients return to a level of activity consistent with their wants and needs. The microskills model can be used successfully to counsel clients with ACL tears.

Study Questions

1. Describe the epidemiologic trends of ACL injuries over the past 20 years.
2. Why are ACL injuries a greater personal and public health problem for girls/women than boys/men?
3. What are the main goals of ACL injury counseling?
4. How is having an ACL injury similar to and different from having a chronic disease?
5. List and describe the risk factors for ACL injuries.
6. List and describe the six phases of ACL rehabilitation.
7. How does the acute nature of ACL injury affect the emotional responses of clients with this condition?
8. How can counselors with a history of ACL injuries use self-disclosure to influence clients?
9. How does changing the focal point help clients view their ACL injuries differently?
10. What are the key directives and logical consequences for each of the ACL counseling goals?

References

Adams E (2002). *An Increased Risk of ACL Rupture in Female Athletes.* Cincinnati: Midwest Institute of Sports Medicine, Epidemiology.

Andrews M (2000). *The knee.* In Swedan N (Ed.), *Women's Sports Medicine and Rehabilitation*, pp. 55–89. Gaithersburg, MD: Aspen Publishers.

Brandon R (2004). Anterior cruciate ligament (ACL) knee injury. *Peak Performance Online*. www.pponline.co.uk/encyc/0150.htm.

Brock C (January 22, 2001). An epidemic of injuries: recent rash of knee injuries in high school stem from inadequate training, physical play and gender. *News Tribune Tacoma*, p. B21.

Cincinnati Sports Medicine Research and Education Foundation (2000). *Sports Injury Test*. Cincinnati.

Cross MJ (February 26, 1998). Anterior cruciate ligament injuries: treatment and rehabilitation. In Fahey TD (Ed.). *Encyclopedia of Sports Medicine and Science*. Internet Society for Sport Science, http://sportsci.org.

Ford I, Gordon S (1999). Coping with sport injury: loss and the role of social support. *Journal of Personal and Interpersonal Loss* 4:1–13.

Griffin LY, Agel J, Albohm MJ, et al. (2000). Noncontact anterior cruciate ligament injuries: risk factors and prevention strategies. *Journal of American Academy of Orthopedic Surgery* 8:141–150.

Hewett TE (2000). Neuromuscular and hormonal factors associated with knee injuries in female athletes: strategies for intervention. *Sports Medicine* 29:313–327.

Hewett T, Lindenfeld T, Riccobene J, Noyes F (1999). The effect of neuromuscular training on the incidence of knee injury in female athletes. *American Journal of Sports Medicine* 27:6.

Hobfoll SE (1988). *The Ecology of Stress*. New York: Hemisphere.

Hospital for Special Surgery (HSS) (January 14, 2003). *Anterior Cruciate Ligament Tears*. http://orthopaedics.hss.edu/services/sports/acl_tears/index.asp.

Ireland ML (2002). *Why Are Women More Prone Than Men to ACL Injuries?* Hughston Clinic, www.hughston.com.

Ireland ML, Gaudette C, Crook M (1997). ACL injuries in the female athlete. *Journal of Sports Rehabilitation* 6:97–110.

Ivey AE, Ivey MB (2003). *Intentional Interviewing and Counseling: Facilitating Client Development in a Multicultural Society*. Pacific Grove, CA: Brooks/Cole.

Kubler-Ross E (1975). *Death: The Final Stage of Growth*. Englewood Cliffs, NJ: Prentice Hall.

Kujala UM, Orava S, Parkkari J, et al. (2003). Sports career-related musculoskeletal injuries: long-term health effects on former athletes. *Sports Medicine* 33:869–875.

Mausner JS, Kramer S (1985). *Epidemiology: An Introductory Text*. Philadelphia, PA: W. B. Saunders.

Smith I (2000). On bended knee: more girls are tearing ligaments in their knees. Here's what they can do to prevent it. *Time* 156:20.

United States Department of Health and Human Services (USDHHS), Office of Disease Prevention and Health Promotion (ODPHP) (2003). *Healthy People 2010: A Systematic Approach to Health Improvement*. www.healthypeople.gov/Document/html/uih/uih_bw/uih_2.htm#obj.

Wiese-Bjornstal D, Smith A, Shaffer S, Morrisey M (1998). An integrated model of response to sport injury: psychological and sociological dynamics. *Journal of Sport Psychology* 10:46–69.

Wojtys EM, Huston LJ, Boynton MD, et al. (2002). The effect of the menstrual cycle on anterior cruciate ligament injuries in women as determined by hormone levels. *American Journal of Sports Medicine* 30:182–188.

Woolston C (2000). Weak in the knees? An innovative fitness program is helping female athletes stay healthy. *WebMD Medical News*.

Yourmedicalsource.com (January 31, 2004). *Anterior Cruciate Ligament Tears: Diagnosing ACL Injuries*. yourmedicalsource.com/library/acltears/ACL_diagnosis.html.

Learning Objectives

By the end of the chapter students will:

1. Compare and contrast sexual disorders, sexual problems, and sexual worries

2. Describe the different DSM categories of sexual disorders

3. List and describe three common sexual problems

4. List and describe three common sexual worries

5. List and describe four common obstacles to discussing sexual concerns

6. Describe one approach to managing sexual concerns

7. Explain how the medicalization of sex counseling affects both clients and counselors

8. Differentiate the role of the sex counselor from the role of the sex therapist

9. Describe the application of the PLISSIT model to sex counseling

10. List and describe the goals of sexuality counseling

11. Describe the role of introductory skills in assessing clients' sex problems, concerns, and worries

12. Explain how body language is related to sexual communication between counselors and clients

13. Discuss the importance of language when discussing sexual issues

14. Describe how to use sexual self-disclosure appropriately

15. Discuss how changing the focal point can help clients view their sexual concerns from a different perspective

16. Describe the key directives for sex counseling

Introduction

Few areas of human behavior are more difficult to discuss than those involving sexual behavior. Patients are often very awkward and shy about discussing their sexual concerns. For many, it seems so private to discuss such matters, and many likely have had little practice in discussing these concerns with anyone—even their closest friends, family, or lovers. Nevertheless, while patients may find this topic to be a difficult area for discussion, they both want and need to be able to discuss such issues with their healthcare professionals. According to Candace Risen (2003), "They dread being asked, but they long to be asked."

It is not, however, only patients' discomforts that may impede the discussion of sexual problems and concerns. Many—if not most—health professionals have had little training and practice in discussing such matters. While most colleges and universities in the United States now offer a course in human sexuality, it is not a required part of the curriculum for many medical schools and other health-related professional programs. In addition, many of the biases and values that each of us holds regarding sexual behavior are not likely to have been examined in a thorough manner. As a consequence, healthcare professionals may subtly *discourage* patients from revealing what they may need to discuss most. According to William Maurice (1999), "Listening and talking skills in relation to sexual issues did not arise (unfortunately) from my medical school education or my specialty training in Psychiatry. Instructors in both settings were tongue-tied when considering anything sexual, but then again, this was the rule rather than the exception during those years."

Patients, although somewhat reluctant and fearful, really do want to discuss their sexual concerns. In one of the largest and most respected studies of sexual behavior in the United States, Laumann et al. (1994) concluded that adults are quite willing to talk about their sexual behavior providing that the interview is conducted in a respectful, confidential, and professional manner.

Overview of Sexual Concerns

According to psychiatrist Stephen Levine (2003), sexual concerns are classified into one of three broad classifications: sexual disorders, sexual problems, or sexual worries.

Sexual Disorders

Sexual disorders refer to those difficulties listed in the *Diagnostic and Statistical Manual of Mental Disorders* (DSM-IV-TR) of the American Psychological Association (2000). The DSM-IV-TR classifies sexual disorders as being either sexual dysfunctions, paraphilias, or gender identity disorders.

According to Wincze and Carey (2001), most sex therapists agree that sexual functioning comprises three primary stages: desire, arousal, and orgasm. **Sexual dysfunction** consists of an impairment or disturbance in one of these phases. For example, hypoactive sexual desire disorder, in which an individual complains of a low or absent level of sexual interest, and sexual aversion disorder, in which an individual complains of an aversion or avoidance of sexual behavior, would be considered disturbances of the desire phase of sexual response. Disorders such as female sexual arousal disorder (inability to attain or maintain sufficient vaginal lubrication) and male erectile disorder (inability to attain or maintain an adequate penile erection) would be considered disturbances of the arousal phase of sexual response. Disorders such as female orgasmic disorder (absence of female orgasm), male orgasmic disorder (absence of male orgasm), and premature ejaculation (lack of orgasmic control resulting in a rapid ejaculation) would represent disturbances of the orgasm phase of sexual response. In addition, the DSM-IV-TR lists sexual pain disorders such as dyspareunia (recurrent genital pain) and vaginismus (recurrent and involuntary vaginal spasms that make vaginal penetration unattainable) as sexual dysfunctions, inasmuch as they interfere with one's ability to engage in or enjoy sexual activity even though they are not related to any particular phase of the sexual response cycle.

Paraphilias are those sexual disorders in which an individual experiences recurrent and intense sexual urges and fantasies involving either nonhuman objects (i.e., a fetish), suffering or humiliation of oneself or one's partner (i.e., sadomasochism [see **Figure 12.1**]), or nonconsenting partners (i.e., pedophilia, exhibitionism, voyeurism, or frotteurism). This section of the DSM has received a great deal of attention recently because many sexologists consider it to be overly judgmental and unscientific. Moser (2001), for example, believes that individuals who have nonstandard sexual interests continue to be pathologized in the DSM, despite a lack of research establishing a difference in psychological functioning between those so diagnosed and "normal" individuals. Moser adds that little evidence suggests that those diagnosed with a paraphilia experience any distress or dysfunction except as a result of societal condemnation of their sexual interests and desires. Moser and other critics of the DSM are careful to point out, however, that they do not excuse illegal behaviors that intrude on or assault nonconsenting partners. Most sex therapists report that the majority of those patients seen in treatment for paraphilic

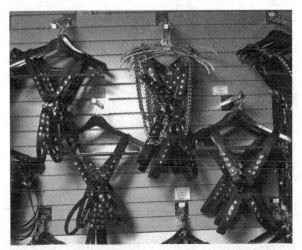

Figure 12.1 Paraphilias can take many forms including sadism and masochism. (© Cindy Charles/PhotoEdit)

disorders are not distressed by their behaviors. Indeed, many have no desire to stop engaging in such behaviors. Rather, they are dealing with *partners* who find the behavior distressing.

Gender Identity Disorder

Gender identity disorder (GID) is also known as transsexualism. Gender identity disorder is characterized by four criteria:

- a strong and persistent cross-gender identification
- persistent discomfort with his or her sex or a sense of inappropriateness in the gender role of that sex
- the absence of any genetic or physical abnormality (intersex condition such as androgen insensitivity)
- significant accompanying clinical psychological distress and impairment in social, occupational, or other functioning

Leavitt and Berger (1990) identified two forms of transsexualism: primary and secondary. Primary transsexuals are individuals who feel strong cross-gender identification from their earliest recollections of their childhood. Often, these individuals have clear cross-gender identification by age three. Secondary transsexuals begin to develop strong cross-gender identification in adulthood. Because secondary transsexuals have gone through infancy, childhood, adolescence, and early adulthood with same gender identification, shifting to their new cross-gender identification is more difficult.

There is much controversy surrounding the classification of GID, especially among secondary transsexuals. Transgender activists and those who serve transgendered clients claim that the "significant enough emotional, social, occupational, or other distress" that "interferes with their daily functioning" (quotes indicate DSM-IV criteria necessary for diagnosis) experienced by most transgendered men and women is not due to their gender identification but by societal reaction to it (Carroll et al., 2002; Klein, 2002; Isay, 1997). Citing this and other controversies surrounding the diagnostic category, Isay (1997) appealed to the American Psychiatric Association for the removal of the classification Gender Identity Disorder. In a rebuttal to Isay (1997), Friedman (1998) acknowledges the problems associated with misdiagnoses of some transgendered persons (especially adult homosexual men) but supports the continuation of the inclusion of the classification in the DSM-IV. Friedman (1998) cites that in comparisons of children with Gender Identity Disorder to others, the children with GID have much more psychopathology. Elimination of the GID classification, Friedman (1998) claims, would cause these children to fall through the cracks and not receive the psychiatric care they need.

Sexual Problems

Sexual problems are situations that, while not officially recognized as disorders in the DSM, may nevertheless cause significant distress for individuals experiencing them. For example, people who are distressed because of relationship problems may find that their stress interferes with their own or their partner's interest or willingness to engage in sex. Concerns and conflicts about one's sexual orientation or sexual interests would also be included in this category. In addition, men and women who have difficulty dealing with and accepting the age-related changes and challenges that their bodies experience—such as vaginal dryness or less firm erections—can be considered as having sexual problems.

Sexual Worries

Sexual worries are those concerns that Levine (2003) considers inherent in the experience of being human. Worries focus on issues such as the following questions: Will I be able to function adequately? Will my partner think well of me? Am I normal? Do other people feel/behave this way? Does my partner love me? Do I really love my partner? Will I be rejected if I express my interest in a particular sexual behavior?

While the treatment of sexual disorders may likely be beyond the scope of training for many sex counselors, helping patients deal with their sexual problems and worries is covered by the skill set of most well-trained counselors using the microskills approach. According to Weinstein and Rosen (1988), "One basic way of differentiating sexual dysfunctions (disorders) from sexual problems (and worries) is by ruling out a (DSM) dysfunction. That is, if an individual (or couple) experiences no difficulty in the desire, excitement (arousal), or orgasmic phases, then a dysfunction (disorder) is not present." However, even though counselors may wish to refer those clients experiencing sexual disorders to those trained in sex therapy, we can still prove quite helpful by being willing to listen to their sexual stories, offering encouragement, and assisting in making referrals to the appropriate resources.

Obstacles to Discussing Sexual Concerns

As mentioned previously, many patients may initially be shy and reluctant to discuss their sexual concerns with anyone, including healthcare professionals. Nevertheless, because of the trust and confidence that our patients place in us, we are in a particularly advantageous position to assist them in discussing such matters. It is, therefore, of the utmost importance that we be willing to ask our patients if they have any sexual questions/concerns. We have the opportunity, and the privilege, of being in a position where patients are willing to open up and share many of their innermost concerns, fears, and conflicts. As counselors, we are let into our patients' lives in a way that no others may be permitted entry. They tell us their "stories" and hope that we will listen in an open, accepting, and nonjudgmental manner.

Unfortunately, many healthcare professionals are uncomfortable with topics related to sexuality and "hide behind" the discomforts of patients in an attempt to rationalize not delving into such areas. According to Risen (2003), health profes-

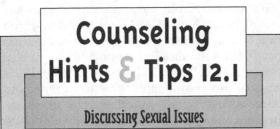

Counseling Hints & Tips 12.1

Discussing Sexual Issues

Many counselors who have not had much experience in discussing sexual issues with clients worry that they will be too embarrassed talking about sexual material, or that they won't know enough about sexuality to effectively address their clients' needs. If you have this concern, here are a few simple tips that you might find helpful.

1. Recognize that sexuality counseling is not much different from other types of health counseling in most ways.
2. You are probably better able to deal with these situations than you realize.
3. Try to listen to what the client is saying and remove the "sex" from the story. You will probably see that the underlying issue is really related to something you are quite familiar with (i.e., fear, anxiety, rejection, trust).
4. As long as you have practiced your microskills and can use them effectively, you will be able to assist your clients, at least somewhat, by just allowing them to tell their stories to someone who responds in a warm, supportive, and nonjudgmental manner.

Remember, the counselor's job is to assist clients in telling their stories and exploring ways to cope with their difficulties and concerns. Counselors are not expected to have all the answers and solve their problems for them!

sionals typically cite several reasons for not wanting to discuss sex with their patients:

- I'm not used to talking about sex—my discomfort and awkwardness will be obvious.
- I don't exactly know why I am asking or what I want to know.
- I won't know how to respond to what I hear.

- I may be unfamiliar with or not understand something my patient tells me.
- I may offend or embarrass my patient.
- I may be perceived as nosy or provocative.
- I won't know how to treat any problem I'm told about.
- I'll be too embarrassed to consult with my colleagues.

While this list is hardly exhaustive, it highlights some common concerns and fears of many members of the healthcare professions. While there are no easy "cures" for relieving these discomforts, listening to sexual stories and discussing sexual issues does become easier with training and practice. Also, even if we don't have the "answers" we think we should have, we can do a great deal of good by simply allowing clients to express their sexual fears or concerns to an authoritative and accepting person. We can often help simply by listening, making suggestions, or normalizing the concerns of patients. Remember, many patients really *want* to discuss sexual issues; they just need us to supply the opening for them to do so.

Helping Clients Manage Sexual Concerns

Throughout this chapter, the emphasis will be on reminding counselors that we are dealing with more than just "sexual problems." That is, we are dealing with *people* who are *experiencing* sexual difficulties and concerns. While this may seem like an obvious distinction, many sex counseling texts, while giving lip service to the notion of treating people instead of problems, have, in effect, reinforced the opposite view.

Many other sex counseling texts have devoted separate chapters to the treatment of a variety of sexual *problems,* thereby giving readers the impression that a particular problem, disorder, or syndrome should be treated with a standard protocol that is specific to that symptom or disorder, *regardless of how the individual or couple may experience the problem.* This approach suggests that one's sexuality or sexual functioning is separate and apart from the rest of one's personality or lifestyle. According to psychologist Peggy Kleinplatz (2001), "Perhaps one of the obstacles to broadening sex therapy has been the notion that it is somehow unique. The belief that dealing with sexuality is intrinsically different from dealing with other human issues and concerns has restricted our field." Accepting the notion that sexuality is not connected to the totality of the human experience prevents us from viewing a person's or a couple's sexual experience within the context of their life or relationship. In other words, if we focus solely on behavior, we miss the essence of the sexual experience for our patients as well as the most essential elements of the stories they are trying to relate to us.

The authors of this book have opted to view sexuality within the context of patients' larger life pictures. For that reason, we have not created separate sections covering topics such as "counseling the gay/lesbian/bisexual patient." This is not to say that a counselor doesn't need to know a bit about the lifestyle, culture, or community within which our patients exist, but rather that we must always remember that our patients are people first, as opposed to merely a constellation of symptoms.

Another problem with the creation of separate sections covering specific sexual concerns is that this approach tends to minimize, marginalize, and trivialize the individual experiences of our patients. For example, a separate chapter on treating gays/lesbians/bisexuals implies that (1) gay/lesbian/bisexual patients are somehow different from other patients, (2) the essence of their being is defined by their sexual orientation, (3) a standard set of therapy protocols should be used and applied in the same manner with all gay/lesbian/bisexual patients, and (4) all gay/lesbian/bisexual patients experience sexuality in the same way simply on the basis of having a particular sexual orientation. This would be akin to saying that all heterosexuals experience sexuality and sexual difficulties the same way simply because they are attracted to members of the opposite gender!

In this chapter, our focus is on more than just "sexual functioning" and "body parts." All too often, sexual counseling/therapy has focused on sexual "performance" as opposed to sexual "pleasure." Psychologist Sharon Nathan (2003) identifies two classic approaches to defining and understanding sexual problems and disorders. The *objective approach* compares sexual behavior with established standards of sexual functioning, identifying a point where good functioning ceases and dysfunction begins. The *functional approach* is not concerned with how a person's sexuality compares with that of others, but rather with how it promotes satisfaction or causes problems. According to Kleinplatz (2001), "As such, the major criterion for effective outcome remains performance. The focus is still on parts, not people; techniques rather than ways of being intimate in relationships." Clearly, both Kleinplatz and Nathan advocate an approach to sex counseling that focuses on the unique needs of each individual/couple seen by the counselor. They remind us of the importance of seeing our patients as *people* first and foremost, and listening carefully to the stories they tell us. Only by understanding sexuality in a context that is larger than just penises and vaginas will we become able to truly assist our patients in living more sexually satisfying lives.

The Medicalization of Sexuality Counseling

Recent years have resulted in many new medical treatments that are designed to assist patients with certain sexual problems, especially sexual dysfunctions/disorders. While a complete review of these discoveries is beyond the scope of this chapter, there is little doubt that the medical advance that has had the most significant impact on sexuality and sexual functioning has been the discovery of oral medications, such as sildenafil citrate (Viagra, see **Figure 12.2**), for the treatment of male erectile dysfunction. The introduction of Viagra and its competitors to the sex therapy scene has produced both positive and negative effects on how we conceptualize and treat sexual problems. On the positive side, we have been able to offer new and effective treatments to many men experiencing erectile disorders. The success of Viagra, and other drugs with similar effects, has spurred much-needed new research into the causes and treatments of many sexual dysfunctions. In addition, the advertising of these medications to the general public has made it much easier for patients to feel comfortable about bringing up their sexual concerns with their physicians or other healthcare professionals.

On the negative side, the intensive focus on the medical treatment options for sexual dysfunctions, or what has come to be referred to as "the **medicalization** of sex therapy," may reinforce the counterproductive notion that sex is merely a mechanical process (Watter, 2001). This idea has led many healthcare professionals, as well as the lay public, to assume that sexual problems are amenable to a "quick fix." The emphasis on a "simple" solution such as a pill has great appeal, but overlooks the complexities of the human condition. As psychologist Leonore Tiefer (1995) points out, "The primary disadvantage of med-

icalization is that it denies, obscures, and ignores the social cause of whatever problem is under study." Kleinplatz (2001) adds, "We continue to focus on symptoms rather than the context in which sex disappoints us, and in which we disappoint our sexual partners and vice versa."

When entering into a counseling relationship with patients who are experiencing sexual conflicts and concerns, counselors want to be sure that they are not tempted into looking too soon for the "quick fix." This is not to say that we do not want to encourage medical treatments for those patients who would truly benefit from them; indeed, many clients will be quite satisfied and happy with such options. However, even Pfizer Pharmaceuticals, the company that developed and sells Viagra, has admitted there are limits to medical treatments for sexual difficulties, especially with regard to the sexuality of women. In a recent *New York Times* article (Harris, 2004), Pfizer announced that it was abandoning its effort to show that Viagra would improve sexual functioning in women. After years of research, the company concluded that its data did not support the hypothesis that Viagra would improve sexual functioning for those women who were experiencing difficulty. In fact, the Pfizer researchers found that the sexual satisfaction of women was determined by many more factors, and was much more complicated, than focusing solely on genital responses would suggest (Salerian, Deibler, Vittone, et al., 2000; Basson, 2000).

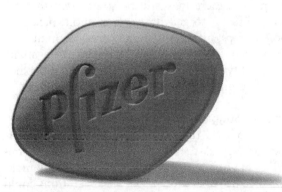

Figure 12.2 Viagra is one of the most widely prescribed drugs in the United States today. Reprinted with permission from Pfizer, Inc.

Counseling Clients with Sexual Concerns

As mentioned earlier, while the sexual disorders may be best handled by those with specialty training in sex therapy, sexual problems and worries can be well managed by the skilled health counselor. Being able to sit and discuss such private concerns with an attentive, accepting, and nonjudgmental professional can often be healing in and of itself. Unfortunately, many healthcare professionals are so busy and harried by the demands of their practice that they "rush" people through their sexual stories and miss the essential ingredients of what they are being told. For example, many patients have reported that they wanted very much to discuss their sexual concerns with their physicians, but the physician either seemed too busy or impatient to allow the story to unfold. Also, many in health care have been too narrowly trained in their approach to dealing with sexual issues and rush to fix "technical" problems, rather than remembering that they are dealing with "human" problems.

As sex counselors, we know that the majority of those who seek us out need to *talk* more about their sexuality and their sexual relationships. They may begin their discussions by talking about body parts, or the *mechanics* of sex, but they often really want and need to talk about the process of sex, or the *meaning* of sex in their lives. For many, when the "parts don't work," their bodies are telling them something. Our patients, at some level, know this, and we need to help them articulate their concerns and be willing to listen as they tell us their sexual stories.

The PLISSIT Model

Referring back to Risen's comments earlier in this chapter, we can consider some of the reasons why health counselors seem reluctant to discuss sexual matters with their patients. Some counselors are, perhaps, uncomfortable discussing sexual material, while others may be unsure how to respond or how far to take their responses.

In 1976, psychologist Jack Annon described a particularly helpful approach for addressing sexual concerns known as the **PLISSIT model**. The PLISSIT model describes several levels at which counselors can choose to respond to the concerns that patients bring to them. In the acronym PLISSIT, "P" stands for *permission,* "LI" stands for *limited information,* "SS" stands for *specific suggestions,* and "IT" stands for *intensive therapy.*

Permission

Some patients need only someone's permission to move past their sexual concerns. This statement does not mean that the health counselor makes judgments or acts in an overly authoritarian way to decide for patients which sexual behaviors are allowed. Rather, counselors can give clients "permission" to *speak* about their sexual concerns by listening in an active, accepting, and nonjudgmental manner to the stories that they tell. While this may not sound like a particularly powerful intervention, keep in mind that many patients have never felt comfortable with discussing, or been "allowed" to discuss, their sexual concerns with anyone before. For many reasons, they may have considered such topics to be too personal or embarrassing to bring up. It can be quite therapeutic just to let clients know that someone is willing to hear them and enter into a discussion of matters that may have been kept closeted for quite some time. Indeed, counselors' willingness to actively listen and not judge may be one of the greatest strengths of the counseling process.

Limited Information

Limited information refers to counselors' ability to assist patients in learning more about sexual functioning and behavior. We may be able to provide information about resources such as books, websites, and organizations (see **Figure 12.3**). While it is easier than ever before for people to access sex information, there may still be some areas that are more difficult to get information about (i.e., support groups, alternative sexual lifestyles), and patients may have little idea about how to evaluate the quality/credibility of the sex information they may find on their own.

Specific Suggestions

Depending on their level of comfort and expertise, as well as the needs of their patients, counselors may be able to assist some clients by making specific suggestions. Specific suggestions could include the use of a lubricant for vaginal dryness, vibrator, or other sexual aid, or a referral to another healthcare professional who may be more

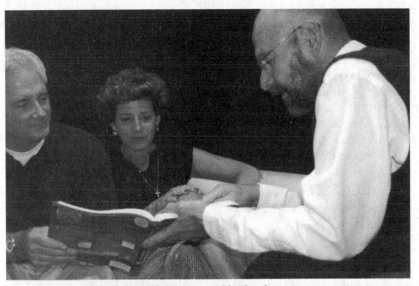

Figure 12.3 Therapist giving pamphlet/book. (Photo by Michael Blonna)

knowledgeable or skillful in treating or addressing a specific sexual concern.

Intensive Therapy

For those patients who may be experiencing a sexual disorder/dysfunction or who may be experiencing **co-morbid conditions** such as depression, anxiety, or relationship problems, intensive therapy may be indicated. This level of intervention is likely beyond the scope of practice and training of most health counselors, so it would be wise to refer patients in such situations to a qualified sex therapist. A listing of trained sex therapists can be found from organizations such as the Society for Sex Therapy and Research (SSTAR; www.sstarnet.org) and the American Association of Sex Educators, Counselors, and Therapists (AASECT; www.aasect.org).

Many health counselors will find the PLISSIT model to be useful. Quatman (1997) cautions, however, that the PLISSIT model, while helpful, skips over an essential set of interpersonal realities involved in handling sexual material. Specifically, sex often takes place within the context of a relationship, so focusing on body parts, or the *mechanics* of sex, can cause counselors to miss key components of their patients' sexual stories. More often than not, patients need to talk about how they *feel* about sex and sexuality; what sex and sexuality *mean* to them; and how sex and sexuality *affect* their daily lives, relationships, and sense of self.

Sexuality Counseling Using Microskills

Overall Goals of Sexuality Counseling

According to Weinstein and Rosen (1988), the goals of sexuality counseling are similar to the goals of counseling overall. That is, counselors seek to assist patients in enhancing coping skills, promoting decision making, improving developmental potential, and effecting positive behavioral change. In terms of sexuality counseling specifically, counselors seek to assist patients in becoming more comfortable with their sexuality, overcoming barriers and obstacles to sexual expression, improving communication about sexual matters, and coping with sexual difficulties. These goals are achieved through counselors' willingness to assist patients in speaking about sex and sexual difficulties, and through their ability to listen to clients' sexual stories without being critical, judgmental, or rejecting.

As mentioned previously, sexuality counseling presents a challenge to many health counselors due to the discomfort that many counselors and patients feel with regard to discussing sexual material. Many will find these topics to be extremely personal, perhaps embarrassing, and rarely discussed with others. While the PLISSIT model may be a good guide, the effective use of the microskills approach will ultimately allow counselors to establish effective therapeutic alliances with their patients.

Case Study 12.1
Mark

Mark is 20 years old, single, and heterosexual, and he identifies as Caucasian. A college sophomore, Mark was concerned about situational difficulties regarding his ability to maintain penile erections. Specifically, while he rarely had difficulty achieving erection with a partner, he would often be unable to maintain his erection long enough to have sexual intercourse. This situation would improve as Mark became more comfortable and familiar with his partner. As the relationship continued, Mark would find that his ability to function sexually during intercourse would gradually improve. After a few weeks to two months, there were no noticeable difficulties. Mark was concerned, however, because this pattern made him very reluctant and anxious about beginning new relationships. As a result, he often found himself either avoiding opportunities to meet new partners or avoiding opportunities to be sexual, even though he may have desired to do so.

Mark consulted with a nurse-practitioner at the college health center. While she did not suspect that there was anything medically wrong with Mark, she suggested a consultation with a local urologist who was knowledgeable about male sexual disorders. Mark met the urologist, who examined him and found him to be in good physical health. The urologist suggested that Mark might want to try some oral medication, such as Viagra, and consult with a counselor who was familiar with sexual

problems and concerns. Mark took the prescription for Viagra, but didn't feel comfortable with the idea of taking medication as a permanent solution.

Mark regularly exercised aerobically, watched his diet, smoked cigarettes, drank alcohol socially, and used marijuana occasionally. He was both relieved and perplexed to hear that there was nothing wrong with him physically. While pleased to know that his body was healthy, he worried that he might have a "psychological" problem, was concerned that it might mean he was "crazy," and was unsure how his condition could be treated. Mark was considerably distressed about his sexual function and decided to seek the assistance of a counselor.

Introductory Skills

As mentioned previously, topics related to their sexuality are among the most difficult for clients to discuss. Few subjects are considered more private, personal, and intimate. For this reason, counselors need to be cognizant of the importance of making clients feel as comfortable as possible from the outset. It is essential to set a tone that is encouraging, accepting, and nonjudgmental.

Identify Yourself

While it is important that counselors "experiment" and find a style of relating that is comfortable for them, I usually begin with a smile and a firm handshake, identifying the client by his or her full name.

Example

Counselor: (Smiling, extending hand) Mr. James, please come in. My name is Dan Watter.
Mark: Hello.

Note that I refer to the client as "Mr. James" and identify myself as "Dan Watter" as opposed to "Dr. Watter." Until I develop a relationship with the client, or unless he or she asks me to do otherwise, I use a title of Mr., Dr., Ms., and so on to convey an important degree of respect. In addition, note that many clients are somewhat intimidated by healthcare professionals, even though we may try our best to not come across as authoritarian. There is an inherent *power imbalance* in the relationship between patient and professional by virtue of the differences in their roles. As healthcare professionals, we are seen as people who are knowledgeable and in a more powerful position. Clients are coming to us for assistance; as such, they are likely to feel vulnerable and anxious. Therefore, using their surname helps to make them feel at less of a power disadvantage.

I also begin by using my first and last name instead of my professional title to help clients relax and feel more comfortable with me. I then allow them to choose how they would like to refer to me. Some appreciate the opportunity to call me by my first name; others prefer the more formal "Dr. Watter." I let them know that whatever makes them feel most comfortable is fine with me.

Following the introduction, invite the client to sit and begin with some basic, nonthreatening questions to allow them to ease into the session.

Example
Counselor: Did you have any difficulty finding my office?
   (If the client is wearing an interesting piece of clothing, such as a Knicks shirt, I might inquire if he or she is a basketball fan.)
Counselor: I notice you are wearing a Knicks jersey. Are you a Knicks fan?
Mark: Yeah, I've followed them for the past 20 years. I like to watch basketball on TV to relax.
Counselor: I know what you mean. I'm a Nets fan myself, but I really am more a fan of the game. I like to go out and shoot baskets in the driveway just to unwind.
Mark: Yeah, there's nothing like hoops!

Explain the Nature of Counseling, and Clarify the Client's and the Counselor's Roles
Following the exchange of pleasantries, begin by explaining a bit about the counseling process. This step is especially important for those clients who have not had any prior exposure to counseling. Explain that conversations between a client and a counselor are confidential, and identify the limits of confidentiality with regard to the counselor's particular discipline, state of practice, or policies of the agency/clinic or other healthcare setting. Also, explain to patients that it is not your job to pass judgment or impose your values on them, but rather that you want to help them to learn more about themselves and assist them in finding a way through this difficult time. Encourage clients to be as open and honest as possible, but tell them to feel free to proceed at a pace that is comfortable for them.

Example
Counselor: Mr. James, before we talk about what brought you here today, I'd like to go over a few things regarding my counseling methods and how we will work together.
Mark: Okay, but can you please call me Mark?
Counselor: Okay, Mark. Tell me about your experience with counseling.
Mark: I've never been in counseling before. I don't know what to expect.
Counselor: Let me start by saying that everything that we discuss is confidential. In my practice we stick to the following practices and policies [hands Mark a written copy of practice standards].
   It is not my job to pass judgment or impose my values on you, Mark. I am here to help you learn more about yourself, and to assist you in finding a way through this difficult time.
   For this to happen, I need you to be as open and honest with me as possible, but to feel free to proceed at a pace that is comfortable for you.
Mark: That seems fair, Dr. Watter.
Counselor: Great, Mark. If it makes you more comfortable, you can call me Dan.
Mark: It feels a little strange. Do you mind if I call you Dr. Watter?
Counselor: Not at all.
Mark: Is it all right if I smoke? I am pretty nervous and it helps calm me down.
Counselor: I'm sorry, Mark, but I don't allow smoking in my offices. If you wish, you can

step outside into the smoker's lounge for a few minutes.

Mark: Okay, I'll be right back.

Counselor: (When Mark returns) Mark, because smoking is implicated in erectile disorders in men, I am going to give you this material to read. I'd like to talk to you a little about your smoking during future visits. If you would like help in quitting, I know some excellent resources for doing so.

Mark: Thanks.

While counselors hope for complete honesty and openness from their patients from the outset, this will often not be the case. Sexual concerns, like many other concerns of counseling clients, are difficult to talk about with anyone, especially someone you may have just met and are unsure how much to trust. Clients' stories often evolve over time. As patients become more comfortable, they are likely to reveal more about their concerns.

Set Goals for the Session(s)

Counselors must be patient and not push too much too soon for details. In addition, they need to be careful to not "rush in too quickly" by providing suggestions or "solutions" to clients' problems, as counselors may get the *full* story rather slowly and in bits and pieces. The need to be patient with the *process* of counseling is a point that cannot be emphasized enough.

Transition to the Client's Story

A good way to make the transition from the introduction to getting clients to tell their stories is to use an open-ended question. A question such as "How can I be of help today?" or "Tell me what brings you in today" allows clients to begin their stories at a place that feels comfortable to them. If you know in advance what the client's concern is, you might give a bit more of a leading question—for example, "I understand you have some concerns about your sexual functioning during intercourse. Would you like to tell me about that?" An open-ended question allows clients to begin their stories at a point of their choosing. It also encourages clients to be more expansive in the telling of their stories, so they may have an easier time relating the important details. Beginning counselors often use too few open-ended questions and too many closed questions. Closed questions often cut off the flow of conversation, so that many essential details are never discussed. As with most things in life, practice, practice, practice and you will improve in your skillfulness of knowing when it is appropriate to use both open-ended and closed questions.

Example
Counselor: I understand that you were referred to me by your urologist, Dr. Michaelson. Tell me about the difficulty you've been having, and let's see how I can be of help.

Mark: Well, I'm not sure how to begin. I've been having difficulty with, you know, my abilities.

Clearly, Mark is nervous and unsure how to describe his problem. He also seems somewhat embarrassed about both the problem and the need to discuss such personal material.

Attending Skills
Attending skills set the tone for the session to follow. As mentioned previously, sexual material is among the most difficult topics for clients to address. They are often hesitant about opening up regarding their sexual concerns because they may be embarrassed or guilty about their behavior or afraid of being judged unfavorably by the counselor. Therefore, it is especially important that the counselor set a warm, encouraging, and welcoming tone for the session.

Attending skills are those skills that counselors employ not only to make them better listeners to their clients' stories, but also to better communicate to clients that they are interested, concerned, and *listening*. According to Ivey et al. (1997a), four key dimensions make up attending behavior: eye contact, attentive body language, vocal style, and verbal following. While these are rather simple skills to understand, they only become effective tools with practice, practice, and more practice!

Nonverbal Skills
There is a good chance you will hear stories that stand in contrast to your personal sexual attitudes, values, and behaviors. Some of these stories might make you feel uncomfortable. It is important not to show this discomfort through nonverbal cues related to your body language and eye contact.

Often, when confronted with sexual stories that make them uncomfortable, counselors will inadvertently tense individual body parts or major areas or avert eye contact. For instance, clenching and unclenching the hands may signal the client that something about his or her story is making you uncomfortable.

Avoiding eye contact because dealing with the client makes the counselor feel uncomfortable is another behavior to guard against. While it is normal to look away and periodically break eye contact, averting the eyes when clients are talking may indicate to them that you are having trouble hearing their concerns.

For example, in the case study, the counselor working with Mark may be unaccustomed to hearing about sexual problems from such a young man. The idea that a young man is not "eager and willing to have sex whenever the opportunity may arise" may be quite surprising to some. Counselors need to be sure that if they are, indeed, surprised to hear such a story, they do not display their discomfort or surprise with a tightening body motion or facial expression. Many new counselors worry that they will give too much away with their nonverbal reactions, but it is important to note that we often feel more discomfort on the inside than we display on the outside. Even so, remember that as counselors become more experienced and practiced in handling sexual concerns, they will tend to feel much less discomfort and respond to clients much more effectively.

Example
As Mark begins to describe his reason for coming to see the counselor, his body tenses and he averts eye contact. The counselor senses Mark's discomfort and makes a mental note that this topic is embarrassing and difficult for Mark to talk about.

diverse perspectives 12.1

Sexual Minorities

Typically when we think about "diversity," we think in terms of racial, ethnic, or religious groups. We also need to be aware of individuals who are considered "sexual minorities." We live in a predominantly heterosexual world and are often quite judgmental of those who live sexual lives, or have sexual preferences, that run counter to the "mainstream." It is important to recognize that no valid and reliable psychological measures would suggest any type of psychopathology based simply on sexual orientation or preference. That is, while some individuals may participate in a sexual lifestyle or behavior that we may not feel comfortable with, we need to recognize that this reaction is more a measure of our level of discomfort than it is a measure of their level of sexual health.

In this chapter's case study, Mark is a heterosexual male. Would it be any more difficult for you to help him if he were gay? If so, you need to reexamine the role of the counselor and your own reactions (counter-transferences) to people who may be quite different from yourself. Effective counseling always puts the client first. It does not focus on the counselor and the counselor's own "politics." It is imperative that the counselor stay focused on the client's agenda and needs, regardless of his or her racial, ethnic, religious, or sexual status.

Responding Skills

Nonverbal Minimal Encouragers

When you are uncomfortable with certain issues, your body language and eye contact will often reflect that discomfort. When dealing with sexual concerns, it is crucial that the counselor's body language and nonverbal feedback come across to the client as nonjudgmental. Discomfort about being judged is a major barrier when clients try to tell you about their sexual concerns/problems/conflicts. Try to maintain a relaxed posture, and periodically scan your body for signs of tension that might be transmitted to clients. Chapter 3 showed what open and closed body language looks like. Try especially hard to avoid judgmental poses such as folding your arms over your chest.

Clients also send out nonverbal messages about how they feel when telling certain parts of their stories. Pay attention to the same attributes in your clients that you do with yourself. Aversion of eye contact, tension, and closed body posture all might indicate unspoken concerns that you may need to address at the appropriate time. They could also represent discrepancies between *what* is being said and *how* it is being said.

Example

The counselor, sensing that Mark is uncomfortable, makes sure he is relaxed, faces Mark squarely, and adopts an open, approachable body position. In addition, the counselor nods his head, makes direct eye contact, and maintains a sympathetic look—all signals to Mark that the counselor is approachable and understands how difficult it is for Mark to talk about this topic.

Verbal Minimal Encouragers

Simple "uh huhs," key words, and mirroring are very important tools that can be used to encourage clients to continue their stories. They are especially helpful with sensitive sexual subjects because they demonstrate acceptance and assist in keeping clients talking.

Open Invitation to Talk

Using questions to clarify sexual information is very important because intimate relationships and behaviors are often quite confusing. Making sure that you understand who is doing what with whom on what occasions requires a skillful, nonjudgmental use of questioning skills.

Open-Ended Questions and Statements

One helpful way to clarify sensitive sexual information with clients is to use open-ended statements and questions liberally to create a more re-laxed, conversational tone. It is better to get the answers to a series of individual sexual questions by asking the client one or two open-ended questions than by asking a series of yes/no (closed) questions. The use of open-ended questions is often seen as a less intrusive way to gather necessary data. This technique allows you to listen more and observe how the client comes across. Rather than having to focus on which closed question to ask next, you can sit back and listen to the client. You can always use closed questions to go back and clarify any missing information.

Example

Counselor: Tell me about the difficulty you've been having, and let's see how I can be of help.

Mark: Well, I'm not sure how to begin. I've been having difficulty with, you know, my abilities.

Clearly, Mark is nervous and unsure how to describe his problem. He also seems somewhat embarrassed about both the problem and the need to discuss such personal material.

Counselor: Uh huh.

The counselor nods his head (nonverbal minimal encourager) and uses a verbal minimal encourager to get Mark to continue talking.

Counselor: I know this isn't always easy to talk about, but could you tell me what you mean by your "abilities"?

The counselor uses an open-ended question to get clarification and to give Mark an opportunity to expand on his answer.

Mark: Well, you know, when I want to have sex with a woman, I don't get hard.

Counselor: I see. So when you want to have sex with a partner, you are unable to get an erection?

The counselor uses a minimal encourager ("I see") to let Mark know that he is listening to his story, and follows it with a closed question ("So when you want to have sex with a partner, you are unable to get an erection?") to get clarification that the counselor has understood Mark correctly.

Mark: Yeah, that's right. It's been really embarrassing for me.

Paraphrasing, Reflection of Feelings, and Summarizing

Paraphrasing and reflection of feelings work similarly for sexual counseling clients as they do for clients presenting with most other concerns. The major difference is the wide range of emotions associated with sexual issues and material. Because they often relate not only to the individual but also to a partner, sexual conflicts and concerns may evoke strong emotions associated with a partner and their relationship.

Paraphrasing judiciously throughout clients' stories will help you clarify how they view their difficulty and its relationship to their sexual partners. This technique will also aid you in reflecting clients' feelings toward themselves and their partners. Getting to the feelings associated with having sexual problems can greatly facilitate the counseling process.

Once clients' thoughts and feelings about their situations are expressed, summarization helps clarify what each client is thinking and feeling. It is an opportunity for clients to hear the stories again and decide whether anything needs to be added, deleted, or clarified. It also shows them how well you are following and your assessment of the situation.

Example

Counselor: Embarrassing. I'll bet it's a tough situation for you.

The counselor uses reflection of feeling to let Mark know that he is following him.

Mark: Oh, yeah. I'm so nervous and afraid of approaching women. I just keep thinking, what if they expect to have sex, and I'm unable to do it? When it happens, I get so embarrassed that I just want to disappear. I don't even want to meet people anymore.

Counselor: Tell me, Mark, how long has this been a problem for you?

The counselor uses a closed question to get some specific details.

Mark: It's been a problem ever since I began having sex. I guess that would be about three years.

Counselor: Are there any times when you do not have a problem?

The counselor uses a closed question to get one more piece of information about Mark's story.

Mark: Well, yeah, there are times that I'm fine.

Counselor: Can you tell me about them?

Again, the counselor asks open-ended questions to get more details and to give Mark an opportunity to expand on his story.

Mark: It seems I have the problem only when I'm with women in the beginning of the relationship. After I'm with them for a couple of months, my sexual problems seem to get better.

Counselor: I see. Let me be sure I understand you correctly. You're telling me that you have problems with erections when you want to have intercourse with women, and this has been very embarrassing for you. However, if you are able to spend enough time with a woman—that is, if the relationship continues for a couple of months—your erection problems seem to disappear. Is that right?

The counselor uses a paraphrase to allow Mark to hear what he has told him, and to give him an opportunity to correct any misunderstandings. The use of paraphrasing also lets Mark know that he is listening carefully to his story.

Mark: Yeah. That's it exactly.

Counselor: Okay, good. As a result of this difficulty in the beginning of a sexual relationship, you have become unwilling to get involved in new relationships because you're afraid it will place you in an embarrassing situation if you can't function sexually the way you would like to. That sounds like a lot of pressure!

The counselor uses a summary that includes a paraphrase of the content followed by a reflection of feeling.

Mark: Oh, man, yeah. I feel pressured about it all the time. I don't know what to do anymore.

Influencing Skills

Self-disclosure

As we mentioned in Chapter 5, self-disclosure can be an excellent technique for building confidence in clients regarding their perceived ability to make changes in their lives/relationships. Self-disclosing to clients that you, the counselor, know what they are going through because you have dealt with difficult situations yourself is one way to do so.

It is *extremely* important to remember, however, that any self-disclosure should be done with the client's benefit in mind. You must be careful that you (or your client) do not use this self-disclosure to shift the conversation or focus of the counseling onto you. This technique should be employed solely to strengthen the relationship between you and your client. By self-disclosing, you are merely trying to establish a connection with the client and empower him or her by providing encouragement regarding the possibilities for change.

Confrontation

Confrontation will come into play extensively, especially when responding to incongruities related to clients' stories. Clients may tell discrepant stories for a variety of reasons. Many clients mistrust health professionals and are not sure how their stories will be received. Sometimes, they may be uncertain about whether their confidentiality will be maintained. Clients may also be embarrassed about their sexual activities/concerns and will discuss only parts of their stories and withhold other parts, especially if they sense any judgmentalism coming from the counselor.

Many clients who have discrepancies in their stories are trying to hide some facet of the story that is either too difficult for them to deal with or they feel will lead to too many problems if discussed. However, don't let clients' hesitancy to be all revealing in the early part of counseling discourage you. Counseling requires a great deal of patience, and clients need to feel comfortable with their counselors before they will let us into their lives. Even the most experienced counselors do not get all of the relevant information right away. Clients often hold a bit back until they feel more trusting of the counselor. This tendency explains why trust, acceptance, and a nonjudgmental environment are so crucial for effective counseling work. This is especially true when the concerns deal with the sexual realm. Also, remember that the technique of confrontation is not meant to provoke a conflict with the client. Instead, as Ivey et al. (1997b) remind us, confrontation in counseling situations is designed to assist clients in identifying discrepancies and incongruities in their lives. The objective of confrontation is to help clients see things about their lives and behaviors that they may not have seen before.

Example

Counselor: Mark, I can really sense your frustration right now, because I'm feeling similar emotions thinking about how you are choosing to handle this situation. You seem to be placing yourself in somewhat of a bind. If you are aware that your erectile difficulties seem to improve over time, but you are reluctant to initiate new relationships, you seem to be cutting yourself off from the prospect of finding the person with whom you would like to have a relationship.

The counselor begins with a self-disclosure statement to let Mark know how he is experiencing his distress. He then follows with a gentle confrontation designed to point out to Mark the inconsistency in his approach to the situation.

Mark: I see what you mean, but I just feel so embarrassed. I'm so afraid that women will think I'm not really a "man" or that I'm "weak."

Interpretation of Meaning and Reframing

The art of interpretation and reframing is one of the most powerful techniques a counselor can develop. In the microcounseling model, interpretation is the ability to interpret or reframe a problem or concern so as to redefine "reality" (feelings, attitudes, behaviors, situations) from a new point of view (Ivey et al., 1997b). It does not simply mean that counselors try to put a "positive spin" on whatever clients may be struggling with or try to "talk clients out of feeling a certain way." Rather, counselors try to give clients a new way to interpret, or frame, their experiences through a different lens.

Example

Counselor: (Continuing where Mark left off) I know that puts you in a tough spot, Mark. You are afraid of appearing unmanly or weak. However, did you ever consider that some women might see your patterns as one of extreme "sensitivity and caring" as opposed to something so negative?

The counselor begins with a brief empathic paraphrase, followed by interpretation/reframing to give Mark an opportunity to see his "reality" through a different lens or perspective.

Mark: Well, no, I never considered that possibility. Do you think it might really be seen that way by women?

Counselor: I think many women might see it that way. How do you feel about seeing it that way?

It is very important to check out with clients how they feel about your interpretation/reframing. For it to be helpful, it must resonate with the client.

Mark: I like that. I mean, I think I really am a sensitive person, and I have thought that at least some women would appreciate the fact that I don't sleep around.

Counselor: I think you're on to something there, Mark. Suppose we try an exercise of sorts that is designed to assist you in becoming more comfortable with this new insight?

The counselor wants to engage Mark in the helping process before suggesting any directives.

Mark: What kind of exercise?

Directives and Logical Consequences

According to Ivey et al. (1997b), directive giving is the clearest example of some helpers' desire to influence others. To communicate directives to clients effectively, counselors must remember three basic points. The counselor's directives must (1) have appropriate verbal and nonverbal behavior to support the directive, (2) be concrete and clear, and (3) include a "checking-out" with the client as to whether the directives were understood and agreed upon.

While directives can be quite helpful in the counseling setting, the counselor must be aware that they can be easily overused. In that case, they will compromise the counselor's ability to assist clients in being able to make their own decisions. Remember, counseling is not about making decisions for clients or telling them how best to live their lives. As counselors, we want to empower our clients with the confidence to make life and health-related decisions, and the willingness to be responsible and accountable for those decisions.

The logical consequences are the outcomes clients can expect (both positive and negative) if they follow the directives.

Directive 1: Do Homework to Develop Positive Feelings

1. Have the client visualize the positive aspects of his sensitivity.
2. Have the client repeat how his sensitive nature is a positive sexual attribute.

Logical Consequences of Doing Homework to Develop Positive Feelings

1. Clients will begin to develop a picture of sensitivity as a positive attribute.
2. Clients' inability to develop erections will begin to lessen.

Specific Instructions for Doing Homework to Develop Positive Feelings

1. Have the client close his eyes.
2. Have the client repeat to himself several times that his sexual function is more a reflection of his sensitive side than of any weakness.

Example

Counselor: A type of "homework" actually. How would you feel about taking five minutes, three times a day, to simply close your eyes and repeat to yourself over and over that "my sexual function is more a reflection of my sensitive side than it is of any weakness I may have"?

Mark: Yeah, I could do that. I think I would even like to do that!

Counselor: Great, Mark. I think it could be quite helpful. Let's go over the instructions again. Tell me what you have understood the homework assignment to be.

It is very important to verify that you and your client have the same understanding of the directive.

Mark: I'm going to close my eyes for five minutes, three times a day, and just think to myself, "My sexual functioning is more a reflection of my sensitive side than it is of any weakness I may have."

Counselor: Sounds good to me, Mark. Now let's talk about when we can meet again to discuss this further.

Here the counselor and client confirm their understanding of the directive and make plans for follow-up.

Directive 2: Use PLISSIT to Provide "Limited Information"

Recall that the PLISSIT model describes several levels of possible intervention. In this acronym, "P" stands for *permission,* "LI" stands for *limited information,* "SS" stands for *specific suggestions,* and "IT" stands for *intensive therapy.* The counselor can choose which level of intervention would be most appropriate depending on the client's situation and the counselor's comfort and expertise in dealing with the particulars of the client's problem. In Mark's case, *permission* has already been granted by the counselor's willingness to listen attentively and nonjudgmentally to his story. This activity, in and of itself, can be extremely therapeutic and reassuring to the client. Many clients will be revealing information about themselves that they may never have told anyone before. The act of telling someone who is open and accepting something that they may have been conflicted about can provide almost an immediate relief for many clients.

1. Give the client material to read and websites to visit.
2. Have the client take an erectile dysfunction (ED) self-assessment.

Logical Consequences of Using PLISSIT to Provide "Limited Information"

1. Clients will become more knowledgeable about ED.
2. Clients will realize that their problems are not organic and can be resolved through psycho-education.

Specific Instructions for Using PLISSIT to Provide "Limited Information"

1. Have the client read the pamphlets, reprints, and other materials provided by the counselor.
2. Have the client visit the ED website.
3. Have the client fill out the ED assessment form.

4. Suggest that the client come prepared to discuss this material during the next visit.

Example

Counselor: Mark, sometimes it is helpful to read some material about erectile dysfunction to see that it is very common in men and that you are not alone with this problem.

Mark: What did you have in mind?

Counselor: I'd like you to read these materials [hands Mark a few reprints and pamphlets] and take this self-assessment. It is taken from this website [gives Mark the URL]. When you are done, I want you to write down how your problem compares with that of other men experiencing the same concern. We'll talk about this next week. How does that sound?

Mark: Sounds okay—it reminds me of school.

Counselor: A lot of counseling is like school. Ideally, you will learn a lot of important things about your sexuality, which will help you.

Directive 3: Provide Specific Suggestions Regarding Losing and Regaining Erections

Depending on the level of comfort and expertise counselors may have with the treatment of sexual concerns, they may decide to intervene at the next level, *specific suggestions.* Such suggestions may include behavioral exercises that are designed to build confidence in erections (Zilbergeld, 1992) or cognitive disputing exercises (Ellis, 1973; Beck, 1976) that may assist in dealing with anxiety about approaching new partners and/or coping with erectile difficulties.

1. Suggest a behavioral exercise to practice gaining/losing erections.
2. Explain that the goal of the exercise is to become more confident in the ability to regain an erection if the initial erection subsides.

Logical Consequences of Providing Specific Suggestions Regarding Losing and Regaining Erections

1. Clients will become more confident in the erectile functioning of the penis.
2. Clients will experience less anxiety regarding the possibility of erectile loss.

Specific Instructions for Providing
Specific Suggestions Regarding
Losing and Regaining Erections

1. Stroke your penis with a lubricated hand and focus either on the sensations produced or on an exciting fantasy.
2. When you have an erection, enjoy it for a moment and then stop stimulation.
3. Take your hand away from your penis and let your erection subside completely, which may take from a few seconds to a few minutes.
4. When your penis is soft, resume stimulation and focus on the sensation or fantasy.
5. Most of the time your erection will return, in which case you should again stop and let the penis become soft.
6. Two complete cycles of this sequence—stimulation, erection, stopping, losing erection, stimulation—are sufficient for one session.
7. If your erection does not return within a few minutes after resuming stimulation, ask yourself if there is anything you can do to get into a more relaxed and more arousing frame of mind.
8. Repeat as necessary with at least one day's rest between sessions (Zilbergeld, 1992).

Example

Counselor: Mark, I would like to ask if you would be willing to practice a type of behavioral exercise designed to help you develop more confidence in your ability to regain your erection, even if you should have a problem and lose it.

Mark: Yeah, I guess so. Anything that would make me feel more confident would be good.

Counselor: Great. Let me tell you how the exercise works [give Mark the instructions], and then you can tell me if it sounds reasonable to you.

Mark: Okay. That sounds good to me.

Counselor: I'm glad. Now I would like you to make some notes after each practice session and bring them with you on your next visit.

We can discuss what you noticed, learned, and felt as you worked on this exercise. Is that okay? Is there anything you would like to go over again regarding the assignment?

Mark: No, I think I've got it. I'm ready to proceed!

Counselor: Good, Mark. I will look forward to seeing you next time.

Summary

This chapter provided both information and reassurance for the counselor working with clients who are experiencing sexual difficulties and concerns. While the discussion of sexual issues may be quite difficult for many clients (and counselors), clients really do value the opportunity to open up and discuss such private and personal concerns with an open, accepting, and nonjudgmental health professional.

It is crucial that the counselor view clients as *people experiencing sexual concerns* as opposed to viewing them, and their sexuality, as being simply a set of *functional/mechanical problems*. The use of the microskills approach allows the counselor to attend and respond to clients in an appropriate and helpful manner. The use of Annon's PLISSIT model, which allows the counselor to respond in a manner that is consistent with his or her level of comfort and expertise, provides useful guidance regarding the appropriate level of counselor intervention.

Study Questions

1. How are sexual disorders, sexual problems, and sexual worries similar and different?
2. Describe the three categories of sexual disorders specified in the DSM-IV-TR.
3. Discuss three common sexual problems encountered by counselors.
4. What are the most common sexual worries expressed by clients?
5. Describe three client obstacles to discussing sexual concerns.

6. What approach to managing sexual concerns does this book recommend?

7. What is meant by the "medicalization" of sexuality counseling?

8. How does the medicalization of sexuality counseling affect clients' perceptions of sexuality counseling and dealing with sexual disorders, problems, and worries?

9. How does the nature and practice of sexuality counseling differ from sex therapy?

10. What does the acronym PLISSIT mean?

11. Pick a sexual concern and describe how you would apply the PLISSIT model when counseling someone with it.

12. What are the major goals of sexuality counseling?

13. How are introductory skills used to assess clients' sex problems, concerns, and worries?

14. How do clients communicate sexual information through their body language?

15. How do sexual language and sexual communication differ from other forms of communication between clients and counselors?

16. What are some of the cautions when using sexual self-disclosure with clients?

17. How does changing the focal point help clients view their sexual concerns from a different perspective?

18. Describe the key directives for sex counseling.

References

American Psychological Association (2000). *Diagnostic and Statistical Manual of Mental Disorders,* 4th ed. *Text Revision.* Washington, DC: American Psychological Association.

Annon J (1976). The PLISSIT model. *Journal of Sex Education and Therapy* 2:1–15.

Basson R (2000). The female sexual response: a different model. *Journal of Sex and Marital Therapy* 26:51–65.

Beck AT (1976). *Cognitive Therapy and the Emotional Disorders.* New York: Meridian.

Carroll L, Gilroy PJ, Ryan J (2002). Counseling transgendered, transsexual, and gender-variant clients (practice and theory). *Journal of Counseling and Development* Spring 80(2):131–140.

Ellis A (1973). *Humanistic Psychotherapy.* New York: McGraw-Hill.

Friedman RC (1998). Gender identity. *Psychiatric News: Viewpoints.* January 19. www.payxh.org/pnews/98-01019/gender.html.

Harris G (February 28, 2004). Pfizer gives up testing Viagra on women. *New York Times,* C1.

Isay RA (1997). Remove gender identity from DSM. *Psychiatric News: Viewpoints.* November 21. www.psych.org/pnews/97/-11-21/isay.html.

Ivey AE, Gluckstern NB, Ivey MB (1997a). *Basic Attending Skills,* 3rd ed. North Amherst, MA: Microtraining Associates.

Ivey AE, Gluckstern NB, Ivey MB (1997b). *Basic Influencing Skills,* 3rd ed. (videotape). North Amherst, MA: Microtraining Associates.

Klein JA (2002). A sex of one's own (book review of *How Sex Changed: A History of Transsexuality in the United States*). *The Nation* 274(19):33–39.

Kleinplatz PJ (2001). A critical evaluation of sex therapy: room for improvement. In Kleinplatz PJ, (Ed.). *New Directions in Sex Therapy: Innovations and Alternatives,* pp. xi–xxxii. New York: Brunner/Routlege.

Laumann EO, Gagnon JH, Michael RT, Michaels S (1994). *The Social Organization of Sexuality: Sexual Practices in the United States.* Chicago, IL: University of Chicago Press.

Leavitt F, Berger JC (1990). Clinical patterns among male transsexual candidates with erotic interest in males. *Archives of Sexual Behavior* 19(5):491–505.

Levine SB (2003). Preface. In Levine SB, Risen CB, Althof SE, (Eds.). *Handbook of Clinical Sexuality for Mental Health Professionals.* New York: Brunner/Routlege.

Maurice WL (1999). *Sexual Medicine in Primary Care.* St. Louis, MO: Mosby.

Moser C (2001). Paraphilia: a critique of a confused concept. In Kleinplatz PJ (Ed.). *New Directions in Sex Therapy: Innovations and Alternatives.* New York: Brunner/Routlege.

Nathan S (2003). When do we say a woman's sexuality is dysfunctional? In Levine SB, Risen CB, Althof SE (Eds.). *Handbook of Clinical Sexuality for Mental Health Professionals.* New York: Brunner/Routlege.

Quatman T (1997). Talking and thinking about sexuality. In Charlton RS (Ed.). *Treating Sexual Disorders.* San Francisco, CA: Jossey-Bass.

Risen CB (2003). Listening to sexual stories. In Levine SB, Risen CB, Althof SE (Eds.). *Handbook of Clinical Sexuality for Mental Health Professionals.* New York: Brunner/Routlege.

Salerian AJ, Deibler WE, Vittone BJ, et al. (2000). Sildenafil for psychotropic induced sexual dysfunction in 31 women and 61 men. *Journal of Sex and Marital Therapy* 26:133–140.

Tiefer L (1995). *Sex Is Not a Natural Act and Other Essays.* Boulder, CO: Westview Press.

United States Department of Health and Human Services (USDHHS), Office of Disease Prevention and Health Promotion (ODPHP) (2003). *Healthy People 2010: A Systematic Approach to Health Improvement.* www.healthypeople.gov/Document/html/uih/uih_bw/uih_2.htm#obj.

Watter DN (2001). What's new in . . . sex therapy. *New Jersey Psychologist* Winter:13–18.

Weinstein E, Rosen E (1988). *Sexuality Counseling: Issues and Implications.* Pacific Grove, CA: Brooks/Cole.

Wincze JP, Carey MP (2001). *Sexual Dysfunction: A Guide for Assessment and Treatment,* 2nd ed. New York: Guilford Press.

Zilbergeld B (1992). *The New Male Sexuality.* New York: Bantam Books.

Abortion Termination of an established pregnancy through surgical or nonsurgical techniques.

Abstinence Practicing self-restraint. Abstinence is often taken to mean not having sexual intercourse.

Abstraction ladder The continuum of clarity in clients' thinking. It ranges from crystal clear to very ambiguous.

Action stage The stage in which clients are actively working on changing.

Active listening Listening that requires feedback. Active listeners show that they are listening by providing both nonverbal and verbal feedback.

Actual use effectiveness The percentage of women who get pregnant while using a contraceptive method for one year.

Adherence A measure of how well patients comply with therapeutic regimens that they actively develop with medical professionals.

Aldosterone A hormone that helps regulate the body's sodium and water balance by retaining sodium and water and excreting potassium.

Allergens Particles of protein matter such as pollen or molds, dust mite or cockroach droppings, or dog or cat dander, urine, or saliva.

Amenorrhea The absence of menstruation at some time after a female has reached menses.

Angiotensin A hormone that triggers the release of aldosterone.

Anilingus Oral stimulation of the anus.

Animal dander A protein found in the saliva, dead skin flakes, and urine of fur-bearing animals.

Anterior cruciate ligament (ACL) A ligament that lies in the middle of the knee. It prevents the tibia from sliding out in front of the femur, and provides stability to the knee as it rotates.

Anterior drawer test An ACL injury test that starts with the knee bent to 90 degrees.

Antileukotrienes Oral medications that block leukotrienes, powerful chemicals that are involved in the constriction and swelling of airways associated with asthma.

Atherosclerosis The narrowing and hardening of the arteries caused by the buildup of fatty cholesterol plaques on the inner walls of arteries.

Auditory An orientation to life that describes the world in terms of sound.

Barrier methods Nonsurgical contraceptive measures that prevent the sperm and egg from uniting.

Basal body temperature (BBT) The lowest body temperature of a healthy person during waking hours.

Behavioral intention When clients intend to engage in behavior change activities.

Behavioral theories Theories founded on the belief that insight is not necessary to produce behavioral/emotional change.

Beta-agonists Quick relief rescuers that stimulate beta-receptors, relaxing smooth muscle and opening the bronchioles.

Birth control The broadest term covering all methods designed to prevent the birth of a child.

Body language Nonverbal messages we send through posture, gestures, movement, and physical appearance, including adornment. Our body language intentionally or unintentionally sends messages to receivers.

Body mass index (BMI) A measure of your weight in relation to your height. It approximates your total body fat in relation to being overweight.

Cannula A tapered, strawlike tube used in the vacuum aspiration method of abortion.

Catecholamines Stress hormones that raise blood pressure.

Celibacy Avoidance of sexual relations. The term is usually associated with a religious decision not to marry.

Challenge A stress-like response that mobilizes energy in a similar way to alarm but is accompanied by positive thoughts and emotions and a feeling of being in control (not threatened).

Classical conditioning Promoting new behaviors and positive behavior change by rewarding good behavior.

Closed questions Queries that can be answered yes or no and typically don't motivate clients to answer with much more detail than that.

Codes of ethics   Formal statements, developed by professional organizations, that prescribe standards for practice, state principles regarding responsibilities, and define rules expressing the duties and behaviors of professionals to whom the codes apply.

Cognitions   Another name for thoughts.

Cognitive-behavioral therapy (CBT)   Therapy that focuses on the development of insight through an understanding of current thoughts, feelings, and behaviors.

Collagen   A protein that forms the white, inelastic fibers of tendons, ligaments, and fascia.

Combination pills   Birth control pills that combine synthetic estrogen and progesterone. The synthetic estrogen suppresses ovulation by elevating overall estrogen levels within the bloodstream, inhibiting the secretion of follicle stimulating hormone (FSH), and preventing the release of a mature ovum. The synthetic progesterone provides additional protection by keeping the cervical mucus thick. This makes it harder for sperm to penetrate the cervix.

Co-morbid conditions   Other health problems, such as depression, anxiety, or relationship problems, that coexist with sexual problems.

Compelling indications   Chronic diseases such as diabetes that complicate controlling hypertension through medication.

Compliance   A term currently out of favor with health professionals that essentially means getting clients/patients to do what the health professional wants them to do. It is the "extent" to which a person's behavior coincides with medical or health advice.

Confrontation   Pointing out clients' discrepancies in a way that uses "supportive challenge."

Congruence   A counselor's genuineness based on an awareness and acceptance of one's own feelings.

Contemplation stage   A stage in which clients are at least aware of the need to change behavior and are thinking about making a change in the next six months.

Contraception   Methods designed to prevent conception of a child.

Corticosteroids   A type of steroid used to reduce inflammation and irritation of the airways.

Counseling   An intensive, interactive process characterized by a unique relationship between the counselor and client leading to change in the client in one or more of the following areas: behavior, personal constructs, ability to cope, or decision making.

Cruciate   Cross-like ligaments.

Cues to action   Signals or reminders that prompt people to take action.

Cunnilingus   Oral stimulation of the vulva.

Curette   A long-handled, spoonlike instrument used to scrape out the contents of the uterus in an abortion.

Defense mechanisms   Coping strategies employed by clients to protect themselves and avoid facing painful memories.

Demographic   Information pertaining to the study of populations and trends in populations.

Diastolic blood pressure   The pressure exerted on the artery walls when the heart is at rest, or in between beats when it is filling. It is the bottom number in a blood pressure reading.

Dilation and curettage (D&C)   A surgical abortion procedure that removes the embryo and placenta from the uterus by scraping them out.

Dilation and evacuation (D&E)   A second-trimester abortion procedure in which the cervix is dilated, and then the fetus is removed by suction and curettage.

Directives   Broad, overall strategies or components in therapeutic regimens. Another name for instructions given to clients to help them adhere to parts of their therapeutic plan.

Discrepancies   Internal or external inconsistencies in what is said, how it is said, or what is said and what is actually done.

Distress   Outdated reference to stressors that cause discomfort and lead to GAS.

Dream analysis   A technique used in psychoanalysis to help clients understand the underlying meanings of their dreams and how these meanings relate to their current problems.

Ectopic pregnancy   A pregnancy in a body part outside the womb.

Elastin   A protein that forms yellow, elastic tissue fibers.

Eliciting and reflecting meaning Helping clients uncover the most deeply held thoughts and feelings they have about their health problems.

Emergency contraception pill Commonly called the "morning-after" pill, is a combination of synthetic estrogen and progestin. It is administered under medical supervision within 72 hours after unprotected intercourse. The early administration of the pills works to prevent the release of an ovum, or slow the movement of the ovum, or prevent implantation.

Empathic understanding The counselor's ability to understand the feelings and personal meanings the client is expressing, to "feel with" the client.

Empathy Feeling "sorrow with" someone rather than feeling "sorry for" the person.

Endemic A level of infection in which 20% or more of the population has the condition.

Epididymitis Irritation and inflammation of the epididymis.

Essential hypertension Also known as idiopathic hypertension or systemic hypertension of unknown cause. It appears to be caused by a complex interaction between genetic predisposition and environmental factors.

Ethics A system by which one determines whether an action is moral or immoral.

Eustress Outdated reference to stressors that invigorate or motivate.

Expectancies The values people place on the outcomes of the new behavior. Expectancies are akin to incentives.

Expectation citing Using the power differential in counselor–client or patient–provider relationships in a positive way by stating instructions as counselor expectations.

Explicit The concrete, observable facts of clients' stories.

Family planning Postponing having children until the optimal point in one's life.

Family system A unique structure of human relationships extending beyond the individual to include the entire family, however it is defined and characterized.

Feedback Objective information about how the client is behaving.

Fellatio Oral stimulation of the penis.

Femur The thigh bone.

Fertility awareness Also known as natural family planning and the rhythm method. This strategy is based on avoiding unprotected intercourse during days of peak fertility.

Fertility control A neutral term that refers to all attempts by women to control their own fertility.

Focusing the narrative Changing the focus of the story to help clients see their problems from a variety of different focal points or perspectives.

Forced-choice questions Questions that limit clients' range of options for responding but are valuable for helping them make decisions.

Free association A counseling strategy that encourages clients to describe their initial, random thoughts and feelings about specific topics introduced by the counselor.

Genuineness Being yourself, and being as open and honest with clients as possible.

Global words Words such as "total," "complete," "should," "must," and "ought," as well as phrases such as "what a complete waste of . . ." and "what a totally useless. . . ." These words and phrases are evidence of illogical thinking and need to be followed up on later in the interview.

Health The state of complete mental, physical, and social well-being; not merely the absence of disease.

Health behavior The things people do or do not do to promote their health and prevent disease.

Health counseling A psycho-educational process that revolves around two primary functions: (1) helping clients understand and cope with the feelings and emotions associated with their health problems and (2) helping clients develop and adhere to their therapeutic regimens.

Health education Any combination of planned learning experiences based on sound theories that provide individuals, groups, and communities with the opportunity to acquire information and the skills needed to make quality health decisions.

Health promotion Any planned combination of educational, political, environmental, regulatory, or organizational mechanisms that support actions and conditions of living conducive to the health of individuals, groups, and communities.

Healthy People 2010   A coalition of national STD stakeholders representing a variety of public, private, and nonprofit groups and organizations.

Holistic transaction   An appraisal process involving the individual, a potential stressor, and the environment.

Hormonal contraceptive patch   A thin, beige, 1.75″-square patch that administers hormones through the skin and is reported to be as effective as birth control pills.

Hormonal contraceptive ring   A plastic ring, similar to the one at the end of the female condom. It is inserted by the woman deep into the vagina, where it remains for three weeks, releasing synthetic estrogen and progesterone.

Hormonal contraceptive shot   A progestin-only hormonal contraceptive injection given every 3 months. Its action is the same as the minipill.

Humanistic school   A theoretical framework, best characterized by the work of Abraham Maslow, that suggests humans maximize their potential by working through a hierarchy of personal and interpersonal needs from birth to death.

Hypertension   Systolic readings above 140 mm Hg or diastolic readings above 90 mm Hg.

Hysterotomy   A surgical procedure in which the fetus and placenta are removed surgically through an abdominal incision.

Illness behavior   The things people do or do not do from the time they suspect that they might be exposed to, infected with, or developing a disease or illness.

Illogical beliefs   Thoughts and feelings about potential stressors that are not based on factual evidence.

Implicit   The hidden meanings of clients' stories.

Incongruities   Synonym for discrepancies.

Insight theories   Theories that are based on understanding the origins of client behavior. Insight theorists believe that behavior change comes about only after clients gain some understanding or insight into the origin of their difficulties.

Instructions   The specific details involved in how to implement directives.

Irritants   Substances that "irritate" the lungs, such as cigarette smoke (first- or second-hand), cold air, ozone, paint fumes, and perfume.

Key word   The most important word in the sentence that captures the essence of the sentence. Key words can be either cognitive (thoughts) or affective (feelings) words.

Kinesthetic   An orientation to life characterized by being acutely aware of feelings and movement.

Lachman's test   A ligament stability test.

Laparoscope   A flexible surgical instrument with a cameralike attachment that can be inserted into the abdomen to view the fallopian tubes and other organs.

Lateral collateral ligament (LCL)   A ligament that runs along the outer part of the knee and prevents the knee from bending outward.

Limbic hypersensitivity phenomenon (LHP)   Increased susceptibility to stress-related diseases because of excessive lymbic system arousal.

Limbic system   The part of the brain that lies between the cerebral cortex and diencephalon and is linked to emotional arousal.

Long-term controllers   Medications used daily to maintain the potency of the airways by controlling inflammation.

Macro-environment   The level of well-being at a larger level—state, country, and the world at large.

Maintenance stage   The last phase of change that begins after six months of adherence to the new behavior. It is a period of constant attention to the new behavior to prevent relapse.

Major depressive episodes   At least two-week periods of depressed mood or loss of pleasure.

Mania   A distinct period when a person's predominant mood is either elevated, expansive, or irritable and is accompanied by other manic symptoms.

Mast cell stabilizers   Nonsteroidal long-term controllers that work by stabilizing the membranes of mast cells that produce histamine, a chemical released during allergic reactions that result in the inflammation of airways.

Medial collateral ligament (MCL)   A ligament that runs along the inner part of the knee and prevents the knee from bending inward.

Medial meniscus   One of the shock-absorbing cartilages in the knee.

Medicalization   The intensive focus on medical—rather than counseling—treatment options for sexual dysfunctions.

Micro-environment The most immediate environment consisting of school, home, neighborhood, and work site.

Mini-laparotomy A female sterilization procedure in which the fallopian tubes are cut to block transport of the egg.

Minimal encouragers Techniques in which counselors intentionally use the "minimum" amount of feedback necessary to encourage clients to keep talking.

Minipills Birth control pills that contain progesterone only.

Mirroring Restating the person's exact words while mimicking his or her body posturing. It is done intentionally for impact when dealing with emotionally charged issues.

Mixed messages Client statements that can be interpreted in more than one way.

Morality A judgment about whether an action is good or bad, right or wrong.

Morbidity The number of new cases of a disease within a given time period (usually a calendar year).

Mortality The number of deaths from a disease within a given time period (usually a calendar year).

Open-ended questions Similar to open-ended statements except that they end with a question mark. Often referred to as open-direct questions.

Open-ended statements Queries that cannot be answered with a simple yes or no. Also known as open-indirect questions.

Operant conditioning Extinguishing (eliminating) negative behaviors by punishing bad behaviors.

Palliative Therapeutic regimens designed to reduce pain and suffering but not cure a health problem.

Paraphilias Sexual disorders in which an individual experiences recurrent and intense sexual urges and fantasies involving either nonhuman objects (i.e., a fetish), suffering or humiliation of oneself or one's partner (i.e., sadomasochism), or nonconsenting partners (i.e., pedophilia, exhibitionism, voyeurism, or frotteurism).

Paraphrasing A responding skill in which portions of the clients' stories are restated by counselors in their own words to keep clients talking and to clarify information in their stories.

Passive listening What we do when watching television, a movie, the radio, and so on. The listener merely soaks in what the initiator of the message is sending.

Patient quizzes Verbal requests by counselors for clients to repeat specific parts of the treatment plan.

Pelvic inflammatory disease (PID) A catch-all term used to describe infection of the uterus, fallopian tubes, or ovaries resulting in fever, malaise, pain, and other symptoms.

Perceived barriers The things that people see as standing in their way when trying to change their behavior.

Perceived benefits The benefits that people feel will come from changing their behavior.

Perceived seriousness The extent to which individuals believe or perceive an illness to be serious.

Perceived susceptibility The extent to which individuals believe they are at risk of contracting a disease or developing a health problem.

Performance accomplishments Outcomes that occur through personal mastery of specific skills or tasks.

Permission-asking questions Open-direct questions that end in a question mark and are asked in such a way that clients perceive that they are being asked their permission to answer.

Pivot shift test An ACL injury test that puts greater stress on the knee as it is straightened by the physician from a bent and inwardly rotated position.

PLISSIT model A sex counseling model. "P" stands for *permission,* "LI" stands for *limited information,* "SS" stands for *specific suggestions,* and "IT" stands for *intensive therapy.*

Post-abortion syndrome (PAS) Long-term negative psychological effects of abortion.

Posterior cruciate ligament (PCL) A ligament that works in concert with the ACL in preventing the tibia from sliding backward under the femur. The ACL and PCL cross each other inside the knee, forming an "X."

Pre-contemplation stage The initial stage of change where no serious thought is being given to behavior change within the next six months.

Pre-hypertension Systolic blood pressure of 120–139 mm Hg or diastolic blood pressure of 80–89 mm Hg.

Preparation stage   The planning stage where clients focus on making the desired behavioral change as quickly as possible.

Primacy   Assessing the client's most important (primary) issue.

Primary prevention   Activities designed to reduce the likelihood that the person ever develops the health problem.

Principles   Responsibilities to clients and others that are set by the code of ethics.

Prophylactic treatment   Treatment given prior to (or in the absence of) obtaining definitive diagnosis of a condition.

Psychoanalysis   A type of insight theory that seeks to probe conflicts in the unconscious minds of clients and bring them to light.

Psychogenic   Psychosomatic illnesses without a causative organism.

Psychosomatic   The interaction of the mind and body in the disease process.

Pulse   Systolic blood pressure minus diastolic blood pressure.

Punishment   A negative consequence; giving something that is not wanted or taking away something that is wanted.

Quick relief rescuers   Medications (usually inhalers) that treat an asthma attack by relaxing the constricted muscles of the airway, increasing breathing potency and thus relieving symptoms.

Reciprocal determinism   A principle stating that a change in one factor related to a behavior change modifies all other factors.

Reflection of feelings   Similar to paraphrasing except that the focus is on feelings (the affective domain) instead of thoughts and facts (the cognitive domain).

Reinforcer   A positive consequence, a reward, or something that is pleasant or wanted.

Rennin   An enzyme that triggers production of angiotensin.

Repetition   The planned verbal and written repeating of specific instructions during the client's visit to increase the client's adherence to them.

Responding skills   Verbal and nonverbal techniques used to keep clients talking and to clarify issues in their stories.

RU-486   The "abortion pill"; mifepristone, a drug used to induce menstruation by blocking the absorption of progesterone, thereby preventing the uterine lining from supporting implantation of an embryo.

Rules   Spell out the actual behaviors deemed appropriate and inappropriate by the code of ethics.

Safe zone   A fertility awareness concept that considers ovulation and the length of time sperm and eggs can live when determining a time to avoid intercourse.

Secondary hypertension   The elevation of blood pressure associated with having another illness or condition or using certain medications or products.

Secondary prevention   The early detection and prompt treatment of health problems.

Self-control   The extent to which the client has control over a behavior.

Self-disclosure   Counselors' *intentional* disclosing of information about themselves in an effort to connect with clients in a deeper, more personal way.

Self-efficacy   The personal belief in one's ability to accomplish something.

Self-monitoring   The use of devices (e.g., medication packaging, logs) to help patients keep track of components of their therapeutic plan.

Self-talk   The subvocal, inner dialogue that people carry on with themselves when thinking about situations.

Sexual disorders   Those sexual difficulties listed in the *Diagnostic and Statistical Manual of Mental Disorders* (DSM-IV-TR). The DSM-IV-TR classifies sexual disorders as being either sexual dysfunctions, paraphilias, or gender identity disorders.

Sexual dysfunction   An impairment or disturbance in one of the three phases of the sexual response cycle: desire, arousal, or orgasm.

Sexual problems   Situations that, while not officially recognized as disorders in the DSM, may nevertheless cause significant distress for individuals experiencing them.

Sexual worries   Common, everyday concerns—Will I be able to function adequately?, Will my partner think well of me?, Am I normal?—that are inherent in the experience of being human.

Sexually transmitted disease (STD) Any disease capable of being transmitted through any type of sexual contact (oral, anal, vaginal, heterosexual, homosexual, bisexual) between two or more people.

Sick role behavior The things people do or do not do from the time they are diagnosed with a condition to the time they are cured or their condition is in a maintenance stage.

Somatogenic Psychosomatic illness that involves a causative organism.

Sphygmomanometer Blood pressure cuff.

Standards Criteria that set levels or degrees of quality.

Sterilization Techniques (vasectomy and tubal ligation) that prevent sperm from reaching ova.

Stress A holistic transaction between the individual, a stressor, and the environment, resulting in a stress response.

Stress response A set of physiological adaptations of the body to regain homeostasis in the face of threat, harm, or loss.

Stressor Any stimulus appraised by the individual as threatening or capable of causing harm or loss.

Summarizing Restatement of clients' stories that covers more information and a longer span of time. Summarization differs from paraphrasing and reflection of feelings in that it combines the two into a statement of both fact and feeling.

Sympathetic nervous system The branch of the nervous system that controls many involuntary functions, including the stress response.

Synergistic effect An effect that occurs when all of the levels of coping are working together simultaneously. The combined result is much greater than the sum of the individual parts.

Systems theory Also referred to as structural theory. A theory that looks at the structure of human relationships as people relate to others in their environments. Systems theory believes that a change in any one member of the social system affects the nature of the social system as a whole.

Systolic blood pressure The pressure exerted on the artery walls when the heart beats. It is the top number in a blood pressure reading.

Tailoring Modifying components of the therapeutic plan (e.g., medication taking, engaging in physical activity or exercise) to fit the client's lifestyle rather than to match a predetermined schedule.

Termination stage The stage where behavior change is completed and maintenance comes to an end.

Tertiary prevention Limiting disability and premature death of clients who have had the health problem for a while and are suffering from complications associated with the problem.

Theoretical effectiveness The lowest expected percentage of women who will get pregnant while using a given contraceptive method.

Theoretical framework A context, also known as a theoretical perspective, that unifies and organizes how counselors view client behavior and counseling practice.

Theory A set of interrelated concepts, definitions, and propositions that presents a systematic view of events or situations by specifying relations among variables in an effort to explain and predict the events of the situation.

Tibia The shin bone.

Transference A technique used in psychoanalysis to help clients project their thoughts and feelings about others onto the therapist.

Triggers Stimuli that initiate an asthma episode or attack.

Tubal ligation A female sterilization procedure in which a surgical instrument is used to cut and tie back the fallopian tubes to block passage of the ova, thereby preventing fertilization.

Unconditional positive regard The counselor's willingness to be warmly accepting of the client, regardless of the counselor's liking or not liking the client's behavior.

Urethritis Discharge and burning upon urination.

Vacuum aspiration Induced abortion procedure in which uterine contents are removed by suction; used for early abortions.

Vasectomy A male sterilization procedure in which the vas deferens are cut and tied to block the transport of sperm.

Verbal persuasion Encouraging, coaching, and re-assuring clients that they can achieve their desired outcomes.

Verbal tracking Literally, following clients' stories. The goal is to keep the dialogue going where clients lead rather than where counselors want to go.

Vicarious experience The learning that occurs as a result of watching others perform a desired behavior.

Virulence The strength of an organism; related to its ability to infect a susceptible person.

Visual An orientation to life that describes the world in terms of sight.

Wellness An approach to health that focuses on balancing the many aspects or dimensions (physical, social, spiritual, emotional, intellectual, and environmental/occupational) of a person's life through increasing the adoption of health-enhancing conditions and behaviors rather than attempting to minimize conditions of illness.

A

AAHE (American Association of
    Health Education), 5
Adherence, 34
    adherence theory, 34-39
Anterior Cruciate Ligament (ACL)
    injuries
    anatomy and physiology, 257
    diagnosis, 257-258
    epidemiology, 255-256
    overview, 255
    treatment, 258-261
ACL injury counseling
    attending skills, 263-265
    directives, 271-277
    goals, 261
    influencing skills, 267-277
    introductory skills, 262-263
    logical consequences, 271-277
    responding skills, 265-267
    specific instructions, 271-277
Allergens, 165
Alcohol reduction, 218
Ardell, Donald, 5
Asthma
    control and prevention, 168-169
    diagnosis, 164-166
    epidemiology, 164
    long-term controllers, 166
    peak flow meter, 167-168
    quick-relief rescuers, 167
    treatment, 166-167
Asthma counseling, 170-191
    attending skills, 173-176
    directives, 180-191
    goals, 171
    influencing skills, 178-191
    introductory skills, 172-173
    logical consequences,
        180-191
    responding skills, 176-178
    specific instructions, 180-191
    triggers, 185-191
Asthma treatment
    hypo-sensitization, 167
    long-term controllers, 166
    quick relief rescuers, 166-167
Attending skills, 47-55
    body language, 52

culturally appropriate eye
    contact, 48-49
    verbals, 51-54
    visuals, 48
    vocals, 49-51
Attending skills
    in ACL injury counseling,
        263-265
    in asthma counseling, 172-173
    in birth control counseling,
        149-150
    in chlamydia counseling, 237-241
    in hypertension counseling,
        205-206
    in stress counseling, 108-110

B

Bandura, Albert, 23-25
Beck, Aaron, 31
Becker, Marshall, 22
Behavior change theories, 22-29
    health belief model, 22-23
    self-efficacy theory, 25
    social cognitive theory, 23-24
    stimulus-response/behavior
        theory, 28-29
    theory of reasoned action, 27-28
    transtheoretical/stages of change
        theory, 25-27
Behavior theory, 28-29
Benson, Herbert, 102
Birth control, 130
Birth control counseling, 146-161
    attending skills, 149-150
    directives, 157-161
    goals, 146
    influencing skills, 153-161
    introductory skills, 146-149
    logical consequences, 157-161
    responding skills, 150-153
    specific instructions, 157-161
Birth control methods, 134-145
    birth control pills, 141-142
    celibacy/abstinence, 135
    cervical cap, 139
    chemical spermicides, 140-141
    coitus interruptus, 136
    contraceptive patch, 142
    contraceptive ring, 142

    contraceptive shot, 142
    diaphragm, 139
    female condom, 138-13
    fertility awareness, 136
    intrauterine devices, 141
    kissing/hugging/massage, 136
    male condom, 137-138
    masturbation, 136
    mechanisms of action, 134-135
    medical abortion, 144
    oral-genital behavior, 136
    sex toys, 136
    surgical abortion method,
        143-144
    tubal ligation, 143
    vaginal contraceptive film, 141
    vaginal contraceptive sponge,
        139-140
    vasectomy, 142
Blood pressure, 193, *see also*
    Hypertension
    high blood pressure, 194-195
    measurement, 194
Blonna's Five R's of Coping, 104-106
Body language, 52
Body weight, 218

C

Chlamydia trachomatis, 227-253
    diagnosis, 229-230
    epidemiology, 228-229
    prevention, 230-234
    treatment, 230
Chlamydia trachomatis counseling,
    236-253
    attending skills, 237-241
    directives, 245-253
    goals, 236
    influencing skills, 244-253
    introductory skills, 235-237
    logical consequences, 245-253
    responding skills, 241-244
    specific instructions, 245-253
Challenge, 100
Client observation, 61
Client orientation, 61-62
    auditory, 61
    kinesthetic, 62
    visual, 61

Index

Closed, or yes/no questions, 69
Cognitive behavior therapy,
    31-32
Compliance
    compliance (factors related to),
        37-39
    compliance (factors unrelated
        to), 36-37
    compliance theory, 34-39
    definition of, 34
Communicating about sexuality,
    145-146
Contraception, 131
Confrontation, 76-80
Counseling
    definition, 9
Counseling theories, 29-34
    behavioral theories, 32
    insight theories, 29-32
    Ivey's Microskills, 32-34
Counselor-client relationship, 13
Counselors
    characteristics of, 9-11
Culturally appropriate eye contact,
    48-49

D

Dimensions of wellness, 5-7
Directives, 89
Disorders of arousal model, 103
Dunn, Halbert, 4

E

Egan, Gerald, 9
Effectiveness of birth control,
    131-133
    actual use effectiveness, 131-132
    pregnancy risk, 132-133
    theoretical effectiveness, 131
Eliciting and reflecting meaning,
    87-88
Ellis, Albert, 31
Ending counseling, 16-17
Eroticizing condom use, 138
Ethical issues in counseling, 14-16
Ethical dilemmas, 14-15
Everly, George, 102

F

Family planning, 131
Feedback, 80
Female condom, 138
Fertility control, 131
Focusing the narrative, 81-86
    culture/environmental focus,
        86-88
    family focus, 82-83
    helper focus, 85-86
    mutuality focus, 84
    other individual focus, 83-84
    problem and individual
        focus, 82
Forced choice questions, 69-70
Folkman, Suzanne, 100
Fowler, James, 6-7
Freud, Sigmund, 29-30

G

GAS (General Adaptation
    Syndrome), 99
Gender differences
    in ACL injuries, 255-256
    in communication styles, 140
Gonorrhea, 2
Greenberg, Jerrold, 14-15

H

Health, 4
    components, 5-7
    definition, 4-5
Health behavior, 20
Health counseling
    definition, 11-12
    for primary prevention, 12
    for secondary prevention, 12
    for tertiary prevention, 12
    practice of, 12-13
Health education, 7-8
Health promotion, 7
Healthy People 2010, 8-9
    access to health care, 36
    alcohol and substance use, 77
    environmental air quality
        and asthma, 168
    immunization, 44

injuries and violence, 259
    mental health, 105
    overweight and obesity, 208
    responsible sexual behavior, 234
    smoking, 290
    unintended pregnancy, 144
High blood pressure (*see*
    hypertension)
Hypertension, 194
    as a risk factor, 199-200
    controllable risks, 198-199
    diagnosis, 194-195
    epidemiology, 196
    essential, 195
    overview, 193-194
    prevention and control, 200-202
    secondary, 195
    uncontrollable risks, 196-198
Hypertension counseling, 202-224
    attending skills, 205-206
    DASH eating plan, 212-214
    directives, 210-224
    goals, 202
    influencing skills, 209-224
    introductory skills, 204-205
    logical consequences, 210-224
    medication taking, 222-224
    responding skills, 206-209
    specific instructions, 210-224
Hypertension risk factors
    (controllable)
    alcohol, 199
    obesity, 198
    sedentary lifestyle, 198
    sodium and potassium, 199
    stress, 199
    tobacco use, 198
Hypertension risk factors
    (uncontrollable)
    age, 196
    family history, 197
    gender, 196
    race, 197

I

Illness behavior, 20-21
Influencing skills, 74-95
    confrontation, 76-80

directives, 90-91
eliciting meaning, 87
feedback, 80
focusing the narrative, 81-87
information giving, 89-90
instructions, 91-94
interpretation of meaning, 88
logical consequences, 94-95
reflecting meaning, 88
reframing, 88-89
self-disclosure, 80-81
Influencing skills
   in ACL injury counseling,
     267-277
   in asthma counseling, 178-191
   in birth control counseling,
     153-161
   in chlamydia counseling,
     244-253
   in hypertension counseling,
     209-224
   in sexuality counseling, 294-298
   in stress counseling, 113-128
Information, 89
Information-giving, 89-90
Injuries (ACL)
   career ending, 261
   epidemiology, 255-257
   serious, 259-260
Insight theory, 29-31
Instructions, 91-94
   in asthma counseling, 180-191
   in birth control counseling,
     157-161
   in hypertension counseling,
     210-224
   in stress counseling, 119-128
Introductory skills, 44-47
   describing roles, 46-47
   exchanging names, 46
   handshake, 45-46
   smile, 44
   touch, 54-55
   transition to client's story, 47
Introductory skills
   in ACL injury counseling,
     262-263
   in asthma counseling, 172-173
   in birth control counseling,
     146-149

in chlamydia counseling,
   235-237
in hypertension counseling,
   204-205
in sexuality counseling,
   288-291
in stress counseling, 107-108
Irritants, 165-166
Ivey, Allen, 32
Ivey's Microskills model, 32-34

K

Kasl, George, 19
Key words, 64
Kübler-Ross, Elisabeth, 261

L

Lazarus, Richard, 100
Leading health indicators, 8
Listening, 49
Logical consequences, 94-95

M

Macroenvironment, 6
Medicalization of sexuality
   counseling, 284-285
Microenvironment, 6
Minimal encouragers, 62-64
   key words, 63
   mirroring, 63-64
   non-verbal, 63
   verbal, 63-64
Minimizing distractions, 51
Mirroring, 63-64
Multicultural issues
   language level, 62
   space requirements, 52

N

Non-verbal communication,
   52, 63
Non-verbal minimal
   encouragers, 63

O

Open-ended statements
   and questions, 68-69
Observational skills, 61-62

P

Pain management, 277
Parallelism, 81
Paraphilia, 281
Paraphrasing, 70
Pavlov, Ivan, 32
Pavlov's dogs, 32
Peak flow meter, 167-168
Personal space needs, 55
Personality and stress, 101-102
Physical activity, 214-216
Physical appearance, 52
PLISSIT model, 286-187
   intensive therapy, 287
   limited information, 286
   permission, 286
   specific suggestions, 286-287
Prevention
   primary, 12
   secondary, 12
   tertiary, 12
Primary prevention counseling, 98
Psychoeducator model, 33
Psychoanalysis, 29-30
Psychosomatic disease and
   stress, 102
Psychogenic illness, 102

Q

Questioning, 64-70
   closed, or yes/no questions, 69
   forced choice questions, 69
   open-ended statements, 68-69
   positive uses of, 66
   potential problems with, 66-68
   why questions, 67-68

R

Reflection of feelings, 70-71
Reframing, 88-89

Responding skills, 62-72
  minimal encouragers, 62-64
  paraphrasing, 70
  questioning, 64-70
  reflection of feelings, 70-71
  summarizing, 71-72
Responding skills
  in ACL injury counseling,
    265-267
  in asthma counseling, 176-178
  in birth control counseling,
    150-153
  in chlamydia counseling,
    241-244
  in hypertension counseling,
    206-209
  in sexuality counseling, 292-294
  in stress counseling, 110-113
Risk tolerance, 132-144
Rogers, Carl, 9, 29

S

Self-efficacy theory, 25
Self-disclosure, 80-81
Seligman's ABCDE Model, 125
Selye, Hans, 99
Sex partner evaluation, 248-249
Sexual concerns, 280-282
Sexuality
  communicating about, 145-148
  guidelines, 148
  vocabulary, 145-146
Sexuality counseling, 284-298
  attending skills, 291-292
  directives, 296-298
  goals, 287-288
  influencing skills, 294-298
  introductory skills, 288-291
  logical consequences, 296-298
  responding skills, 292-294
  specific instructions, 296-298
  the medicalization of, 284-285

Sexuality counseling concerns,
    280-282
  helping clients manage, 283-284
  obstacles to discussing, 282-283
  sexual disorders, 280-282
  sexual problems, 282
  sexuality worries, 282
Sexually transmitted diseases,
    226-227
Sexually transmitted disease (STD)
  counseling, 227-228
  goals, 227
  guidelines, 235
Sexually transmitted disease (STD)
  prevention, 230
  a pyramid of risk, 230-234
  sexual behavior, 231-234
  sexual relationships, 231
Sodium reduction, 216-218
Space
  intimate, 52
  personal, 52
  public, 52
  social consultive, 52
Sick role behavior, 20
Silence, 52-54, 59
Skinner, BF, 28-29
Social–cognitive theory, 23-24
Somatogenic illness, 102
Stimulus-response behavior theory,
    28-29
Stress
  definition, 98
  effects of, on disease, 103-104
  personality and, 101-102
  psychosomatic disease and,
    102-103
Stress counseling
  attending skills, 108-110
  directives, 119-127
  goals, 104-106
  influencing skills, 113-128
  introductory skills, 107-108

logical consequences, 119-127
  responding skills, 110-113
  specific instructions, 119-127
Stress transaction model, 100
Summarizing, 71-72
Surgeon General's Report
  on Physical Activity
  and Exercise, 127

T

Termination of counseling, 16-17
Theory of reasoned action, 27-28
Theoretical basis of counseling,
    29-34
Theoretical frameworks, 21-22
Time frames, 52-54
Touch, 54
Trans-theoretical model, 25-27
Triggers, 185-191

U

Universal stressors, 108

V

Viagra, 284-285
Videotaping sessions, 50
Visuals, 48-49
Vocals, 49-51
Verbals, 51-52
Verbal following, 51
Verbal minimal encouragers, 63-64

W

Wellness
  components, 5-7
  definition, 5
World Health Organization
  (WHO), 4